GETTING OUT

Failing to Survive Surgical Residency Training

Virginia Adams O'Connell

University Press of America,® Inc.
Lanham · Boulder · New York · Toronto · Plymouth, UK

Copyright © 2007 by
University Press of America,® Inc.
4501 Forbes Boulevard
Suite 200
Lanham, Maryland 20706
UPA Acquisitions Department (301) 459-3366

Estover Road
Plymouth PL6 7PY
United Kingdom

Library of Congress Control Number: 2006937932
ISBN-13: 978-0-7618-3662-9 (paperback : alk. paper)
ISBN-10: 0-7618-3662-4 (paperback : alk. paper)

Dedication

This book is dedicated to the memory of my parents,
Rosemarie Chesney Adams and Edward Arthur Adams,
and to my wonderful family: my husband, Stephen Austin O'Connell;
my daughter, Hilary Rose O'Connell; my son, David Adams O'Connell;
and my sister, Mary Kay Adams.

Your love and unwavering support made this possible.

Contents

Tables

Foreword

Priority fights in science are often intense, protracted, and bitter affairs. When such struggles involve new treatments, technologies and the profits that trail in their wake, when something tangible is at stake, then the contested nature of discovery, the charges and counter-charges that are exchanged, and the general sour atmosphere that trails in the wake of the resolution of such contests are understandable. But, even when nothing much is at stake save prestige, honor, and the approbation of one's peers, priority fights over exactly who deserves credit for discovering what still retain their rancorous nature. As Merton so long ago pointed out, scientific reward systems depend upon the proper crediting of intellectual achievements.

So, when Virginia Adams O'Connell, first proposed using these materials to produce her own manuscript, I was apprehensive on two accounts. First, I was apprehensive that, no matter how much the final analysis was hers, she would not receive the credit that she deserved for the final product. At the outset of her project, we had long discussions of the career problems working on a topic so closely associated with a former teacher might present. Second, and much less nobly, having studied surgical problems for so long, having used them as my particular window into fundamental, recurrent problems of social organization—the management of uncertainty, the high cost seeking an unattainable perfection exacts from members of this occupational community, and the inevitability of failure when one continually tries to beat long odds—I worried that when this work was finished I might be tempted to claim credit for a product not my own. So, when Virginia Adams O'Connell asked me if I wished to be a co-author of this book, her gracious way of acknowledging that I helped with the design of the survey, provided some assistance in securing participation from the associations of program directors in the five specialties that took place in the survey, and helped gather some of the data, I was deeply touched. I was also mindful of mindful of Merton's admonitions about how firmly the integrity of scientific communities rests upon the principle that credit for work be assigned to those who produce it. So I declined the co-authorship and instead offered to write a brief prefatory note signaling how much this is the work of Virginia Adams O'Connell. My own ambivalence about the ownership of this little corner of social life, surgical residency, got the better of me despite the best of intentions. This book has awaited publication for an embarrassing number of months as I have fumbled to put a few brief prefatory paragraphs together. For this delay, I owe an apology not just to Virginia Adams O'Connell but to the entire community of scholars interested in professional socialization, the interplay of race and gender in creating hurdles which need to be cleared successfully in the beginning stages of professional training, and the processes of social control within the medical profession.

So let me state as clearly and as forcefully as I can the following. While I played a role in the design of this study and in the collection of the data, the data analysis, the indices, and the measures are Virginia Adams O'Connell's. The interpretation which is so impeccably grounded in this data is hers as well. I announce this as bluntly as I do not because I want to distance myself from the product; but, rather, because I recognize how important it is that credit goes where credit is due. In fact, there is much here that, if I could but do so honestly, I would love to claim as my own.

There is so much here that precisely details what earlier ethnographic studies have hinted at, and so much that will prove useful in formulating policy to provide safer, higher-quality health-care. For example, O'Connell's work allows us to see some very interesting features of the social organization of success and failure within medical residencies. Her data allows us to see that much of what students of professional socialization have always assumed but never documented with such rigor. First, a significant proportion of residents who fail to complete their training are offered the option of face-saving resignation. There is a structured silence about their observed shortcomings as they shuttle from the programs they leave to those they enter, programs in need of warm bodies to provide the extensive and necessary labor hospitalized patients require. Residents switch programs under a faculty regime of, "Don't ask, Don't tell."

Next, a puzzlingly large number of programs never experience any attrition at all—Do these programs have faculty who are wizards at selecting recruits or faculty that fail to apply standards? Third, once the decision to fire a resident is made, there is a surprisingly large time lag between decision and formal action so that a case justifying the firing can be built. The structured silence that accompanied forced-resignations is heard again when residents are terminated for cause. A disturbingly large proportion of residents fired from one training program enter into another without anyone in the new program making inquiries or seeking references from faculty in the training program from which the resident departed. Also, although program directors fear litigious residents and although many residents who are fired threaten legal action, precious few are able to mount successful problems. Finally, to conclude a partial list, a disturbing number of residents finish their residencies successfully despite reservations of program directors about their fitness for independent practice. Program directors simply pass their problems to specialty boards which are then asked to make the difficult decision (with a much more limited set of data) that program faculty were unable to make.

The concrete and thickly described social dynamics that surround resignation from, termination from, or problematic completion of a residency in a medical specialty is what makes O'Connell's study such a rich rewarding empirical work. Like all complex studies it raises difficult questions that resist overly simple answers. Chief among these are two questions fundamental to the organization of the professions in modern society: namely, does the behavior we observe around the social control of performance justify the large grants of autonomy that we, as a society, grant to the medical profession? Does the profession use its license and mandate with regard to judging those it recruits into its ranks in an even-handed way that promotes meritocratic standards? Or, alternatively, are notions of competence and skill used to introduce and reinforce, through the back door as it were, old prejudices? This is a work that skillfully blends qualitative and quantitative data first to document patterns of behavior that surround the success or failure of recruits into the medical profession and then to raise important questions about the implications of those patterns for the quality of care that we all receive.

Before I shuffle off these pages and allow you to examine Virginia Adams O'Connell's work for yourself, let me make one last point. Since the press releases announcing the Institute of Medicine's report on medical error in the fall of 1999, there has been an enormous amount of effort aimed at improving quality and reducing harm through a focus on the properties of the *system* through which care is delivered. There is no gainsaying that quality can be improved in this manner. However O'Connell's work is a salutary reminder that personnel are a part of the health care system. Any redesign of the system that anticipates improvement in outcomes needs to pay close attention to how personnel are trained, how their inevitable mistakes are managed, and how this management and training conveys or fails to convey a service ethic, a sense of professional integrity, and norms of accountability. O'Connell's work reminds us, at a time when that lesson is in danger of being lost, that system performance is dependent upon the skills, values, and integrity of the personnel who operate it.

Charles L. Bosk, Ph.D.
University of Pennsylvania
Philadelphia, Pennsylvania
September 7, 2005

Preface

The national attrition rate from medical school averages about 1%, but attrition from surgical residency programs is much higher, roughly 16%. The risk of attrition is greater for white women and racial minority men and women than for white males. This research examines the factors which lead to attrition in these graduate residency programs by looking at the dynamic interplay between the institution and individual residents. We collected data from 556 certified residency programs in anesthesiology, general surgery, neurosurgery, orthopedic surgery and plastic surgery, and conducted 75 interviews with the attendings, residents and nurses from five neurosurgery programs. While we analyze the current shortcomings in the process of selection, we also look at how the culture, structure and organization of these educational programs affects the risk of attrition once residents have been accepted. Since surgery is one of the last stalwarts of the "old boy's network" in medicine, an analysis of the culture of these programs helps account for the greater risk of attrition among female and racial minority residents. But an examination of the process of resident evaluation reveals even more. In addition to being graded on cognitive knowledge and clinical judgment, residents are also evaluated on personal characteristics, the most important being "honesty." We demonstrate how the medical faculty's subjective assessment of these elusive and contestable qualities can help identify the morally deficient among the technically proficient. It can also, however, enable discrimination. White women and racial minority men and women are hampered on a number of counts in these training programs, including fewer and poorer interactions with program faculty. The process of resident evaluation must be reviewed for potential abuses.

Virginia Adams O'Connell
Swarthmore, PA 19081
July 15, 2004

Acknowledgements

I want to first thank Charles L. Bosk, Ph.D., University of Pennsylvania, for access to the data on surgical attrition. Dr. Bosk served as the principle investigator on this project and graciously shared his own interview material with me. More importantly, however, I want to thank him for his many years of friendship, support and guidance.

I want to thank Renee C. Fox, Ph.D., University of Pennsylvania, for showing me from the first day of my graduate training the joy of sociological investigation and for her many years of support. Dr. Fox read through many versions of each chapter and always gave timely and constructive comments. As many who have studied with her will attest, she is an extraordinary teacher. I want to also thank Robin L. Leidner, Ph.D., University of Pennsylvania, for her editorial prowess, and especially for her guidance on matters of race and gender.

I also want to thank the Pew Charitable Trust for funding this research on surgical resident attrition. This research was made possible not only with financial support from Pew, but also from the following physicians who served on the project's steering committee: William F. Collins, Jr., M.D. (Yale University), Julian T. Hoff, M.D. (University of Michigan Hospitals), David L. Kelly, Jr., M.D. (Bowman Gray School of Medicine), Edward R. Laws, M.D. (University of Virginia School of Medicine), M. Steven Mahaley, Jr., M.D., (now deceased), Robert A. Ratcheson, M.D. (University Hospitals of Cleveland), Richard L. Rovit, M.D. (St. Vincent's Hospital, New York), William Shucart, M.D. (New England Medical Center), and Martin H. Weiss, M.D (USC Medical Center). The idea for this project was driven by these physicians' concerns for their surgical residents. This group represents caring medical educators trying to provide top notch medical education. Their efforts should be commended.

I also want to thank the other two members of the project staff, Deborah Putnam Thomas, and Michael Polgar, Ph.D. Ms. Thomas was the Project Administrator, our link to all of the various programs that participated in this project, and Dr. Polgar was an invaluable contributor to the survey instrument.

A special thanks goes out to the American Association of University Women for awarding me a Dissertation Fellowship during 2000-2001 that provided me with the funds and time to focus on finishing the collection and organization of all the data presented here. I greatly admire that AAUW and its mission and I am proud to have been an AAUW Fellow. Being honored by the AAUW was a crowning moment in my graduate school experience.

And finally, I want to thank my family. Without their love, joy and support, this book would never have seen the light of day. Stephen, Hilary and David give meaning to my life and hope for the future.

Introduction

From the moment of our birth and throughout our lives, we join together with people in various social organizations. We both seek to join and are recruited to various vocational and social organizations. In many instances, the interplay between self-selection and recruitment is a dynamic and complex process. What motivates anyone to seek membership in a particular group? How do the members of that group decide whether to allow that person to join? And how is the "goodness of fit" between the person's talents and values and the group's shared talents and values assessed and evaluated?

In this study, we look at this dynamic process by studying residents in surgical residency programs in the United States. The data for this study come from two sources: 1), a two-part survey on resident attrition that was sent out in 1990, and 2), 75 interviews conducted with the faculty, residents and nurses of five neurosurgery programs. The survey collected data on both the structure and organization of the participating residency programs and on residents from these programs. Five specialties are represented in this sample: anesthesiology, general surgery, neurosurgery, orthopedic surgery and plastic surgery. All of the residents in this study entered into residency training in order to become surgeons or anesthesiologists. After an undergraduate program and another four years of medical school, these graduates pursued residency training in a surgical specialty—they actively sought and were provisionally granted membership in the profession of surgery. Not all the residents in this study, however, remained members of this occupational group. They are the failures of the dynamic process of recruitment and training. While some of them voluntarily resigned from their programs, others were terminated. People in these two categories left for a variety of reasons. The residents who resigned either decided that the work did not bring the anticipated rewards, or felt that they did not have "what it takes" to complete training. The medical faculty fired residents when senior physicians concluded both that these residents did not possess the skills and/or personal traits to be a surgeon, and that the skills and traits could not be taught within the normal context of a residency training program. The resident who resigns typically rejects the group. The group rejects the resident who is terminated.

We will also be looking at a third category of resident—the problematic completer. The problematic completer is the resident who fulfilled all official requirements of the program but about whom the program faculty has reservations. Worried that the problematic completer will make major errors without close supervision, the program director and the attendings are reluctant to see the resident leave the program, but they are unable to force the resident to stay for additional training. The requirement for group membership--the completion of a residency training program--fails to produce the desired product, an independent competent surgeon. But by completing the process, the resident becomes a legitimate member of the group. The problematic completer has become a surgeon, even if he or she is not a very good surgeon.

This study focuses specifically on the failures, on the residents who either resigned or were terminated. Why do we focus on the failures? As Becker noted in his research on medical education:

> "The point of concentrating on instances where things do not work well is that
> it helps one discover when they do work well, and these are discoveries that are
> more difficult to make in situations of harmony because people are more likely
> to take them for granted." (Becker et al, 1961: 21)

We do not often reflect on what makes a successful employee. When a colleague resigns or is terminated, however, our collective attention is drawn to the case. Assessing the reasons why these residents either rejected or were rejected by the community of surgeons sheds light on the nature of the work, on the process of evaluation, on how the medical faculty judges residents' performance. Studying attrition illustrates good performance precisely by contrasting it against unacceptable performance. In this context we pose the question: how are the criteria used to judge performance related to the jobs which these residents perform?

Why else study attrition? Failures in the recruitment process can be costly for both the individual and the group. For individuals who want to join a profession like medicine, the route to membership is typically through an educational program. The residents in this study had already invested quite a lot in their education, having completed both an undergraduate and medical school degree prior to starting the residency program. For the individual who has already paid tuition and/or postponed other pursuits while pursuing a degree or certification, dropping out may engender regrets about wasted time and finances. Leaving the program may also signal for the resident the end of a dream since he or she may be permanently blocked from pursuing a particular career path. The psychological cost may be as great or greater than the financial one. Program faculty may feel similar sentiments, viewing their efforts with and scholarship support of students who drop out as squandered. For the hospital programs in this study, resident attrition is especially costly because it may leave the hospitals understaffed. Studying when the process does not work may lead to revisions in both the recruitment and socialization process that reduce attrition and therefore the costs borne by both the individual and the group.

Specialized education programs like residency programs not only teach a unique body of knowledge and technique, they also convey the morals and values associated with the professional work. In our analysis of the culture of surgery, we will explore some of those morals and values. Students, in this case the residents, demonstrate their mastery of the knowledge by passing tests and performing proficiently. They display their acceptance of the profession's morals and values by adopting certain modes of conduct, obeying certain rules of interaction, and using a specialized vocabulary. Evaluators bemoan the fact that it is much harder to judge trainees on their morals and values than to test their grasp of knowledge, but they claim the former a far more important task. We will explore the different ways the medical faculty evaluates technical proficiency vs. the moral character of the residents, and explore how the residents' race and gender impact the evaluators' assessment of the residents' elusive, contestable, and non-quantifiable moral fiber.

Since we are examining the interplay between the characteristics of the individuals seeking membership and the characteristics of the group, both will factor in our analyses. We will evaluate both the institutional effect and the resident effect on overall attrition rates and on factors related to attrition risk. We will see what characteristics of the residency program are associated with higher and lower rates of attrition and what characteristics of the resident predict whether he or she will successfully complete the program.

The first chapter describes the culture of surgery, focusing on the culture of the training programs, and in particular, on neurosurgery programs. Since both this study and others have indicated that women and minorities are at a greater risk of leaving these training programs, we will isolate features that potentially make these programs inhospitable to women and minorities. In the second chapter, we will describe the application process and evaluation procedures used by educators in surgical programs. This section will be followed by a review of some attrition studies, focusing on attrition in medical education. The analysis of both the culture of surgery and the evaluation procedures will help to decipher both the implicit and explicit "yardsticks" employed by evaluators when assessing a resident's "goodness of fit."

Chapter 3 will focus specifically on the relationship between the culture and organization of the residency programs and attrition rates. How does the presence or absence of social activities affect the rates? Does using a standardized form for evaluation raise or lower problem rates? Who does the evaluating and how does the mixture of people involved affect the identification of problems? Do larger or smaller programs have higher rates of resignation, termination or problematic completion?

In Chapter 4, we will turn our focus on the residents who resigned from their programs. Why did the residents resign? Did men resign for different reasons than women? How were those residents performing compared to their peers at the time of resignation? Did program directors try to convince these residents to leave or to stay? What characterized the resident who was likely to resign? What was the resident likely to do after resignation? How was the resignation process different for the female or minority resident than for the white male resident?

Chapters 5 and 6 will pose many of the same questions as Chapter 4, but these chapters will focus on the experiences of the residents who were terminated or who problematically completed their training. In Chapter 5, we will examine why the residents who were terminated were considered unredeemable in the context of a normal residency training program—what was so bad about their performance that they had to be expelled from the group? In contrast, when we examine the problematic completers, we will see the redeemable qualities these residents displayed despite their poor performance. What kept these residents from being fired? Again, while we raise this multitude of questions, we will also be addressing how race and gender affects the risk of termination and problematic performance.

In Chapter 7, we focus on a particular aspect of the evaluation process that we mentioned earlier—the evaluation and assessment of non-quantifiable traits. In this chapter, we will focus specifically on the evaluation of honesty. Program directors are quick to state that honesty is the most important quality a resident can possess, but what do these directors mean by "honesty" and how are residents judged as "honest" or "dishonest?" We will show that race and gender play a significant role in whether program directors judge a resident as honest or not. Being labeled as honest gives a resident some protection against termination. The poorly performing, honest resident is significantly less likely to be terminated than his or her counterpart who displays equal technical proficiency yet is considered "dishonest." We will show that an honest resident is good at interacting with medical faculty, basically displaying strong interpersonal skills. Honest residents know how to behave in the culture of medicine.

A number of key themes emerged from our analysis. We note that despite some minor changes in the structure of residency training in the last few decades, the education of the surgical resident remains an extremely arduous program and the toxic effects of this environment do take their toll on residents. Although many medical educators believe that a crushing and demanding program produces great surgeons, there is little evidence other than anecdotal accounts to support this theory. Demanding and inflexible schedules cannot continue to be justified on the basis of unsubstantiated claims. Can we make the schedule of residency training more humane and still produce quality surgeons? We cannot know unless we are willing to try.

We also note in our analysis of the culture of the residency program a driving desire for group harmony among the members of the program staff. We find this same desire for group harmony in many different occupational settings. As we will note, however, this desire is heightened by the unique nature of doctoring. Doctors, entrusted with patients' lives, need to trust that each member of the group will provide the very best of care to patients and be willing an able to co-ordinate treatment plans. This is an ideal greatly desired but rarely achieved. In order to create this group harmony and keep the unit running smoothly, program faculty tend to create homogenous groups of white male residents. The process of producing homogenous and harmonious groups, however, leads to discrimination and is therefore inherently unjust.

Ironically, program faculty's appetite for harmony leads to attrition and will continue to feed attrition as the pool of medical students continues to become more and more diverse. If women and racial minorities are at a greater risk for leaving simply because of their race and gender, as they continue to represent a greater proportion of potential candidates for residency posts, we will see an increase in attrition rates across surgical specialties. Program faculty are challenged to keep units running smoothly while also insuring fairness in selection and training. The solution may be re-organizing residency programs in such a way to facilitate harmony among a diverse staff.

We also note that wider social forces and pressures affect the experience of both faculty and residents in these residency programs. We cannot leave our non-professional identities at home when we come to work. Our views about men and women, whites and other racial categories, and what characterizes a "good person," affect how we think and function in our work settings even if we try to limit their effect. We hope that our demonstration of how race and gender impact the interpersonal contacts between faculty and residents, and the assumptions about goodness of fit, will lead to a self-conscious re-evaluation of the process of resident education and evaluation.

Research Population

The data for this study came from two sources: 1) a two part-survey, and, 2) interviews with a sample of 75 attendings, residents, and nurses from five neurosurgery programs. The interviews were conducted by Dr. Charles L. Bosk, principle investigator on a resident attrition project funded by the Pew Foundation and the Society of Neurological Surgeons (SNS).[1] The interviews were conducted at five different hospitals in the Northeast and Mid-Atlantic.

The grant staff designed the surveys with guidance from nine neurosurgeons who served on the project steering committee.[2] Survey I gathered information about the overall rates of resignation, termination, and problematic completion for five different specialties: anesthesiology, general surgery, neurosurgery, orthopedic surgery, and plastic surgery. The first survey collected data about sup-

1. Pew Charitable Trust Grant No. SNS-01
2. The staff included Charles L. Bosk, PhD, Deborah Putnam Thomas, Virginia Adams O'Connell, MA, and Michael Polgar, MA. Our thanks to William F. Collins, Jr., M.D. (Yale University), Julian T. Hoff, M.D. (University of Michigan Hospitals), David L. Kelly, Jr., M.D. (Bowman Gray School of Medicine), Edward R. Laws, M.D. (University of Virginia School of Medicine), M. Steven Mahaley, Jr., M.D., (now deceased), Robert A. Ratcheson, M.D. (University Hospitals of Cleveland), Richard L. Rovit, M.D. (St. Vincent's Hospital, New York), William Shucart, M.D. (New England Medical Center), and Martin H. Weiss, M.D (USC Medical Center) for their assistance and support.

port systems available in the programs and other hospital characteristics. Survey I also gathered information on the process of selection, specifically information on what traits, aptitudes and characteristics are sought in new recruits. We also learned about the forms and frequency of resident evaluation, as well as pay structures. At the time the survey was sent out, 767 programs in these five specialties qualified to be included in the study. Of these, 625 (81%) returned Survey I. Of these, 69 of the surveys were unusable (blank, incomplete or filled-out incorrectly), so the final return rate was 556 (72%).

Survey II was sent to the 418 programs (75% of our final Survey I respondents) that reported any resignations, terminations or problematic completions on Survey I. A separate survey was mailed for each resignation, termination or problematic completion so we could gather specific information on each resident. A total of 2153 second surveys were sent out. We gathered demographic information on the residents as well as background information on training and on the dynamics of each resident's experience. The total response rate for Survey II was 53% (n=1144). There were no systematic differences between the programs that returned either Survey I or II and those that did not.

Both Survey I and II were completed by program directors. In many cases, this was not problematic since program directors can accurately report on program characteristics, hospital structure, and other factual information. Program directors are also the appropriate respondents when we are seeking information on how programs select and evaluate residents. However, in Survey II, program directors were also called upon to report on the residents' perceptions of problems and stresses. We are aware throughout our analysis that our data suffer from not having a better representation of the residents' voices. We are aware that some of our findings may represent the selective (biased) recall of program directors rather than the truth about residents' performance and/or experience. We try to make this prospect apparent throughout our analysis. From a review of the surveys, however, it is our opinion that many program directors did try to fairly represent residents' perspective when asked. We still proceed with caution.

Our data also suffer from a lack of information about the residents who successfully completed their programs without being labeled a problematic completer. In Survey II, program directors were asked to compare the problem resident with his or her successful peers, but this indirect measure does not give us a rich picture of the comparison group's experience. We do not know, for example, how much of what we describe as the experience of these problem residents is also experienced by the successes. For example, do successful residents not have problems, or is the difference between the successful and the problematic resident a matter of degree? Numerous studies on the experience of residency training suggest that the latter is a more accurate perception of the reality of graduate medical education (for example, Bosk 1979, Mizrahi 1982, Marion 1989). Even successful residents have their fair share of trouble, but we surmise that their troubles are less frequent and less severe.

We conducted interviews with the staff of six prominent university-based neurosurgery programs on the East Coast. These programs were in varying stages of development. Some were already well-known while others were trying to make a name for themselves. The number of interviews at each institution ranged from nine to 17. In three of these programs, we interviewed nurses as well as residents, attendings and program directors. Overall, we collected interviews from six program directors, 19 attendings, 34 residents and 12 nurses. All of the program directors were white males, reflecting the majority of neurosurgical program directors. All of the attendings were also white males. The residents were predominately white males with the exception of one white female and two non-white males. The nurses were all white females.

I

The Culture of Surgical Residency Programs

Why Study Surgery?

The reasons we chose to study surgical specialties are multiple. The first is that the study was initiated by the Society of Neurological Surgeons (SNS), whose members were concerned about the high rate of attrition in neurosurgical residency programs. At the time the study was begun in 1990, the rate of attrition from neurosurgical programs was hovering around twenty-five percent. Dr. Charles L. Bosk was approached by the SNS because he had done ground-breaking work on the definition and management of mistakes in surgical residency programs in the 1970s. He noted in his classic study, *Forgive and Remember*, that there were two kinds of errors that residents committed: errors in technique and moral errors. Errors in technique, according to Bosk, were of two varieties. Residents either failed technically or made a wrong judgment about a course of action. Bosk similarly separated moral errors into two types, normative and quasi-normative. Normative errors were a breach in the "code of conduct on which professional action rests" (Bosk 1979:168). Quasi-normative errors involved failing to meet the particular conduct demands of a particular attending or group of attendings, a subset of the greater professional culture. The surprising result of Bosk's field work was that breaches in moral conduct were treated much more harshly than breaches in technical performance—in fact, technical mistakes were expected within the normal context of residency training, but moral breaches were not tolerated:

> "As far as the control of performance is concerned, we would expect impersonal evaluations of technique to have priority over personal judgments of an individ-

ual's moral performance. How are we to account for the fact that the opposite is
the case?" (ibid: 169)

Bosk concludes that the explanation for this discrepancy lies in the "nature of the
professional-client relationship." As we will discuss in greater detail below, doctors
have special privileges in our society and with those special privileges come unique
responsibilities. In order to fulfill their professional duties, doctors must honestly
and conscientiously do everything within their power to help their client, the vulnerable patient. Residents-in-training must demonstrate through their words and actions
that they are honest and conscientious, ready and able to assume a physician's responsibilities. Among the pool of residents in this study who left, just under 25%
left their programs because of an inability to master surgical techniques. The remainder left because of social and behavioral problems that rendered them unfit in
the eyes of teaching faculty to assume the professional duties of a physician. What
Bosk found in the 1970s still rings true today.

A second reason for studying surgery is that surgical errors are at least theoreti-
cally more obvious than errors made in other realms of medicine (Hafferty 1991: 9).
Morbidity and mortality statistics can be calculated not only for organizations but
also for individuals. The time spent with a surgeon is often of short duration. The
kind of care and treatment a surgeon provides is time-bound—"quick and episodic"
(Rosenberg 1992:328)—therefore the effect of the care is more directly related to
the surgeon's intervention. When something goes wrong during an operation, it is
hard for the surgeon to claim that he or she had no hand in the outcome, even if the
surgeon was not directly responsible for the bad turn of events (Parmer 1982:2). As
stated by one of the residents in our sample, "you feel like if there is one false
move, it's like leaving a trail of blood on the water" (R27).[1] This more direct level
of intervention imposes a heavier burden on the surgeon, suggesting that a surgeon
needs to be even more scrupulous in his or her work than the internist. Shoddy surgical work risks far greater damage to the integrity of the patient's body than other
less invasive medical procedures—"the potential for a major disaster from a brief
error in judgment or technique is ever present" (Spencer 1989:141). As one attending commented:

"The stakes are just too high to have anyone in the field who is not conscientious."
(A14)

Errors in technique should be more obvious in surgical fields than in other medical
fields that rely more on pharmacological interventions.

Surgery also occurs in a surgical theater. In this forum, the surgeon's performance is accessible to colleagues and support staff. The internist consulting with his

---

1. Respondents have been coded as follows: A=attending, R=resident, and N=nurse. The
number that appears after this identifier is randomly assigned and does not correlate with
a particular institution. This random assignment was done in order to assure anonymity.

or her patient behind closed doors does not perform as "publicly" as the surgeon does. Therefore by studying surgeons, we expand the number of respondents who can comment on the quality of a surgeon's work. This does not mean that respondents necessarily agree on what constitutes a good performance, only that a larger network of people is involved in the evaluation.

But even with this direct link of the surgeon's intervention and the patient's outcome, we are left with the ironic but reassuring result that the majority of residents in this study who did not complete their programs was not terminated because residents were leaving a trail of dead bodies in their wake, but because they had failed to convince their teachers that they could assume the responsibilities associated with surgical work.

We will now take a look at the culture of surgical work in America.

Section 1: The Culture of Medicine and Surgery

> *"Do not go gentle into that good night,*
> *Old age should burn and rave at close of day,*
> *Rage, rage against the dying of the light"*
> *Dylan Thomas*

This stanza captures the sentiment toward death held by many in modern Western cultures, including American culture. We strive to extend our lives by investing great sums of money and energy in scientific attempts to thwart and overcome death. The group in our society that best embodies this sentiment is our medical practitioners. In fact, one cannot understand the behavior of doctors without understanding their internalization of the value of life and the fight against death. Doctors believe that "human life is precious, that it is better to search and improve than to accept what is, that scientific investigation is good, and that human suffering should be alleviated" (Mumford 1970: 19). Not only is human life precious, but doctors hold "reverence for life above everything else" (Hafferty 1991:40). Socialized to believe that death is the ultimate failure (Swazey 1985: 48, Rhoden 1988: 379), physicians protect life without necessarily questioning the quality of the life they are saving (Bosk 1995). Numerous physicians and other healthcare workers express this reverence for life in their reflections on medical work:

> "Where there's life, there's hope." (Nolen 1968:199)

> "To think that patients can go through hell…can go through everything people go
> through when they are sick and have terrible things happen to them and still have
> life—well, it's really magnificent." (Anderson 1978:294)

There is an active inculcation of this sentiment during the young physician's training. In many biographical accounts of residents' experiences, we are exposed to story after story of the young resident being ordered to do everything feasible to keep a patient alive (for example, Shem 1978:286, see also Glantz 1985: 65). This view about and proactive stance toward life result in part from a physician's direct experience with the "dramatic save." Every physician will have had at least one direct or indirect experience with the dramatic save—when the procedure, the code, worked and saved the life that would have otherwise been lost (Bosk and Frader 1992). Just as every non-physician knows at least one account of a person who has been saved by a dramatic medical intervention (Dubos 1959), so too, the physician who has had this experience is unlikely to forget it. As Shem points out, all the futile attempts are to help you prepare for the one time that it is not futile (Shem 1978:50). As reported by some of our respondents, the dramatic saves are the best moments in their careers:

> "We got them to CT scan and to the OR, got the blood clot out, got the brain decompressed and they wake up the next day and they're talking to you and the girl is twenty-three years old who is a nursery school teacher in the community and you get a card from her students, or you see the cards from the students up there on the wall and you just sort of feel you brought this person back from the dead and that feels good..." (R15)

> "I sort of feel close to her because I feel that I played an important role in allowing her to be here today. I think that is probably one of the most rewarding things about this profession—when you can take someone who is near death, or there is a very good likelihood that they will be dead, and help bring them back, or allow them to recover. That to me is the single most rewarding thing." (R13)

This reverence for life motivates doctors' work, especially when they are working against all odds for success.

Doctors hold not only a reverence for life, but also a reverence for activist therapy and the positivistic pursuit of cures and understanding, a value again shared and supported by the wider culture (Starr 1982:3).

> "I'm just talking about the culture, the civilization of Western Hemisphere...doctors are forced to do instead of standing back and letting nature take its course." (A22)

Coupled with these values is doctors' focus on individuality and the ideal of the traditional doctor/patient relationship. Taken together, the activist approach and the centrality of the individual, the culture of medicine ideally epitomizes the interests and values of the middle class in modern Western cultures (Haas and Shaffir 1987:20).

As is characteristic of professions in general, physicians believe that their work is special and worthy of note and esteem. Laymen also accord it prestige, treating physicians, even if unknown as individuals, with an "awe and reverence" (Light 1980: 301) that testify to the authority of the medical profession. Doctors are given special privileges because of the special nature of their work:

"Taboos that exist for all other members of society are put aside for physicians--they alone are entitled to authorize the injections of poisonous substances, to cut into living flesh, to cause disability in the pursuit of cure. The primary value is health, physicians are taught, and all values must give way to this one." (Glantz 1985:63)

Doctor's work is thought by doctors and by many laymen to be of special benefit to society in a way that is superior to other occupations, even to other professions (Freidson 1986:26-28, Fox 1974). Doctor's work is especially altruistic, and it is unique in its joining of the exercise of power with intimate care. We look to physicians to make sense of the world of illness that we will inevitably experience as mortal creatures, although scientific and technical explanations are often insufficient (Illich 1976). The physician's understanding and mastery of information about the workings of the human body enables us to feel more secure and less vulnerable in our world (Gerber 1983:30), which feels all the more frightening when we are ill. Medical practice consists of numerous rituals, procedures and techniques that combat our sense of helplessness and ambiguity in the face of illness (Hafferty 1991:13). The doctor's advice is "a shortcut where reason is expected to lead" (Starr 1983:15).

The prestige associated with medical work can be seductive for practitioners. Gerber reports that the physicians he studied felt insulated from the mundane problems and issues of everyday life and protected from the feeling that their work had no meaning and made no difference in the world (Gerber 1983:166). Our respondents expressed the view that doctors, and surgeons in particular, are special in ways that are exalting:

"Because you realize, I mean you are like god, and you just try to do what you can and you work your hardest." (R38)

"It takes enormous ego to be a physician. It takes an even bigger ego to be a surgeon. And to be a neurosurgeon, the ego is phenomenal...that does lead them to look at other people as mere mortals...patients feel like this man sits on the right hand of god, obviously, or he wouldn't be doing this." (N20)

Living a life imbued with meaning and importance is enviable, but it comes with a price. The price the physician pays for the prestige is high and many who have studied medical education have questioned whether the cost is too great for any individual. The work of the physician is all-consuming and relentless. The period of training is arduous and long. After completing a competitive four-year undergraduate degree, the doctor-to-be enters a grueling four-year graduate program at medical school. The pressures of medical school are great. As early as the 1950s, medical students complained that they were being forced to learn more than they could possibly absorb in four years of study (Starr 1982:355). The curriculum has grown geometrically since the 1950s. Upon receiving his or her MD degree, the young doctor enters a residency program. Residency training for a primary care specialty lasts an average of three to four years. For those people seeking specialty training, the residency program is even more extensive, running from six to ten years if you include post-residency fellowship training. The young doctor-in-training lives a life so arduous that no self-respecting physician would prescribe the life to any patient. It is a life of self-abuse (Starr 1982:206).

The period of training not surprisingly occurs when the individual has the physical stamina to endure such a taxing educational process. Some descriptions of a typical work week for surgeons show just how taxing that process can be:

"When you're at (institution name), you are on call 24 hours a day, seven days a week...It's almost impossible to have a normal life outside this institution. We'll start at six in the morning and you're lucky if you are home by nine at night. That means going home, saying 'hello' to my wife, eating dinner and going to bed." (R44)

"Some weeks, I have to work 120, 130 hours without much sleep. I find it very much to be a physical strain, an emotional strain to have to do that for years at a time. I've been doing it for a few years now and I don't enjoy it because I don't feel well. I feel sick a lot. When I go home, I fall asleep with my clothes on in bed....I don't get to see my family very much...All I get to do is work." (R30)

"It's hard to be a good neurosurgeon and not spend three-fourths of your time in the hospital." (A14)

And life near Olympus is not colored by one medical miracle after another. In addition to the dramatic save, the job well done, and the grateful patient and family are the failures—the patients who did not make it, or who were damaged by the medical treatment. There are also difficult patients who present a variety of challenges to the young doctors.

"And we see people, you see some of the pits of society, right in off the streets, that came in the emergency room that are sociopaths. Clearly, are just out of jail, whatever. You have to be nice to them. I don't think there are too many other fields where you really have to, absolutely have to be nice to people who are so clearly distasteful not only to me, but to society." (A36)

"Sometimes you get called in the middle of the night to take care of someone who just, you know, is an IV drug user, just got drunk, is throwing up all over everybody, throwing punches..." (R42)

"A lot of patients I've disliked. A lot of very rude people in the world. I've had patients spit at me, vomit on me, punch me, pinch me, kick me, swear at me. No one likes that, but that's the world." (R30)

This time of life also corresponds with the period when many other people the same age who are not in these educational programs are beginning their families.

This is also the time of a woman's peak childbearing age (Martin 1998: 229, Cassell 1998: 111). Many surgeons-in-training feel that they cannot start their own families due to the demands of their educational programs. Gerber (1983) has looked at the consequences in the psychological and social development of the young doctor since he or she puts all of these other life events on hold in the name of medical education. The young doctor may excel in cognitive development, but not in personal development. In a number of studies, Gerber and others find that the interpersonal development of medical students and residents is stunted, and it is thought unlikely that the time will ever be made up once the difficult training program has ended:

> "One now wonders whether this new practicing physician can allow himself time to grow in this most important but postponed area of development...But if he does not allow himself time, what are the personal costs to him, his family, his patients, now and in the future?" (Gerber 1983:111)

The following statistics shed light on the cost of a professional life that is so demanding as to be all-encompassing. Physicians are more prone to suicide, alcoholism and drug addiction than the rest of the population (Gerber 1983:45, Konner 1987:28, Ruddick 1985:211, Vaillant 1979: 372). Among a group of surgical residents, 16% reported having used illicit drugs during their residency training (Schwarz 1992). In our sample, three percent of the residents were reported as having serious and sometimes fatal addictions to drugs and alcohol. Doctors in general are more likely to use psychotherapy than the general population (Vaillant 1979: 372, Konner 1987:371). Doctors also have higher rates of troubled marriages than other professions. In one survey, 40% of the residents reported having trouble with a spouse or partner, and of those, 72% stated that their problems were related to the stress of residency training (Landau 1986: 654). Seventy percent of medical marriages have been classified as dysfunctional (Iverson 1996:294). Cassell offers this anecdote to show that a failed marriage is not necessarily a sign of failure for a physician:

> "Surgeons tell of a celebrated chief of surgery whose program was so rigorous and time-consuming that the marriage of every surgeon in his department dissolved." (Cassell 1998:100)

The amount of time that a physician typically has to devote to his or her work means that other life pursuits are sacrificed or put on hold. Part of the stress associated with the medical practitioner's life style is related to this narrow spectrum of social roles. Although the doctor may be a successful physician, he or she may feel like a failure as a spouse, parent, sibling and/or friend. Becoming a physician often results in the pursuit of one social identity at the cost of all other social identities.

The surgeon is the most esteemed member of the medical hierarchy (Dunn 1997). In addition to the prestige, surgeons earn twice the median net income of general and family practitioners, despite the possibility that the primary care specialist has a greater impact on the overall health of the general population (Weitz 1996:247, Daniel, Kennedy and Ikawachi 2000). Why does surgical work command such prestige and financial reward? Surgery has been described by many as the most aggressive and dramatic example of medical intervention, the field that most closely enacts the activist and therapeutic ideal.

> "Of all the doing that had attracted me to medicine, the surgeon's was the most impressive, not because it necessarily worked better, but because it was so drastic an intervention." (Konner 1987:185)

As Rosenberg has noted, sickness that is episodic and technical garners much more public support than chronic conditions (Rosenberg 1992: 328). Unlike many other specialists, surgeons are not trained to patiently manage patients' conditions with various pharmaceutical agents. Surgeons identify the problem and cut into the human body to remove or repair the offending substance. The limits of the human body to tolerate repeated trauma constrain surgical work—it must be "precise and definitive" (Bosk 1979). Because the surgeon's work is seemingly so much more well defined than the tasks of other physicians who manage a greater number of uncertainties in the practice of pharmacology and pathophysiology, surgeons are "the epitome of competence" (Good 1995: 66).

> "Surgery attracts a different sort of person than does medicine. The guy that goes into surgery is the fellow who doesn't want to sit around waiting for results. He wants the quick cure of the scalpel, not the slow cure of the pill. What he lacks in patience he makes up for in decisiveness." (Nolen 1968: 204)

Described in these terms, surgical work sounds deceptively appealing—a well-defined task, a heroic effort, and a cure. But even surgeons, like all medical practitioners, are plagued by uncertainties in their work (Fox 1989). Much remains unknown about the human body and various disease processes, but physicians must act even in the face of uncertainty. Freidson describes the motivating force behind this work imperative for all physicians:

> "...since its focus is on the practical solution of concrete problems, it is obliged to carry on even when it lacks a scientific foundation for its activities: it is oriented toward intervention irrespective of the existence of reliable knowledge." (Freidson 1986: 163)

Ladd (1985) points out that the what the patient wants is "comfort, solace and freedom from fear and anxiety" (ibid:27). In order to fulfill his or her professional obligations, the physician must intervene. The physician is "expected to do anything possible to return the patient to health" (Glantz 1985:65).

There is uncertainly when confronting the unknown boundaries of medical knowledge, but there is also uncertainty in the practice of "textbook" surgery. Surgery even in its most basic form "is not an exact science" (AMA 1989: 33). Surgery is actually a mixture of technical and scientific knowledge and the art of practice.

"To me, surgery is a fusion of art and science. Science because it's exact, it's like pottery you know. It's fashioned art, yet it is very methodical and very scientific." (R20)

The general body of knowledge and technique must be adapted to every individual patient and this is where the "art" of surgery, the inherent uncertainty, is manifested (Burkett and Knaff 1974: 87).

"There are standard treatments which are pretty straightforward, but in many cases, it takes some ingenuity of fashioning a particular treatment." (A27)

It is hard to imagine, even at a time in our history when we are dreaming about "designer drugs," that medical technology will ever be so precise as to overcome the uncertainty inherent in adapting the general to the specific, whether medical advances come from developments in genetics or better procedures. Because medicine is an art *and* a science, seniority is based on both educational credentials *and* experience. It is only through experience that physicians learn how to apply the general to the specific, how to adapt and change to the needs and peculiarities of each individual patient. Although the young doctor fresh out of a residency program may have been exposed to all the latest developments in the field, he or she does not have the amount of practice in the application of that knowledge that a more senior physician can claim. It is because each patient is truly an individual, a unique organism, and the surgeon must adapt to the unique characteristics of that patient, that the profession claims that surgery cannot be standardized. And there are many different ways to adapt the general to the specific. As one of our respondents noted, "there is more than one way to skin a cat."

"They [the doctors at another hospital] do things radically differently than we do here, and they do just as well." (R17)

Similarly, an attending noted that:

"Each institution has a special flavor, or a way. You have to go to different places to have the opportunity to see what other institutions are doing." (A30)

Individual practitioners can become attached to some adaptations in the same way that people get attached to other routines in their lives, like sitting in the same seat in a meeting room, or at the kitchen table. For example, some surgeons like certain types of aneurysm clips and will refuse to use any other kind even if another clip works just as well (N14). Even within the same institution, there can be significant variations in the ways patients are managed, even after controlling for the severity of the illness (Griner 1988: 49-51). In these situations, the individual practitioner's experiential comfort with a particular mode of practice and/or adaptation is more determinative than any scientific justification for its use.

Surgeons contend that because surgery involves both the application of knowledge and an ability to uniquely adapt that knowledge during an operation, the quality of surgical work can only be evaluated by another experienced surgeon (Wilson 1985: 38) who can assess both technique and the management of unexpected factors. The focus on the differences between patients rather than on their similarities thwarts the establishment of a scientific standard or a scientific evaluation since it can be argued in every individual case that something slightly unique was needed (Millman 1977: 241). This sentiment directly conflicts with current demands both within and outside of medicine for accountability and greater reliance on evidence-based medicine, much to the dismay of many of our respondents who defend this view of the essential nature of medical practice.

Traits of A Surgeon

What traits must an individual have to be a surgeon, to master the techniques and adaptations of surgical practice? Kaufman proposes that surgeons need "the integration of muscle strength, speed, precision, dexterity, balance and spatial perception as well as poise and endurance in the execution of surgical procedures" (Kaufman 1987: 1). But as we cited earlier, these traits were not lacking among the majority of the residents in our sample. In addition to the basic physical talents, those in the medical profession and those who study the practitioners profess that surgeons also need a lot of self-confidence. Few people, these same folks claim, can actually do what a surgeon does. Many argue that it takes a special kind of self-confidence to overcome the more potent "taboos" in our society in order to cut open a human body, to so tangibly have another person's life in your hands:

> "There is hubris in surgery; there is hubris in cutting open, removing, rerouting, or transplanting body parts in order to effect cure." (Bosk 1997: 7)

> "It is cutting, not sewing, that is central to surgery, and cutting into a human body is . . . terrifying. To take a knife and cut into human flesh takes courage, nerve: one has to have an invincible belief in oneself. . . ." (Cassell 1987: 233)

> "...optimism, self-confidence, and resilience in the face of adversity do not seem a list of traits exclusive to surgeons, but without them, they will have difficulty in coping with the pressures of surgical practice." (Hayward 1987: 375)

Nicholas Fox suggests that the draping of the patient's body except for the surgical site not only provides an antiseptic field, but also a psychological field that helps the surgeon overcome the taboo against cutting into human flesh:

> "...covering all body parts except for the site of operation helps remove the sense that there is a person under all that green cloth." (Fox, N. 1992: 11)

Fox also makes the case that surgeons take more risks than other medical practitioners by the very nature of their enterprise (ibid: 93), since their interventions are so direct and dramatic. Risk also results from the greater visibility of surgical work. As noted earlier, there is a theatrical component of surgery that opens the surgeon's work to greater scrutiny than many other medical practitioners. The public's fascination with and support of activist therapies like surgery also result in greater expectations for success. The higher the expectation, the greater the potential fall. To accept all of these risks requires a large amount of self-confidence.

All medical training programs, both undergraduate and graduate, provide opportunities for physicians-in-training to overcome the taboos that prohibit the kinds of physical contacts and invasions of privacy central to medical work (Parsons 1951). Surgical training programs have their own ways of socializing their initiates into the work of surgeons. Socialization is accomplished in part through role-playing even prior to matriculation (Hafferty 1991: 178) and the stereotypical surgeon has historically been a colorful character indeed. The stereotype is telling since it portrays an arrogant individual.

A belief widely bantered about in the literature is that in order to "cut," one has to possess a "macho mentality." Surgeons have been depicted as gun-slinging cowboys. "The archetypal surgeon is invulnerable, untiring, unafraid of death or disaster" (Cassell 1987: 231). In a guide for choosing surgical residency programs written by two physicians, the following stereotype is presented in a tongue-in-cheek fashion, yet its presence in this guide illustrates the power of the image for surgeons:

"It is thought that one should be male, athletic, anal-compulsive, addicted to locker room humor, possessed of a vocabulary of single syllables . . . , have the endurance of a marathon runner, and maintain a political, social, and sexual orientation somewhat to the right of Attila the Hun." (Heimbach and Johnson 1986:3)

Similar portrayals can be found in other writings about hospitals settings:

"I have to admit, my time in surgery made me feel that I was finally discovering what it was like to be part of a boys' athletic team. The locker-room camaraderie. The insults to each other's masculinity (including mine). The poopoo jokes. The nicknames. The boasting about the highly improbably conquests, medical, sexual, or other. The highest praise: "Awesome!" (Klass 1988: 95)

"There are a lot of stereotypes about surgeons. All of them are true. Surgeons are narrow-minded...bigoted...stupid. We're very stupid, all we know is cut, cut, cut, tie, tie, tie...We're nasty to our wives and kids. And we don't know any medicine. All the stereotypes are true. Oh, yes. And we're male chauvinist pigs....Even the women. Fortunately there are few of those. We've managed to keep most of 'em out. And you know, none of 'em are any good." (Konner 1987: 45)

The self-confident surgeon sounds arrogant, but this is the way that the mythical surgeon demonstrates his or her command and proficiency. Merton states that there is "little evidence of a connection between personality and the choice of different kinds of medical careers. But this has not prevented the emergence of a distinct student lore about the type of personality required for each kind of specialized practice" (Merton 1957: 68). This lack of a correlation has been found by others as well (Bosk 1984, Lorber 1984: 33). Despite the lack of a significant correlation, the myth of the surgical personality is alive and well, as these quotes from our respondents show:

> "I have what I consider to be a surgical personality. It's more active, looking for short term results." (R12)

> "I'm somewhat of a true surgical personality. I like to get things done, do things." (R18)

> "I met Dr. X who is a pediatric neurosurgeon and he said that he thought I had the personality for this. He asked me to do what was a sub-internship at the time for six weeks initially. It was great. It was better than sex for those six weeks." (A33)

Note that in the first two quotes, the residents cited specifically that they are more "active" and "like to get things done," which corresponds to our earlier depiction of surgery as the most activist medical intervention. Their interpretation of the surgical personality, however, is more staid than the quotes we provided earlier.

Later in this chapter, we will discuss the effects this stereotype has on the women who attempt to enter surgical specialties. The world of medicine is becoming more diverse with every passing year, and in light of the changing demographic composition of the population of medical students and medical residents, some within the culture question whether these old stereotypes have a place in the modern hospital setting:

> "None of this macho stuff...you're rough, you're tough. It's not 1880 where there are holsters... I think that really has to go...very macho, it's not productive." (R20, male resident)

Putting the gunslinger image aside, Heimbach and Johnson (1986) agree with Kaufman (1987) that a surgeon needs good manual skills, spatial dexterity and endurance. Heimbach and Johnson believe that a surgeon also needs impatience, an ability to make decisions with an incomplete data set, a less-contemplative mind-set, and an ability to sublimate outside personal needs (Heimbach and Johnson 1986: 3). While we may question the existence of specialty "personalities," we may agree that these attributes, considered important for the work of surgery, are not necessarily the same traits that would be sought in trainees for other specialties (Bucher and Stelling 1977: 23)—impatience would be undesirable for a pediatrician.

These ideas about the personality traits and characteristics required for the job are the "idiom" (Milkman 1987) of surgery. This idiom can be so potent that it is unquestioned. Bosk, however, has spent a lot of time questioning the idiom and has a different list of important qualities for the surgical resident: "quickly recognizing a complication, promptly seeking appropriate help in treating a problem, and consistently improving performance over successive trials" (Bosk 1984: 73):

> "A superior surgical resident may be outgoing or contemplative, brash or shy, humble or arrogant; these individual characteristics count for little as long as the resident, in dealing with others, displays thoroughness, dedication and commitment. Therefore, although there is a great deal of discussion about 'a surgical personality,' the individuals who are considered 'superior' actually vary to a great extent." (ibid)

Bosk's definition of the superior resident is certainly more gender-neutral than the gun-slinging stereotypical surgeon, but it is also more gender-neutral than Heimbach's and Johnson's description. Impatience, good manual and spatial dexterity, staying power, ability to make decisions with an incomplete data base, a less contemplative mind-set, and an ability to sublimate outside personal needs have been historically considered masculine traits, while "a pleasing personality . . . ability to approach people, make friends, [and] work harmoniously with various classes of people" (Thomas 1990:221) have been characteristically female traits. As numerous authors have found, men tend to be engaged in occupations requiring them to be "cool, impassive or stern" (Cockburn 1991: 150). Specifically in the medical domain, some researchers have found that "women physicians and midwives were identified as having intuitive, qualitative, and experiential knowledge and the men were considered masters of technical and specialist expertise" (Good 1995: 66). In medical education, "[m]en consistently received higher scores from residency program evaluators for medical knowledge and technical proficiency, while women received higher marks for humanistic attributes" (Martin 1988: 338). As mentioned earlier, we will explore these issues in greater depth when we discuss women's experiences in surgical residency programs. We will note here, however, that the idiom still appears to affect both the self-selection of medical students into surgical programs as well as their subsequent acceptance by program faculty. Not only are men more inclined to apply for surgical residency posts, they are also more likely to match. Twenty-five percent of women who apply fail to match, while the comparable rate for men is only 15% (Iverson 1996: 290).

Having discussed some of the broad themes in the culture of surgery, we will now turn our attention to the culture of surgical residency programs. This section will be followed by a more in-depth look at the culture of neurosurgical residency programs.

Section 2: The Culture of the Residency Program

The Residency as a Total Institution

In 1961, Goffman published, *Asylums: Essays in the Social Situation of Mental Patients and Other Inmates*. In that book, he described certain institutions in our society as total institutions, which he defined as "forcing houses for changing persons" (Goffman 1961:12). Examples of total institutions ranged from the military training camp, to the monastery, to the mental institution, the site of Goffman's primary observations. A total institution was described by Goffman as a place of work and play separated from larger society. In a total institution, a group of recruits (either voluntary or involuntary) undergo a life administered by a single administrative authority. The purpose of this orchestrated life is identity change. In the military camp, the civilian is changed into a soldier. In the monastery, the layman becomes a cleric, and in the mental institution, the insane (it is hoped) find sanity. Caretakers and teachers in total institutions strip the inmates of their previous modes of relating to the world in order that a new identity can be constructed and internalized. One of the ways in which this stripping of the old and building of the new is achieved is that the inmates are immersed in new modes of behavior. Old ways of dressing, of speaking, of interacting with others are taken away from the inmate and new codes are adopted—a new uniform, a new vocabulary, a new way of interacting. Little time if any is left over for leisure. The construction of a new identity becomes an all-encompassing task.

Although not a total institution in the strictest sense of the definition, medical and surgical residency programs do share some of the characteristics of total institutions (Light 1980, Bosk 1984). The resident dons a new uniform, trading in his or her short medical student white coat for the longer resident's coat. The resident also assumes greater responsibility for patient care than she or he ever had during medical school rotations. But perhaps the aspect of residency training most characteristic of the total institution is the seeming total immersion of the resident into the role of doctor. Although some residency programs are surely less demanding than others, a common characteristic of almost all training programs is that the young resident-in-training is expected to devote virtually all available time and energy to the program.

> "I used to love sports, go out with the guys, you know, for either a racquetball match or something like that. I think that what I get from the job is worth foregoing a large part of that." (R23)

Some residents will find that they are working over 100 hours a week despite legal restrictions on doing so. The new doctor will learn as a resident that being a doctor means always being on call. The residents will discover that pursuing a life in medicine requires the relinquishment of other pursuits, be they professional or personal. From the beginning until the end of training, the resident's time will be controlled by hospital schedules.

Goffman believed that many aspects of the total institution he studied, and the character of total institutions in general, were oppressive to the human spirit. For example, he noted that the time spent in the total immersion of one identity meant that other aspects of a total life experience suffered. Recall from our earlier discussion that recent research on medical students have raised similar fears that the medical student is an emotionally stunted individual who has little time for full social development (Gerber 1983). Goffman, like Gerber, also doubted that the inmate of the total institution could ever make up at a later phase of the life cycle such activities as "courting," or "rearing one's children" (ibid: 15). In addition to his concerns about this lost time in the inmate's life, he also questioned the detrimental effects of a period of life in which there are no opportunities for entertainment, or "release activities," that are important in helping individuals cope with the stresses and stains of everyday life—"movies, TV, reading (for pleasure), smoke and drink" (ibid: 70).

Goffman also noted that within the confines of these institutions, inmates were constrained not only to comply with rules and regulations, but also to demonstrate an internalization of these rules and regulations. As we noted earlier and will explore throughout this study, we find a similar demand placed on the residents in these training programs. This demand to demonstrate a conversion basically quashes the potential for individuals to have a unique and personal response to the institution. It also, therefore, quells the potential for innovation and change. We will discuss this aspect in greater detail when we describe the obstacles facing medical educators who attempt to change the structure of the residency training programs.

In a final note, Goffman reminds us that although we are social beings, "the practice of reserving something for the self is a basic component of human life" (Goffman 1961). This is necessary for all of us, in and out of total institutions.

Other Characteristics of the Residency Program

The residency training program is, like a total institution, a changing house of sorts—the young medical school graduate is being changed into an independent specialist. We know from our discussion above that the demands of residency training are typically so arduous as to be all-encompassing. But we need to look at other aspects of the culture of these programs to understand how this transformation from student to physician takes place. When we looked at the broader culture of medicine and surgery in the United States, we discussed some of the beliefs that motivated doctor's work—their proactive attempt to overcome disease. We will now take a closer look at the structure and function of the residency training programs to see how doctors' work is accomplished in this particular work and training setting. The culture of the residency program shares many aspects of the general culture of medicine and surgery outlined above, but some unique characteristics shall be highlighted.

When we talk of the setting of residency training, we are not just talking about the physical plant or the number of surgeries performed, but also the rules governing interactions, codes of conduct, dress and behavior (Jacobs 1994:67). During a residency program, the initiates are not only being taught surgical techniques, but also the activist mentality that informs medical work, as well as professional standards, goals, attitudes and styles (Cassileth 1979:283, Stelling and Bucher 1979: 140). Through these training programs, the specialties reproduce themselves (Light 1980:40). The programs produce the professional offspring that will carry on the groups' traditions. We will see how, through both selection and attrition, the profession creates the next generation of practitioners and how certain aspects of the program culture are almost synonymous with a male culture.

Although there are many different programs, the residents in each of these programs must complete a curriculum before they become surgeons. They must pass a number of cognitive tests and, depending on the specialty, they must perform a designated number of different surgeries. The Resident Review Committee (RRC) oversees and accredits the various residency programs in the United States, so there is some standardization among the various programs in each specialty. There are many similarities among the programs.

But there are also many differences. For example, each program is given a certain amount of autonomy in deciding how to evaluate the residents in their programs separate from the national standardized tests. We found great variation both between specialties and among the specialties in how often evaluations were done and whether or not written evaluation forms were completed. As some researchers have noted, within a program there are as many modes of evaluation as there are faculty members (Anwar, Bosk and Greenburg 1981:27).

Procedural differences distinguish programs from each other, but so do a host of other variables including size of institution, character and size of patient base, level of trauma, number of residents in each post-graduate year (PGY) year, subsequent size of faculty, and facilities. Although a program's certification by the RRC suggests that each of the programs in our survey produced on average competent surgeons, we also assumed that some programs would be "better" than others—not only better at transforming the young initiate into a competent surgeon, but also better in facility management, overall reputation, reputation of the teaching faculty, etc. It was very difficult, however, to develop any ranking of these residency programs. There was reluctance even among our respondents to rank the programs other than dichotomously: certified or uncertified. We found only one publication that attempted to provide some sort of ranking of surgical residency programs—the Heimbach and Johnson (1986) book cited earlier. Our attempts to rank programs by how many of their residents were able to pass the boards (a restricted measure of quality for sure) were thwarted since neither the different specialty boards nor the individual programs would share this information.

Ranking the Programs

Why is it so hard to rank the programs, and why did we find this reluctance to rank? The first roadblock is that all residency programs want to be considered prestigious—they want to be considered among the best by their colleagues and by their patients. The faculty members at one program are reluctant to claim that their staff is any less competent than their colleagues within the same specialty. This is not to say that the physicians would be reluctant to refer cases outside their scope to other specialists, only that within a specialty, all ideally want to think of each other as peers.

There is also "professional courtesy," as well as a Hippocratic injunction, which constrains directors of one program (and doctors in general) from criticizing or defaming the program director of another program (or other doctors). The medical culture treats physicians as a fellowship of professionals, and fellows do not criticize other fellows in front of people outside that professional circle (Friedson 1970, 1986). Those within the profession will acknowledge that among their colleagues, everyone "knows" who has the best reputations, but they tend not to share this information with people outside of the profession.

And, just as surgeons contend that the success of an operation can only be judged by an experienced surgeon, so too there is a professional ethos that believes that any attempt to reduce doctor's work to a number of measurable traits and characteristics, i.e. some ranking system, will always be flawed and incomplete. The list of variables to be considered can never be exhaustive. There are always unique considerations that have to be taken into account. There is the art of medicine, and within that realm is the art of resident training. The professional conviction that no adequate ranking system can ever be achieved prevents those within the profession from making a concerted effort to develop a potentially flawed but useful system.

The Workday

We have already stressed the point that the work of a resident is all encompassing and arduous, but it is useful to review some of that information again. Of all the specialties, surgical residents report the greatest workloads, both by average hours per week on duty and by maximum number of consecutive days on duty. In a study of residency programs, surgery residents were found to be working over 100 hours a week (Greene 1999, Shapiro and Driscoll, 1989). Some of the respondents we quoted earlier put this number up closer to 120-130 hours a week. We need to keep in mind as we review this information that these surgical residents are working these tremendous hours every week over the course of a minimum of five years.

> "There is tremendous time constraint and you have to be willing to spend five or six years, with every third night being up all night." (R18)

> "...working over a 100 hours a week, and being here until nine, ten, eleven o'clock every night and wearing a beeper on your weekends off because you really want to keep an eye on your patients and know that if there are any questions, they can reach you to find out what is going on." (R27)

Working such long hours and being up all night on such a regular basis leads to chronic sleep deprivation, a recurring problem in residency programs:

> "You never get a decent amount of sleep when you are on call. I know you're not supposed to be on call and get sleep, but having to do it for six years, I mean every third night..." (R21)

> "I can remember falling asleep while as an intern, retracting somebody's liver, hallucinating from lack of sleep, and that was the day I was supposed to be learning something in the OR." (A28)

Recent research has shown that "individuals who are sleep deprived are more likely to make mistakes in a variety of areas essential to complex decision making" (Daugherty and Baldwin 1996: S93, Ratnoff in Cousins 1981: 2141). If a sleep-deprived state makes good doctoring harder, why do these intense schedules persist?

The justifications for an arduous training program are many. First, the volume of medical knowledge is enormous (Hanlon in Singer 1989: 25), and for one individual to master even a portion of what is known in one specialty would take more time than any residency program allots. Secondly, the residency program is a time of transformation when the individual adopts a new identity. As Goffman found, for this transformation to be successful within a certain time frame, the individual must be immersed into the new role. In the medical literature it is professed that the time of residency and its tough schedule teaches the resident to sublimate his or her personal needs in order to serve the patient (Cousins 1981, Anonymous in Cousins 1981:2142). The program creates a "battlefield" condition (Bosk 1979) to test whether the residents are capable of dealing with the crises which are part and parcel of medical practice (Reitz in Cousins 1981:2141). If they jump this hurdle, the medical educators believe that the residents are transformed into independent and competent practitioners.

The faculty in these programs also argues that the long hours allow for continuity of care (Hanlon in Singer 1989: 25). They allow the young resident a chance to see the full course of a mode of treatment or progression of a disease process. Although this belief is well entrenched in the medical literature and in medical folklore, research has shown that continuity of care is experienced by no more than a small percent of residents (Anderson et al, 1996).

Others offer the argument that the suffering that these residents endure during this time of their training elevates their work to a moral calling. Interns and residents are seen as "martyrs to virtue, sacrificing their personal lives and their youthful years to alleviate pain and disease" (Groopman 1987:222).

> "Although lack of sleep directly deprives the self, it tends to cast the day-to-day routines of patient care in the light of a higher calling." (Daugherty and Baldwin 1996:S93)

The doctor is an esteemed member in our society. Max Weber, writing on the social psychology of religion, wrote:

> "The fortunate is seldom satisfied with being fortunate. Beyond this, he needs to know that he has a right to his good fortune. He wants to be convinced that he 'deserves' it, and above all that he deserves it in comparison to others…Good fortune wants to be 'legitimate' fortune." (Weber 1993: 40)

Groopman (1987) sees the suffering endured by the interns and residents through abstinence from food and sleep as one of the means they use to transform their own good fortune into legitimate fortune.

> "Interns often remark that they are 'paying their dues ' in advance, and they expect to reap the benefits of their sacrifices in terms of social and economic privilege." (ibid:222)

A resident in our sample said:

> "I think my life will hopefully get better because my life will be compensated and I won't have to live in poverty. I'll buy a home and take a vacation, pay off loans, that kind of stuff. I'll live what I would consider a middle-to-upper middle-class existence." (R12)

Gerber also found that the students she interviewed took pride "in comparing how much they have suffered and how hard they have worked throughout their medical lives" (Gerber 1983:60). An attending in our study commented, "I'm proud of the hours we keep" (A31). But Daugherty and Baldwin remind us that the "positive, symbolic aspects of sleep deprivation are counterbalanced by a growing number of investigations dealing with the negative consequences of long-term sleep deprivation on both the providers of health care and their patients" (1996: S93). Mizrahi

(1986) also warned that residents who are abused in this fashion implicitly learn that it is okay to abuse patients.

When we talk about attempts to reform any of the various aspects of residency culture, we will address why, as Daugherty and Baldwin note, "despite a decade-long national debate, sleep deprivation seems to be the norm in almost all medical specialties" (1996: S95).

Interdependence and Esprit de Corps

Zerubavel and others have argued that hospital programs want to maximize the interchangeability of physicians and nurses (Zerubavel 1979:44). This interchange-ability is the counterpart of continuity of care. No one physician can stay on duty 24 hours a day, seven days a week, but there are patients in a hospital who need care 24 hours a day, seven days a week. To meet the medical demands presented by the patients while also minimally recognizing the needs of the providers' bodies to eat and to sleep, the hospital staff works as a team, coordinating medical care. In the hospital setting, physicians are constantly covering each other's patients. Although one physician may be in charge of a certain patient, when he or she is not at work, someone else on the staff will attend to the patient's needs, especially if an emergency arises. Since each physician (and nurse as well) must trust that whoever is on call will provide the same quality care that he or she would provide to the patient, the interconnectedness of the medical staff is based to a great extent on trust—trust that each individual will do his or her best for all the patients. Patients must also share this trust, since the inpatient today will see a variety of physicians even during a brief hospital stay.

Because the attending and resident staff must share both the tasks and responsi-bility of doctoring, maintaining harmony among staff members is extremely impor-tant. Each residency program can be viewed as a collective culture unto itself (Broadhead 1983: 11)—a culture in which camaraderie is ranked as extremely im-portant. As one of our respondents notes, the people in the program are close in ways we typically associate with "family" (R17). As other respondents noted:

> "The most important thing, no question, this one thing, actually one ingredient, that is the ability for the residents and the attending staff to work well to-gether...I think the ability for the residents and the attending staff to communicate, particularly when they have disagreements in taking care of patients." (R35)

> "We are a group of nine-to-ten residents and we band together. If one is sick, we cover him on the call schedule. If a guy is having trouble at home we cover him without it getting to the attending if we can." (R12)

> "The one thing that makes this program what it is...THE thing is the resi-dents...Get a collection of guys who are real people, there are no assholes in the

group and everybody supports everybody else." (R18)

"Our chairman likes to think that the residents are 'the boys.' 'The boys' will take care of each other, you know, to use that phrase." (R32)

When the group works well together, the program is said to have a great personality, an "esprit de corps" (Iverson 1996: 204, Miller and Donowitz 1997:65)—a common spirit among the members of the program staff. What predicts the presence of this esprit de corps? We can offer theories to explain what elements make a harmonious program, but even the physicians in these programs confess that sometimes what makes a good program is an elusive quality that cannot be articulated (Bowen and Rudenstein 1992):

"Some programs just feel right, and you may not be able to articulate why..." (Miller and Donowitz 1997:79)

"When visiting the programs, ask yourself, 'Do the residents seem happy and satisfied?'"(AMA article)

One thing many analysts agree upon is that the faculty makes each program unique and sets the tone of the program (Tinto 1990:53, Iverson 1996: 204, Nolen 1968: 50). Each program has a unique combination of personalities that must somehow fulfill the obligations of the medical and surgical staff, and this "chance factor of combination of personalities can have a considerable effect" (Mumford 1970:88) on the unit's ability to perform. The chance factor noted by Mumford suggests that a bit of luck is needed to bring together the right collection of personalities to comprise a good group. As we will discuss later in the section on choosing residents, this is a great challenge to the units that support residency programs, since these groups must choose new members every year.

Another factor is the particular mixture of personalities and characteristics. Kanter (1977) has argued that proportions have an effect on group processes. The more homogeneous the group, the more likely there will be group harmony. The more similarities between two people, the more likely will they feel that they implicitly know and trust each other. People also feel more capable of assessing the "qualitative" characteristics (i.e., honesty, integrity, personality) of people just like them as opposed to of people who are different from them. In fact, Kanter found that in order to reduce uncertainty in the workplace, people tended to hire people just like themselves. This is not limited, however, to recruiting people based solely on race or gender or educational background. Some groups try to maximize the number of similarities. For example, when studying physician recruitment in the late 1980s and early 1990s, O'Connell found that doctors in group practices preferred to hire physicians who played the same sports as the other members of the practice (personal correspondence, O'Connell). So in addition to good letters of recommendations and other professional accolades, the group also wanted to hire a colleague who played tennis or golf.

Until fairly recently, all of medicine was a white man's world in the United States, and surgery was no exception. In light of Kanter's work, we can posit that this homogeneity facilitated the harmonious functioning of the staff and the engendering of trust. Being very much alike, the residents did not have to spend much time learning to trust, making friends, adapting to differences in speech, dress, mannerisms and styles of communication. The shared context for social and professional interaction is already well in place when a group is as much alike as possible. With the growing number of women and minorities entering medical training and practice, diversity threatens group harmony (Bosk 1997b). Galanti (1991), a nurse, wrote a book addressing many of the issues associated with trying to take care of a culturally diverse patient population. She mentions everything from problems with communication, to the troubles adapting to various prohibitions on dress and exposure of the body. There are questions of personal space, tones of speech and respectful behaviors. All the issues she raises illustrate the rules governing human interactions in different settings and also apply to a diverse work environment. Who speaks to whom, in what tone, and in what manner? Do individuals tend to touch each other on the arm when telling a joke? What is a joke? Do you look someone in the eye when speaking to him or her, or should you avoid making direct eye contact? Is it taboo to discuss certain issues with some members of the group? All of these questions and others are raised when working with fellow employees who are not like you. There is a certain amount of interpersonal stress that everyone works through when negotiating rules of interaction (see also Bosk 1997b: 30).

Race and gender are prominent traits in this analysis of group harmony, so much so that they will be discussed separately below. But there are other traits that are associated with race and gender that we can note here. For example, we have already implicitly referred to one earlier in this analysis--the positive view toward medical intervention. Some of the residents in our attrition groups were specifically cited as being too passive. A passive mentality is associated with international medical training, especially training that occurs in developing nations. In a medical residency "how to" book, it was specifically noted that having done a stint in a developing country was not an asset to a residency application since you may have acquired a "third world" mentality while abroad. This caution even referred to volunteer work:

> "...it may teach you some thought processes and methods that are frowned upon in the United States (at a time in your training when it may be hard to distinguish these adequately)..." (Iverson 1996:158)

Some similar sentiments were expressed by some of our respondents. In describing a foreign resident who was terminated, one attending told us:

> "There were some cultural problems, almost a third world ethic in terms of 'people live and people die and you can only take care of people, and what can be done can be done...'"(A17)

And a quote from a minority resident:

> "I've been told that I'm generally not a type-A personality. And you know my attitude is a little laid back compared to some people...I guess they would like to see me push things a little faster...being laid back probably comes from my background." (R26)

Mumford states that there is probably some "optimum number of American-trained interns that will give the highest odds for a good high-morale house-staff in a particular hospital" (Mumford 1970:88), for they will maintain the ethos of an aggressive American medical practice. Again, proportions affect group processes.

The activist approach is one component of medical culture in the United States, but other non-medical aspects appear important as well. We noted earlier that the medical culture in our society reflects the general culture of middle-class America. Program directors and other medical faculty evaluate residents' goodness of fit within the wider culture in part by evaluating how many middle-class American behaviors and sentiments they express. We will pick up this discussion in our later chapters when we provide explicit examples from our surveys that demonstrate that program faculty used information about residents' behavior outside the context of the residency program (i.e. in their home, their relationships with spouses, etc.) to judge the residents' fitness for training. But even in the hospital setting, program faculty are evaluating residents over the coffee pot, in seminars, at departmental social functions, looking to see if they demonstrate "the interests and values that characterize the middle-class" (Haas and Shaffir 1987:23). As stated by one minority student interviewed by Haas and Shaffir (1987), the hardest thing to learn in medical school was "the wine and cheeses" (ibid: 23). Having certain social knowledge and certain modes of behavior suggest that you hold similar values, outlooks, and a proper work ethic. Being able to distinguish between cheddar and brie, a Chardonnay and a Merlot, demonstrates that you have the values that a competent doctor needs.

Before we discuss the different experiences of women and minorities in surgery, we will take a closer look at the culture of neurosurgery programs. The neurosurgery programs in our sample had the second highest rate of resignation after general surgery. A description of the experiences of practicing neurosurgeons helps explain why about one out of every ten residents who join these programs leave to pursue a less stressful specialization. It is not an easy job, and although the saves may be dramatic, there are a lot of tragedies along the way.

The Neurosurgery Program

> *"I said to Resident X, you are going to be absolutely astonished like I was that people are paid to do this. You would do it for free. It's a lot of fun, a great way to spend the day. Some poor bugger will pay you a lot of money to do it. I would do it for free it they asked me. Pleasure and challenges all wrapped up in one. You can't ask for a better life." (A23)*

> *"How many people in the world have a job that allows them 1) to meet nice people, and 2) commit assault and battery on a daily basis...to be allowed to operate on someone, that person has to have enormous confidence in you and enormous trust, and that's a great feeling I think. I like it. I think there is nothing like medicine." (A13)*

In his book on choosing residency programs, Zaslau describes the stereotypical neurosurgeon as the physician who is "rich and prosperous and works over 100 hours a week" (Zaslau 1994: 5). There is a certain amount of glamour associated with the image of the neurosurgeon, who is considered as close to a "god" as any physician can be.

> "Neurosurgery tends, to people who aren't in it and even to people who are, tends to be kind of a glamorous, sexy-sounding specialty..." (A19)

The neurosurgeon works on the brain, the control center of the body:

> "I think neurosurgery is life surgery." (R35)

The neurosurgery training program is considered one of the toughest programs to get through by medical educators. It is also one of the hardest programs to get into.

> "We have two positions we offer every year and for that we probably have between 40 and 50 serious applications." (A14)

For what lifestyle are the chosen few qualifying? An arduous tour. The neurosurgery resident can count on working more than 100 hours per week. The program lasts a minimum of five years after medical school and an internship. Knowing that the road to becoming a neurosurgeon was not easy, we asked our respondents why they chose neurosurgery. For some, the mystique of working on the brain was a draw:

> "The highly technical work, dealing with an organ whose function was barely un-

derstood but whose significance was awesome. Simply the prospect of the challenge scared away most people, but I had also wanted to be a Coast Guard Officer and command the ship that pulled people out of the water in the raging storms. It's really not too different from being a neurosurgeon." (A24)

"Somehow, neurosurgery always had a mystique about it. As I advanced through college and medical school, the mystique increased rather than decreased." (A14)

For others, it was the challenge of working on the brain, the complexity of the cases and the intricacy of the operations:

"There is a lot of fun, or return if you will, intellectually from being able to deal with a patient's brain. It requires a high level of, not intelligence, I think, but intensity and I think it requires skills both mental and physical that are not required in other fields." (R39)

"I like the challenge of having something really seriously wrong with somebody and being able to reverse the process." (R27)

"I think what I like best is that it is always a challenge, even the simple cases are challenging." (A15)

Many residents and attendings also stated that neurosurgery was the "cutting edge of medicine." In this field, you can never get bored.

Others were influenced in part by the prestige associated with being a neurosurgeon:

"I suppose I wanted to work hard and be a star. In retrospect, that feeling was awfully silly. But those were some of the initial motivations." (R24)

"It's probably some kind of ego thing. One of the things that's attractive about neurosurgery is that it's dramatic." (R25)

But even with the glamour and the prestige, neurosurgery is a challenging profession. Its patients have an extremely high rate of morbidity and mortality.

"...the first month I appeared on the neurosurgery service they had a lot of trauma and a high mortality rate and by the end of the month the coroner of the county where I worked knew me by my first name and I wondered if this was really what I wanted to do." (A17)

Patients are often suffering from horrible, incurable diseases, or are the victims of tragic accidents. In Morgan's book, only two out of the 20 patients on the neurosurgery floor could speak (Morgan 1980: 181). The morbidity/mortality rate for one neurosurgery unit in our sample was between 50 and 70% (R32). Iverson states that neurosurgeons not only need great manual dexterity but also "a willingness to accept both dramatic successes and long-term failures in patient care" (Iverson 1996:43). Neurosurgeons deal with "high-priced items, spinal chords and brains" (A33). There is not much room for error when dealing with the body's control center. As Scotti states, brain damage is considered by many patients and their families to be worse than death (Scotti 1988: 74). Neurosurgeons live a conundrum—trained to cure patients, to alleviate pain and suffering (Glasser 1973:157)—this is not what they get to do in the majority of the cases they undertake. Here is how some of our respondents described this tension of working hard at the edge of medical technology to help their patients while failing to achieve success so much of the time:

> "A lot of diseases involve patients who are not going to get well…we don't purposely submit somebody to an operation to make ourselves feel good, but often that seems to be the only benefit to come out of the operation. That we beat our chests and work under a microscope and point out the incredible anatomy of the brain, but it is hard to escape the feeling that, 'well that's all very nice, but this guy is going to be dead in a year' whether we dissect that last cranial nerve or not." (R28)

> "Sometimes it can be very depressing due to the condition of the patients. It is hard to deal with the fact that a lot of the patients, their outcome is less than you would like. You know, you work so hard, you put all into it, yet the outcome is going to be poor for them. That can be very depressing. If you start to see that on a day-in, day-out basis, it starts to get to you after a while." (N15)

> "I've treated about 2500 patients, and there are probably no more than a couple hundred that are alive." (A12)

> "I think we have many problems that we can't do anything about. Everyone with a malignant brain tumor dies, no matter what you do for them. There are few problems that we can fix. You know, a benign tumor you can take out, maybe it will fix that completely. Sometimes the aneurysms do well. But the most difficult tumors, the traumatic injuries and so on? While a patient may live a certain amount of time, the end result is bad. And I think we have a large number of these diseases for which we can offer the patients relatively little." (R30)

So how do the residents and attendings handle the disappointment? How do they motivate their work in the face of so many failures and problems? They learn to focus on the cases where things did go right.

> "The view of neurosurgery, at least in medical school, is it is a specialty where you deal with a lot of quirks and a lot of people who have end stage disease who aren't going to get any better and you're just going to round on a lot of vegetative pa-

tients. I found out that it really wasn't that way. And when I realized that you could make some people better and you could do a lot of good in neurosurgery, I felt I could deal with the patients who don't do well." (R25)

"No matter how bad I might have a couple of sick patients dying of head injuries, or something, I know that when I move along the floor later on, I'll come across a whole group of people who had disc surgery or something like that, who feel great now, who are really very happy that they came under our care. And it is nice knowing that no matter how bad it gets, you have some people who are very happy with the result of your surgery." (R32)

But not everyone has the stamina to face failure after failure. For many residents who enter neurosurgery residency programs, the level of stress is overwhelming. Most of the residents in our sample who resigned from these programs left to pursue a less stressful specialization. Neurosurgeons handle the tragic cases, and every time they open up a patient's skull they risk doing irreparable and debilitating damage to the very seat of human intellect, thought and feeling.

Women in Surgery

In this section, we will expand our discussion of the challenges faced by women trying to enter surgical specialties. We have already addressed two issues which hamper their entrance into these professions: the dominating male idiom of surgical work and the need for the program staff to develop an "esprit de corps" which is facilitated by homogeneity. These issues are not unique to women entering medicine but are faced by any woman trying to enter a male-dominated job. In this context, we will discuss some authors' views on why the presence of women in male-dominated work settings unsettles work relationships.

Women in many different work settings where men have historically done the work must challenge the stereotype (the idiom) that defined "maleness" as a necessary component for success. Women entering such varied industries as banking, teaching, factory production, real estate, insurance, law, clergy, computers and medicine have all faced the challenge of redefining the job requirements which have included traits like physical strength and/or rational composure, traits that women have historically been assumed to lack (Thomas 1990: 221, Piller 1998, Reskin and Roos 1990: 221):

"...women don't have the stamina for surgery." (Morgan 1980: 49)

As Jacobs (1989) has shown, however, although occupations have been historically gendered and many occupations remained extraordinarily gendered (nursing, for example), there is not a universal distinction between men and women's work.

Tasks that are "male" and "female" change from society to society (Jacobs 1989:20). In some cultures, women are the farmers. In others, it is the men. Although some physicians might argue that a woman does not have the physical stamina to do surgery, others offer the counter-argument that women have greater and more precise manual dexterity:

> "'Actually,' he said, 'women have better hands for surgery than men, more delicate, but don't tell anyone I said so.'" (Morgan 1980: 55)

There is no standard which predicts whether a man or a woman will perform a job based on the job description. Individuals in various occupational settings argue certain jobs are a better fit for either a man or a woman based on natural abilities programmed by gender (Preston 1995). This argument does not hold up under scrutiny. Those "natural" distinctions are not necessarily related to men's or women's historically domestic roles (Milkman 1987). Lorber has noted that women appear to be "urged into specialties which have high interaction with patients" (Lorber 1984:1), like pediatrics, in response to what is deemed a woman's natural ability for sociability. A counter-argument is that women would be terrible pediatricians since they would be loath to perform medical procedures on a child that might cause pain and discomfort given their "natural" instinct to care for and to protect children. In a similar vein it has been argued that women migrate to specialties that have schedules that have hours and demands compatible with family responsibilities (Lorber 1984: 1), even though research has not supported this hypothesis (Spenner 1995). It is hard to explain women's overrepresentation in the field of obstetrics and gynecology—few would consider the unpredictable schedule of an OB/GYN to be compatible with a stable home life. Carter and Carter suggest that women find themselves tracked into the least prestigious specialties (Carter and Carter 1981), and the number of women in a specialty actually lowers a specialty's perceived prestige. Pediatrics is one of the lowest-paying specialties and OB/GYNs pay some of the highest malpractice premiums.

Not only must the women pioneers overcome stereotypes and try to fit into the group, they must do so with few if any role models preceding them. As we will address below, the presence of role models has a significant effect on students' ability to achieve in many academic and non-academic settings.

What is unique for women looking to pursue a professional path like medicine, however, is the duration and oppressiveness of the training program. For example, delaying childbearing has more negative consequences for the female resident who wants a family than for the male resident since attempting childbearing outside of the peak reproductive years increases the risk for birth defects and difficult pregnancies. Given the demanding schedule of the typical residency program, female residents find it exceedingly difficult to manage pregnancy (Lorber 1984: 80). We will present some of the experiences of women residents who did get pregnant to show that the time they took for early childrearing was viewed as a shirking of duties by the program staff and by the profession in general. Cassell sums up this dilemma in this manner:

> "Female trainees often put their lives on hold for the duration...Married men have the same punishing schedule, but it is taken for granted that a resident's wife will be patient and understanding, care for the children, send his clothes to the cleaners, see that the house is clean, and have dinner waiting when he comes home ready to crash. A husband who provides *any* of these services is considered a saint—or a wimp." (Cassell 1998: 111)

The idiom of surgical work, the desire for staff camaraderie, the high levels of stress, the lack of role models, and the conflicts between professional training and childbearing all contribute to raising the stakes and lowering the likelihood that women wanting to become surgeons will complete training. We will look at all these challenges separately to get a richer picture on all the separate effects on women's experiences in surgical residency programs.

The Idiom of Medical and Surgical Work and Women's Fitness

We noted earlier that the idiom of surgical work historically has been quite male. The stereotypical surgeon has been portrayed as the gun-slinging cowboy. Not only in surgery, but also in medicine as a whole, the idiom of modern medical work has been "male." For example, it has long been thought that emotional displays by physicians were a sign of weakness—"tendency toward emotionalism renders one unfit to be a physician" (Hafferty 1991: 127)—and emotionalism has typically been associated with women. Emotionalism hampers the doctor's execution of his or her duties (Daniels 1961). The tragedy of human suffering seen by the medical practitioner was and is undeniably very great, and the physician has to control his or her emotions, otherwise those emotions can overwhelm him or her. Men were considered better than women at keeping their emotional responses in check, just as they were considered to have greater stamina (Cockburn 1991: 150).

The Numbers Game

The male idiom of medical practice has only recently begun to be challenged by the influx of women medical students and residents (Reskin 1990: 318). Kanter (1977) believed that as the ratio of women to men rises in any social grouping, we should expect to see a shift in the social relations of men and women as well (Kanter 1977: 209). Similarly, Reskin and Roos (1990) argue that as more and more women enter what was traditionally a male occupation, the idiom of the occupation changes and the work is deemed more appropriate for women. As we shall see below though, although women represent between 45-50% of the current medical school graduates, they are not equally represented among all specialties, and therefore not every specialty is seen as an "appropriate" choice for women doctors. Because women now comprise almost 50% of the medical school class, mid-level medical professionals believe that discrimination in medicine is a thing of the past. However, recent data from the AAMC Data Book shows that women are significantly over-represented in two specialties in particular—OB/GYN and pediatrics—comprising over 60% of the resident slots. There is some "occupational feminization" (Roos and Jones 1995) happening in medicine, but only in certain specialties.

Table 1.1. Percent of women among medical school graduates compared to the percent of women among the pool of surgical residents in four surgical specialties.

	1982/83	1985/86	1989/90	1992/93	1996/97	Change from 82/83 to 96/97
% Women graduating medical school	24.9%	30.8%	33.4%	36.1%	42.6%	+17.7
Surgical Specialty						
General surgery	9.6%	11.8%	13.6%	15.5%	18.2%	+8.6
Neurosurgery	5.3%	6.1%	7.4%	7.7%	9.0%	+3.7
Orthopedic surgery	3.0%	4.1%	5.2%	5.6%	7.1%	+4.1
Plastic surgery	9.0%	13.2%	14.3%	14.8%	16.4%	+7.4

In fields like surgery, the male idiom remains almost unchallenged since few women enter the field. Although it is not unusual to think of a woman doctor, it is still unusual to think of a woman surgeon. Only about 17.2% of all surgical residents are women, and of the 34,882 female residents in the country in 1997, only one-tenth of one percent were in the surgical subspecialties (Steinhauer 1999). Jacobs (1989:75) has noted that women aspire to occupations whose composition is about 60% women, while men aspire to occupations comprised of 20% women or less. The sheer majority of men still occupying the ranks of surgical residents will continue to discourage women from considering surgery as a career choice while they are medical students, creating a "Catch-22" situation—the idiom will not be effectively challenged until more women enter these residency positions (Kuczynski 1999).

From the early 1900s up until only about three decades ago, medical educators believed that investing in a woman's education was wasteful since it was unlikely that she would continue to practice after she got married and started a family (Starr 1982). After the Flexner Report of 1910, enrollments of women in medical school fell to 5% and only recently reached close to 45%. But despite the increasing enrollments, the fear that a woman's education is in part wasted is still expressed today by medical educators. Analysts note that female physicians are significantly more likely to work part-time than their male counterparts. Across specialties they occupy the "pink collar" level of medicine, working 9% fewer hours than males (Iverson 1996:292, Steinhauer 1999). Some argue that women are willing to take a pay-cut in order to work flexible hours and have time to meet family as well as professional demands. Others suggest that women are simply not being offered the full-time and top-tier positions. The overriding belief among medical practitioners, however, is that women are "unwilling or unable to find a balance between the years of study [some] specialties require and a life outside of medicine" (Steinhauer 1999: 1). Kuczynski found that similar sentiments rolled off the tongues of the people he interviewed—"the rigors of training are too intense—women cannot balance training, family, and/or a husband" (Kuczynski 1999: 6). These conflicting views demonstrate the difficulty of deciphering the various influences on people's personal and professional decisions throughout their lives. People's choices are affected by what they perceive as their options, and their choices simultaneously affect their range of options—there is constant feedback. Emphasizing women's choices also puts the focus (and burden) on individuals rather than on the structural constraints that hinder their participation.

Working part-time for women doctors can be particularly damaging to the reputation of a female surgeon. Among surgeons, there is a belief that one must work full-time in order to keep skills sharp:

> "It's hard to be a good neurosurgeon and not spend three-fourths of your time in the hospital…I think no matter how good you are, someone is doing an operation, taking care of a problem 50 times a year and you are doing it once a year. The guy doing it 50 times a year is probably doing it better." (A14)

Surgeons who take time off to raise a family, take care of personal problems, or pursue other medical training risk skill atrophy. Only the individuals willing to invest 100+ hours a week will be considered truly skilled and will be truly respected by his or her colleagues. It is these dedicated and committed practitioners who will get the best appointments and the best referrals. The suspicion that women in general are less committed, less dedicated, more easily distracted by family responsibilities and obligations will likely bias faculty appointments and referrals.

It remains true today that women do assume more responsibility for family issues than men even when controlling for employment (Harrison 1982: 205, Young 1987: 642, Steinhauer 1999). Even if an individual women decides to forego a family and keep the same schedule as her male colleagues, the assumption that she is somehow potentially less involved can hamper her reputation (Hass and Shaffir 1987:31). This sentiment was surely felt by Conley (1996) in her experience as a neurosurgeon. The individual woman maverick who wants to pursue the life of a top-flight surgeon not only has to prove her own dedication and fitness for the job, she also has to free herself from the expectations associated with womanhood—she can feel trapped in a stereotype (Morgan 1980: 308). She has to prove that unlike so many other women, she will not bear the primary responsibility for her family. "Commitment" becomes today's substitute for "maleness" as a necessary trait. Fitness is not spoken of in such obviously masculine terms as stoicism and prowess, but couched in terms like "commitment" which deem that men are still better suited for the job.

Even if a woman makes it clear that she is not interested in having a family, her gender can still be troublesome in the surgical residency program. Although she can challenge the idiom of the work ("I can do this job as well as any man"), her femininity can interfere with the work environment in ways separate from the idiom of surgical work per se. Although her gender may not affect her ability to perform surgery, it may hinder her interpersonal relationships with the members of the department. It is to this topic that we now turn our attention.

A Body Out of Place

Men and women are different in many ways, both biological and social In some realms of our social life, we celebrate these differences and take pleasure in the contrasts. This celebration is most obvious in our cultural preoccupation with romantic love and heterosexuality. In almost every realm of popular media, we are bombarded with images of happy heterosexual couples, and our modern fairy tales involve the search for our romantic mate. In these formats, we cry out, "Vive la difference!" But our gender identities are not just personal identities—they inform and reflect social organization. We expect men and women to behave differently and to occupy different social roles. We judge the appropriateness of each others' behavior based on the presumed correlation of that behavior and actors' gender (West and Zimmerman 1987). We expect women to act feminine and men to act masculine. The categories of "man" and "woman" help structure our everyday lives (Bartley 1998: 39). Our gender identity is a more basic cognitive category than our work roles (Gutek and Morash 1982: 59). Sexual identity makes a difference in virtually every domain of human experience (Jacobs 1989: 103).

We can celebrate the differences, but in some realms of social life, we bemoan the differences. Feminists rail against the fact that gender affects paychecks, opportunities for education and employment, health and wealth, and overall life chances. On average, being female decreases opportunities for wealth, education, employment, and medical care. Women in the workplace continue to make less than men do even when controlling for age, education, and job performance. Women physicians make 40% less than their male counterparts. This difference is only partially explained by differences in specialty, practice setting, age and productivity. The exact amount varies by specialty, but the trend pervades all areas of medical practice (Iverson 1996:292).

Toleration of differences in some realms and intolerance of differences in other realms create an unavoidable tension between the various domains of our social lives. There is bound to be what Gutek and Morash (1982: 58) call "sex-role spillover." The alleged differences between men and women, and the rules governing interactions between men and women in the personal, private, and sexual realms of our society cannot help but spill over into the employment sector and affect the interactions between men and women in the workplace. The effects will be felt in the development of working relations among co-workers, between employers and employees, and in this case, between faculty members and residents. Although more enlightened medical educators would state that there is nothing inherent in a women that makes her less qualified to be a physician, we will show how the more basic concept of gender spills over into the residency program and affects levels of interaction between colleagues and the process of evaluation.

Women who pursue a career in surgery are already challenging some of society's sex-role stereotypes since they are choosing to pursue a career in which women have been quite under-represented. In the current climate of residency training, they cannot completely escape the expectations associated with their gender. Although they are already outside the mold of the typical woman, program faculty's interpretation of their behavior and choices are often framed within more traditional social perceptions of expected female behavior. We will pick up this analysis in our later discussions of program faculty's assessment of residents with family or marital problems.

Relations Among Colleagues

As we noted earlier, the residents in a surgical training program rely on each other to coordinate work schedules and cover for each other in order to meet the demands of residency training curriculum. They have to trust that each has the same commitment to good quality patient care in order to share responsibility for patient care. The residents must believe that each resident will be able to pull their own weight so that the work does not get unfairly distributed among the group members. Camaraderie is very important. The group of residents will spend the bulk of the next five to seven years together, spending more time per week with their colleagues than with their spouses, children, and significant others.

Developing trust and friendship more readily occurs among people who are more alike than not, since many aspects of the wider culture and modes of communication are already shared. The woman who joins a residency program comprised of a majority of men will find it harder to fit in the group, formally or, more importantly, informally. Jacobs and others have noted that informal job training is a vital part of the socialization process into a new job situation (Jacobs 1989: 62). Important information gets shared over a drink after work or during a sporting event (Goldstein 1995). Men are more likely to socialize with other male colleagues after work, when this informal information swapping session occurs. Thus women are excluded from this vital interpersonal interaction and are left without information that can make their transition into the male-dominated, work setting easier. This is true not just for medicine but for many different work settings. The entrenched males pass down important "tricks of the trade" to the younger cohort of males and leave the females without critical information. One female orthopedic surgeon shared the following story with us. It was customary for her department to go out together to a strip joint after a particularly difficult rotation. Her male colleagues in the program refused to change the tradition so that she could attend (since she refused to go to a strip joint). She felt excluded from what was an important rite of passage in her program. Exclusion from particular social events or from the "tricks of the trade" sessions is nothing less than a form of sexual discrimination (Jacobs 1989:152). No acclimation to a new work setting can be successful without the kind of help that only co-workers can provide.

Women are often excluded from informal gatherings outside of work hours, but they can also be excluded from social activities at the work site. Residents experience a great amount of stress from dealing with life and death issues on a daily basis. Residents engage in a variety of behaviors during the workday to deal with and relieve some of that stress. Traditionally in the surgical theater, this has meant a great deal of locker-room humor and other bantering. Recall an earlier quote:

> "I have to admit, my time in surgery made me feel that I was finally discovering what it was like to be part of a boys' athletic team. The locker-room camaraderie. The insults to each other's masculinity (including mine). The poopoo jokes. The nicknames. The boasting about the highly improbable conquests, medical, sexual, or other." (Klass: 95)

This form of the humor reflects a couple of themes—that men have traditionally been the surgeons; that there is an irreducible physicality of surgical work; and that surgery consistently breaches the boundary of the sacred and profane. It demonstrates as well the prowess and self-confidence that is needed to regularly take someone else's life into your hands. It also demonstrates that some forms of humor and bantering are sex-role specific. Humor between men and women typically has a different character than the humor among a group of men or among a group of women. Again we make note of some of Jacobs' findings. Camaraderie and all its forms helps people cope with the stresses of the workplace. In male-dominated settings, this camaraderie has taken the form of bantering, and yet men feel the need to alter their behavior in the presence of women (Jacobs 1989: 154). Women may find it difficult to accept and to participate in the locker-room humor (Conley 1996). We find that the different rules of interaction that we acknowledge in polite discourse spill over into the workplace, upsetting what was an acceptable mode of interaction, and an acceptable coping mechanism, among male residents. The residents may still need to blow off steam, but they will do so out of sight of the other gender. Again, for the female resident in a predominantly male program, this means that she has fewer people available with whom to banter.

Relations Between Supervisors and Subordinates

In the residency program, the supervisors are the program directors and attending faculty and the subordinates are the residents. Since only a small proportion of surgical faculty are women (only 6.6% according to the AAMC Data Book, January 1998), most of the women entering a surgical residency program both at the time of the study and today will be evaluated by only male faculty members, a traditional power relationship. But the medical faculty/resident relationship is not simply an employer/employee relationship—it operates as a mentor/mentee relationship. At some point in the mentor/mentee relationship, the mentee becomes a colleague of the mentor and no longer a subordinate. It is because of this maturation of the mentee that the male/female dynamic threatens the traditional subordinate position of the woman. We should also note that male surgeons have traditionally worked with female nurses, professionals whose power in the workplace is not equal to their own. It is not that male surgeons are unaccustomed to working with women; they are unaccustomed to working with women as peers.

Subordinates typically have very little leeway to question the authority of their supervisors, but peers often do question each other, bounce ideas off each other, and consult each other. Men are more comfortable being challenged by men than by women:

> "'Don't yell at me young woman,' he bellowed, 'I don't allow that! Perhaps these young men will, but you've got to know your place.'"(Cassell 1991: 139)

The place that women are supposed to occupy in the residency program setting is subordinate even while they are training to become professional peers. The rules of interaction both historically tolerated and currently tolerated have spilled over into the residency program culture. And program faculty members are not the only ones who have trouble with challenges to traditional boundaries. Nurses working in male-dominated medical and surgical fields have reportedly had trouble accepting orders from female doctors. Here we find the reverse effect—the women, accustomed to taking orders from males, find it hard to take orders from females who are supposed to be their peers and not their superiors. Cassell reports that nurses reprimanded women residents who threw tantrums in the operating theater, but tolerated the same behavior in men. The nurses purportedly "cull out the weak and the sick" (Cassell 1998: 97) with their behavior toward the women residents.

Morgan also offers an example of how her female colleagues who acted "feminine" were treated differently in her residency program. The male medical faculty considered their behavior appropriate:

> "I felt betrayed that another woman surgeon wept and complained when things got tough." (Morgan 1980:226)

She relays a story about a female colleague who elicited sympathy from male surgeons when she behaved "like a woman," while Morgan, who toughed it out, acted more like her male counterparts.

> "Don't you see, Patsy's turned many of the men against you. She behaves the way they expect a woman to behave, so when you demand that she behaves like any other surgeon, as you do, they take her side." (Morgan 1980: 308)

In the medical field, as well as in almost every occupational category, few men are subject to female authority (Boyd, Mulvihill and Myles 1995). The woman's body is a symbol of sexual and social submission in our society.

> "That same body can therefore be 'out of place' in the workplace when placed in a position of power over a man. The subordinate man can react to the woman in authority as 'teacher, mother, 'bitch.''" (Cassell 1998: 82, see also Goldstein 1995: 1006)

Men are reluctant either to be reprimanded by a woman or be reprimanded in front of a woman. Morgan noted in her account that the men in her program were very concerned about "being ripped apart in front of a woman" at the Mortality and Morbidity rounds (Morgan 1980: 64). Again, we cannot leave our gender identity at home when we go to our work site. Gender identity and career identity become inextricably intertwined.

Sexual Harassment

Men have been accustomed to privilege and authority in the medical world and the rights and privileges associated with their dominance in fields like surgery are typically not given up without a fight (Rosenberg 1992: 341). Researchers in many different occupational settings have found that outright hostility toward women has been a common response to the influx of women into male-dominated settings. In fact, the forms of sexual harassment experienced by women in traditional and non-traditional work settings are very different. Carothers and Crull found that for women in traditional settings, sexual harassment took the form of sexual advances. Women in non-traditional settings like medicine, law, and other professional settings were more likely to face a demeaning work environment (Carothers and Crull 1984: 222). Gutek and Morasch found that women in male-dominated work settings actually experience more sexual harassment than women in neutral or female-dominated environments (Gutek and Morasch 1982: 152). Like Carothers and Crull, Gutek and Morasch found that sexual harassment in the former setting takes the form of a demeaning work environment, which might include sexual jokes, slurs, unwanted physical contact, and sabotage of women's work. Jacobs (1989) also found that in male-dominated settings, sexual harassment took the form of hostility rather than sexual advances (Jacobs 1989: 153). The effect of a hostile environment cannot be underestimated. Studies of women leavers from graduate training programs have found that women in non-traditional areas of study tend to leave because of perceived hostility and lack of support, not because of family responsibilities (Scott , Burns and Cooney 1996: 257). The hostility can be extreme enough to force women to abandon their educational and professional pursuits.

Sexual harassment of the female trying to enter medicine begins not when she enters a residency program, but during her tour at medical school. As Daugherty, Baldwin and Rowley have documented, 69% of women (as compared to 25% of men) were sexually harassed at some point during medical school (Daugherty, Baldwin and Rowley 1998).

Before women face a hostile residency program environment, they experience discrimination in selection to male-dominated fields like surgery. Iverson found that 25% of females applying to surgical residency programs failed to match as compared to only 15% of males (Iverson 1996: 290). For those who do get accepted into a surgical residency program, the women enerting surgery face the greatest risk for sexual harassment among all the specialties.

> "The American Medical Women's Association states that women practicing General Surgery report the highest rate of sexual harassment at 50%...Harassment included gender-specific and sexual comments, being touched or pinched, and being pressured for dates." (Iverson 1996: 293)

Surgical residency programs have been described as particularly inhospitable to women—a "remarkably hostile environment for women" (Kuczynski 1999).

"I learned that the...exclusion (or at least, distrust) or women were characteristic of surgeons." (Cassell 1987:231)

"The term 'sexism' is too abstract, too disembodied, to describe such a visceral rejection of the wrong body in the wrong place; perhaps 'misogyny' is more accurate." (Cassell 1998: 41)

Descriptions such as these do not encourage female medical students to consider a career as a surgeon, or to persevere in the face of a hostile work environment.

Role Models

Women entering surgery have few role models to emulate during training. Pioneers pave their own way, building upon models established by people unlike them. Pioneers adapt to a new environment with little to no guidance from others who went before them. We have already discussed the importance of informal networks in learning work rules. The female pioneer in a male-dominated setting lacks an informal group from which she can learn these rules. She also lacks mentors of her own gender to ease her transition and teach her the ropes. When available role models are a different gender, that difference acts as a constant reminder of an insurmountable and undeniable difference.

The presence of role models has proven to be very important in predicting the likelihood that a woman pursuing a particular career or education path will succeed in her endeavors. For example, in studies of graduate education, there is a significant positive relationship between the percent of female faculty and the performance of female students (Konrad and Pfeffer 1991). Unfortunately, it is also true that the women in the most prestigious settings have the fewest role models (ibid). In fact, although women now earn 50% of all bachelors' degrees, they still only earn one-third of all PhDs and only one-quarter of professional degrees. These disparities are found in medicine as well as in computer technology, engineering, science, business, etc. (Piller 1998). In medicine, although women make-up 45-50% of the medical school class, women hold very few dean or faculty positions in medical schools (Steinhauer 1999), and they comprise only about 20% of medical school faculty. Their faculty appointments are usually at the assistant professor and instructor levels (AAMC 1998). The lack of role models is just one more challenge for the female surgical resident.

Childbearing and Family Commitments

Many current deans and medical faculty believe that women do not occupy the top tiers of the medical profession because they find it impossible to meet both the rigors of the training program and the demands of having a family. Across employment sectors, employers see childrearing as a lack of commitment (Jacobs 1995: 47). More time invested in raising children translates into less time devoted to career advancement. As we have already discussed, it is assumed that women will bear the brunt of responsibility for family matters, and women generally still do assume primary responsibility for childrearing in our society. In fact, employers view a woman's being married as a lack of commitment since she already has one dependent—her husband. Being single is not much better, however, since the single woman is considered either sexually available (Iverson 1996: 293) or sexually dangerous (Lorber 1984: 11)—a no-win situation.

The program directors in our study feared that women's skills would atrophy if they took time off for childbearing, childrearing, or other family responsibilities. Although particular cases will be discussed in detail in later chapters, some of the comments made about women becoming surgeons, or who had children during their residency training, will be presented here to illustrate the prevailing view about how women's competing responsibilities can interfere with training:

> "She didn't want this job. I think she was bright enough but just didn't do it. She shirked her responsibilities in very obvious ways...Three years she was here. She got pregnant twice in one year of internship. Took a ton of time off and you know when she came back, I think that the powers that be didn't want it to look as though they canned her because she got pregnant." (R36)

From a nurse commenting on the dearth of women neurosurgeons:

> "I'm just as happy that there aren't. That's my own personal feeling. I think it's very strenuous work and I think there is still an awful lot of chauvinism in heads of departments. I don't think it is going to be inundated like anesthesia and pediatrics because those services lend themselves a little bit better to a female, the traditional female role of being wife and mother if you chose." (N17)

And other statements which express program faculty's recollection of bad experiences and fears that a surgical education may be wasted on a woman:

> "We've had very bad experiences with female residents. We've accepted two or three women in the past three-four years. One girl had major marriage problems and family problems. Was a nice kid, but really wasn't the kind of temperament that would have lasted. She basically called up and said, 'I can't be there tomorrow,' her first day. We had another woman who was torn between her boyfriend and time commitments, and so forth, and left us hanging in the lurch. I guess if you get burned a few times, there is a tendency to say, 'They have to be really something special for us to take that chance again.'" (R18)

> "The program director finally took a gal, a very good resident, who then *deliberately* (italics mine) got pregnant in her chief residency year and missed the last

four months and then when she finished, we had a lot of discussion of what to do. Do you say, 'Okay, they have completed their residency?' You can't slide them back because you don't have a slot—the slots beneath are filled. In any event, she finished, went out and just decided that she really wasn't interested in doing neurosurgery because she had a family and all the other stuff. And in terms of when you're going out to select people who are going to make a mark in the field, who are going to do things research-wise or at least contribute to neurosurgery, and then they turn around and they don't really do what you've trained them to do, you have a problem." (A36)

As members of the wider culture, we can empathize with women's desire to have children. Becoming a parent is time-honored role for both men and women in our society. The reasons why anyone brings children into the world are multifaceted. As part of their gender socialization, women generally see childbearing and childrearing as expected social roles. But there are many other reasons for pursuing parenthood. For the women in our sample, there may have been pressure from family and spouses, a desire to complete childbearing by a certain age, or an overwhelming personal desire to have a child. Even these reasons do not exhaust the list. For whatever reason(s) these women chose to become pregnant while simultaneously pursuing a surgical career, we cannot see how the demands of childbearing and childrearing can be reconciled with the demands of a surgical training program unless modifications in the training program are made. How can medical educators modify the programs to allow greater flexibility for both women and men who would like to start their childbearing before they have finished the long and arduous training program. Is it true that skills atrophy as much as is feared, or is there more leeway than is anticipated? Can a year be taken off and training resumed after the birth of a child? Can the match program be revamped to allow programs this kind of scheduling flexibility, basically granting sabbaticals to residents? Can slot-sharing, a rare but available practice in some programs, be adopted more widely by residency programs? The conviction that only total dedication and immersion at the cost of all other life experiences produces skilled surgeons is well-entrenched in the surgical culture, but alternative ways of organizing training can be tested. Those who have written on the stressful and unhealthy lifestyles of physicians have called for changes such as those postulated here (Mogul 1985: 143). Others have been more radical and have suggested a modification of all social and occupational life to accommodate women's biological constraints (Martin, 1998).

One issue that crops up in many of the articles on women in medicine is the conflict between trying to be a competent and well-respected physician and to have a happy family life. In reviewing a typical arduous workweek, it seems unlikely that even the male surgeons are happy with their balance between these two competing forces. Some analysts like Cassell (1998) point out a possible advantage for men— the male surgeon may have a wife who is taking care of the children, and the laundry, and has dinner ready—an advantage few women surgeons have. But we have to ask these additional questions: does that male surgeon have a quality relationship with his spouse, or with his children, if he is spending so very little time with them? Those concerned with equality are clamoring, "Let us in!" to these inner sanctums of surgical specialties, but for what kind of life are they clamoring? Can we organize our work so that both men and women can operate on people's brains and still have rewarding personal lives? Raise children? Have balance and pursue hobbies? In many walks of life, we find that in the name of excellence, whether in the arts, in sports, or in science, some people sacrifice a lot of life experiences in their attempt to be the best at something. The Olympic competitor, the great concert violinist, the scientist who continually runs experiments—all of these people devote the bulk of their energy to one activity. Trade-offs may be unavoidable, no matter how we reorganize our social life. We need to take note, however, that data collected by analysts across occupational settings point to the fact that women trade off more than men. It is the disparity in the amount of trade off between men and women, and not merely the trade off itself, that is troubling.

All Boys Club

In this section we have reviewed a host of obstacles that women face when they try to enter surgical specialties. Underrepresented, they must forge an upstream path against the assumption that "maleness" is a necessary trait to have to get the job done. They enter a world in which they are often kept out of the informal circles of colleague interaction. They face a stressful work environment, and the stress-releasing behaviors in that environment are "macho" and inappropriate for women. And they face all these challenges during their peak reproductive years.

Program directors appear to have a preference for male residents, which is reflected in the greater match rates for men as compared to women. Reskin and Roos might say that program directors are "feeding their own appetite for a boy's club" (Reskin and Roos 1990: 37). Why this preference? The first is that the idiom of surgical work drives evaluators to assume either explicitly or implicitly that men are better equipped to perform the work. Secondly, the desire for great camaraderie encourages program faculty to homogenize the resident pool as much as possible in order to create a well-oiled machine. Thirdly, the traditional behaviors associated with not only surgical work but with the coping mechanisms have produced a "macho" mentality. And there remains in the culture of medicine as a whole a reluctance to "waste" a medical education on a woman who may or may not totally immerse herself in her professional life.

In the next section, we will look at how many of the same issues affect racial minorities. How do the history of surgery, the idiom of surgical work, the desire for camaraderie, the traditional power relations between whites and non-whites, and the lack of role models impact the entry of racial minorities into surgical residency programs?

Racial Minorities in Surgery

The stereotypes and preconceptions that challenge women's participation in surgical training programs also challenge racial minority participation. Residents who are both women and racial minorities face a "double jeopardy." Since surgical residency slots are still filled primarily by white males, whatever makes a resident different from the status quo, whether race or gender, challenges participation. We shall discuss how the idiom of surgical work and the need for camaraderie set up similar hurdles for the racial minority resident in order to complete his or her training.

As Konrad and Pfeffer (1991) note, "[j]obs and occupations come to be seen as typical and more appropriate for men or for women and for Whites or minorities" (Konrad and Pfeffer 1991: 144). Just as the idiom of surgical work has been overwhelmingly male, it has also been overwhelmingly white, so the traditional yardstick for measuring appropriateness has been both "maleness" and "whiteness." In their study of educational institutions, Konrad and Pfeffer found extremely high levels of between-organization ethnic segregation and concluded that "maintenance of social distance between ethnic groups many be more important...than may be the maintenance of social distance between men and women" (ibid: 150). Although contacts between the genders may be strained from the spill over of gender and sexual identity into the workplace, Konrad and Pfeffer suggest that the tension of interactions between those of different ethnic groups is actually more threatening and stressful. They point out that social contacts between ethnic groups is often inhibited and strained by cultural differences. Although there may be sexual tensions and role restrictions, men and women from the same ethnic group share a common social fabric and understand each other's different modes of conduct and speech. Goldstein noted that racial minority students have "academic backgrounds and learning styles, personal and family responsibilities, economic constraints, values and goals [which] frequently contrast with those assumed as normative" (Goldstein 1995:983). All of these differences make interactions between colleagues, as well as interactions between subordinates and supervisors, more difficult. Without a common value system, a common language, a common learning style, meaningful and productive interaction can be almost impossible. Again we note the role of homogeneity in creating an easy, operative work environment. The influx of white women, racial minority women, and racial minority males creates new challenges for the organization and operation of the surgical residency program.

Why Whiteness?

Why is there a continuing preference for white residents? The history of discrimination in the United States offers some insight into the phenomenon. Just as men have traditionally wielded power over women, whites have wielded power over other racial minorities. Belief in the inherent hierarchy of the races (which was systematically challenged less than 40 years ago in this country) is very slow to change and continues to influence how candidates are evaluated for positions. In the history of medical education, African-Americans have faced the most extensively publicly sanctioned exclusion of all racial groups (Smith 1992: 3).

Discrimination not only influences matriculation and evaluation; it also taints the everyday experiences of racial minorities in medical school as well as in the residency program setting. As Iverson tells the racial minority readers of his residency program guide:

> "Yet discrimination does exist within the medical fraternity. As you expand your horizons to search out the ideal training program, be aware that you may have to do more to prove yourself than other candidates." (Iverson 1996: 306)

Sixty-one percent of racial minority medical students in programs in the United States reported at least one experience of discrimination during their tour through medical school (Baldwin et al, 1994). The predominate form of discrimination was racial and ethnic slurs (ibid: 19), however, racial minority students also often reported being denied opportunities and experiencing poor evaluations (ibid: 20). These figures do not apparently reflect a reporting bias since over 60% of all residents, both whites and non-whites, reported personal observations of racial or ethnic discrimination in their places of work (ibid: 21). Discriminatory attitudes are part and parcel of the medical school environment. It is especially interesting to note for our purposes that discrimination is most likely to be observed by residents in the specialty of surgery, followed by those in medicine, pediatrics, and OB/GYN (ibid: 21).

Screening for Academic Excellence

Although few if any medical educators today would outright admit a racial preference, other traits and aptitudes substitute for race in choosing residents. For example, choosing candidates both for medical school and for residency slots based so heavily on academic excellence perpetuates the racial disparities inherent in our primary and secondary school systems in the United States (Elliott , Strenta and Adair 1996: 688). Although 24% of Caucasians attend college, only 20% of African-Americans and 16% of Hispanics do (COGME 1991: 2). For those who make it to college, a far lower percent of minorities pursue majors in the sciences, in part because of their poor preparation for these fields of study in secondary school (Elliott, Strenta and Adair 1996: 700). Since the sciences tend to be some of the most competitive fields of study in college, the minority student tends to feel overwhelmed by the coursework. Although African-Americans and Hispanics comprise about 25% of the current population of the United States, they are sorely underrepresented among the cadre of practicing physicians, comprising only 4.1 and 3.4 percent of the nation's physicians (COGME 1991:3). A number of analysts have challenged medical educators to rectify this great disparity (Baldwin, Rowley, Daugherty and Ray 1995, Jonas, Etzel, and Barzansky 1991: 914). Table 1.2 below shows the distribution of some minority groups in a subset of surgical specialties in 1993-94, the first year that the American College of Surgeons began collecting data on the ethnic backgrounds of surgical residents.

This selection "elitism" (Ludmerer 1985: 183) based on past academic performance and standardized test scores has remained despite the growing evidence that test scores and academic achievement are not correlated with eventual success as a medical practitioner. Minority students will on average not perform as well on standardized tests, but if standardized test performance is not correlated with eventual success in the field of medicine, it is hard to continue to justify choosing residents based so heavily on this criterion.

Unfortunately, this selection elitism has been legally upheld in cases like the Bakke case in California (1978) in which the principle of affirmative action was deemed less important than admitting to medical school only the most qualified applicants (Ludmerer 1985: 121)—the most qualified defined as the highest academic performers. A number of researchers have suggested that racial minority scores on exams have to be judged differently than whites' scores given the poorer quality of their primary and secondary educations (Rolph, Williams and Lanier 1978: 51, Tinto 1993). The question is whether medical schools should be more interested in overall potential than in an applicant's current fund of knowledge. Some analysts believe that many minority applicants may be turned away not because they do not have the potential to become excellent physicians, but because they have not had a quality education prior to applying to medical school. Elliott, Strenta and Adair argue that for non-traditional students, the assessment of non-cognitive traits may be more important than standardized test scores in predicting success in medical school (Elliott, Strenta and Adair 1996: 171) since non-cognitive traits are better at assessing underlying potential. Unfortunately, medical schools and residency programs are not currently organized with the kind of curricular flexibility necessary to bring the poorly prepared students "up-to-speed" with extra support and time for study. The challenge facing medical educators is to revamp a well-established and "rational" system for choosing the future cadre of physicians that perpetuates discrimination while at the same time finding a way to correct the mistakes that have compounded over the course of the minority student's lifetime.

Table 1.2.Ethnic Background of Surgical Residents and Fellows: 1993-1994

Specialty	African-American	Hispanic	Asian [2]	White	Other	Total
General	361	396	1197	5262	325	7541
	(4.79%)	(5.25%)	(15.87%)	(69.78%)	(4.31%)	(100%)
Neurosurgery	36	21	107	654	77	895
	(4.02%)	(2.35%)	(11.96%)	(73.07%)	(8.60%)	(100%)
Orthopaedic	109	69	217	2692	111	3198
	(3.41%)	(2.16%)	(6.79%)	(84.18%)	(3.47%)	(100%)
Plastic	13	10	51	394	7	475
	(2.74%)	(2.11%)	(10.74%)	(82.95%)	(1.47%)	(100%)

Apparently, even four years of medical school does not always succeed in filling in gaps of knowledge:

> "I think the one mistake that we make here and a number of places make is taking minority students because they are minority students. These people are far below the caliber that they should be…We have a couple of people from (prestigious medical school) who are rotating who are dumb." (A26)

Correcting compounded neglect is not an easy task for medical schools or for residency programs.

In light of both the prevailing discriminatory attitudes and poorer preparation, minorities subsequently find it much harder to get into their desired residency program (Iverson 1996) and to stay on track in their medical education program (Babbott, Baldwin, Jolly, and Williams 1988). Although some whites and some racial minorities "change their minds" after pursuing a particular residency program, 78% of whites are on track in their PGY3 while only 65.8% of racial minorities are. The reasons for attrition are many and varied, but many racial minority physicians who drop out of more prestigious specialty programs end up in primary care (Babbott, Baldwin, Killian and Weaver 1989).

The Idiom of Surgical Work and the Wrong Mind-Set

We have already discussed the idiom of surgical work at great length. We noted that women have traditionally not been seen as "man enough" to get the job done. Similarly, medical educators often do not see both American-born and foreign-born racial minorities as having the right work ethic or mind-set to get the job done. An

---

2. The category Asian includes Pacific Islander, Indian and Middle Easterner.

activist/optimistic stance reflects the morals and values of "white" middle-class America. Cassell noted this attitude among a surgeon in her study:

> "The chief was suggesting that the foreign-born and foreign-educated surgeons in that area had lower standards, in surgery as well as morality, than those of native-born and native-educated surgeons such as himself." (Cassell 1991: 91)

Some medical educators fear that foreign-born and foreign-trained students in particular develop a "third-world" mentality about health and illness. They define a third-world mentality as a resigned view of health and illness, not an aggressive, battle-like stance. In contrast, the right mind-set for the medical practitioner in general and the surgeon in particular is that of the aggressive perfectionist—the individual who will upturn every stone to find an answer to the problem, who will use every means to fight against disease and death. Surgeons should have a type-A personality, a non-contemplative, compulsive mind-set.

> "My personal philosophy is everybody, 98% of the people that graduate from medical school really probably have the smarts to be good doctors. I think what the difference comes down to is who is compulsive and who isn't." (R44)

Racial minorities and foreigners have to confront the preconception that they do not have the right "cowboy" mentality to get the job done, and their styles of behavior and interaction may be interpreted as "not compulsive" enough. The "reserved" foreigner may be quite compulsive regarding work, but fairly quiet and reserved in interpersonal relations. For example, one Korean woman in our study initially received poor evaluations because she was "quiet, slow...spoke little." She surprised her program director with the "definite" progress she made during the program.

Noting the low percentages of racial minorities in surgical residency programs in the table above, we can put forth a theory similar to our analysis of women in surgery. Until there are more minorities in these programs, the idiom of surgical work that views "whiteness" as a necessary trait will remain insufficiently challenged since whiteness here is assumed to indicate a proper mind-set and work ethic.

Camaraderie

We have already noted that homogeneity facilitates camaraderie and that residency programs value camaraderie among their residents. We have also noted that ethnic and racial tensions may be more stressful than gender tensions in social and work settings. Minorities, both American-born and foreign-born, therefore have a difficult time adjusting to the culture of medical education in general and to the culture of the surgical residency program in particular. The medical school and residency program environments seem alien to many minorities because they require conformity (Ireland 1979: 256)—the sameness that comes from a white, middle-class upbringing.

It is not just conformity that is disconcerting for the minority student. As we noted above, overt discrimination makes the graduate school environment both *foreign* and *hostile* (Tinto 1993: 73). Cultural differences result in minorities having both less favorable attitudes toward faculty and more difficulty interacting with faculty (Johnson 1978: 136). Conflicts between different ethnic and racial groups are exacerbated by misunderstandings resulting from language deficiencies, differences in communication styles, and other cultural differences (Konrad and Pfeffer 1991: 155). A number of racial minority respondents claimed that language barriers were a significant hurdle that had to be surmounted early in training before they either understood what was expected of them or received fair evaluations.

Because the ability to join group activities can be even more strained for minorities than for whites of either gender, some researchers suggest that social integration may be facilitated for minority students through the implementation of formal social activities rather than relying on informal associations (Tinto 1993: 74). Tinto goes as far as to suggest that social integration may be more important in keeping minorities on track than any cognitive integration (ibid). Given our earlier discussion of the similar problem women have socializing informally with male colleagues, formal forms of association would tend to benefit white women, racial minority women and racial minority men in the residency program culture.

Role Models

Similar to the findings we report above for women in higher education, the percent of minority faculty is positively correlated with the performance of minority students at institutes for higher learning. As was true in our study of women role models, those minority students in the most prestigious institutions have the fewest minority role models available to them (Konrad and Pfeffer 1991). However, even the minority students at the less prestigious institutions have few models available to them. The following table shows the percent of minority faculty at U.S. medical schools in 1997 as reported by the AAMC.

Table 1.3: Percent of Minority Faculty at US Medical Schools

Ethnicity	Distribution on Medical Faculty
Native American	< 0.5%
Asian	9.8%
African-American	2.6%
Mexican-American	< 0.5%
Puerto-Rican	< 1%
Other Hispanic	1.8%

The hurdles facing white women and racial minorities of both sexes are formidable. The residents in this study were trying to enter a world that was still over-whelmingly full of white males. We will keep the nature of the challenges the women and racial minority residents faced in mind as we analyze the reasons the surgical residents in this study left their programs.In the next chapter, we will take a look at the processes of matriculation, evaluation and attrition as they relate to surgical residency programs.

II

Matriculation, Evaluation and Attrition

Matriculation

Looking at the way in which individuals are chosen to begin a training or socialization process can tell us a great deal about the culture of an organization and the criteria members use to judge performance. The individual who either resigns or is terminated from a program had already passed some measure of aptitude in order to be admitted. Since the process of selection had suggested that the individual was an appropriate choice, many people who study attrition have concluded that attrition signals problems with the selection process. Why did the process fail to show that the person who leaves did not have adequate motivation, commitment, or talent? They subsequently conclude that better screening processes can help reduce attrition. In this chapter, we will look at the surgical residency screening process to see how difficult it is to choose candidates for training.

Where do the medical educators begin when choosing residents for training? The doctors we surveyed agreed that the bottom line is some level of intelligence:

> "I think you look for people, first of all, who are bright, intelligent, who can handle the intellectual rigors of learning the subject." (A36)

> "The first cut is that we want to look at the best and the brightest...It is probably smarter and just as easy to hire a student with a 3.7 average who is sweet as a student with a 3.8 average who is crazy. You ought to take the 3.7 student, but there is a floor." (A31)

But deciding what other factors are vital and how to assess those characteristics was a real challenge:

> "The problem is we don't know the criteria to pick somebody. It's not just they are smart. Smart is a dime a dozen. They are all smart and anybody in the upper half of the class is smart. The IQ spectrum is probably not more than 10 points, whatever that means. The question is what are the predictors that this guy is going to be a terrific neurosurgeon or not." (A29)

Matching people with occupations is a complex process that often involves the coordination of a variety of people associated with an organization or institution (Jacobs 1989: 54). Trying to match personality and traits with a job description is a process fraught with trouble. As a culture we are loath to think that people's occupational destiny is somehow embedded in their genetic make-up. We recognize that there are some limits—not all of us can become great athletes—and yet we also celebrate the exception to the rule, the individual who succeeds against all odds of having a particular career. We may think that only one type of individual can perform a job only to be surprised when, due to historical events or other changes in society and culture, a new breed of employee comes forth. And change in one occupation can challenge the assumptions made in others. But changes are often slow to come about, partly because the very uncertainty that makes change possible can make decision-makers fall back on old habits rather than take risks.

Managers and administrators recognize how difficult it is to choose someone to join their group. What criteria are used to judge potential? How can you judge the potential of an individual who has never performed the job in the first place?

> "I don't think anyone really knows what they're getting into until they're here...You don't understand the responsibility until you are in the driver's seat." (R18)

Medical students begin applying to residency programs in their third year of medical school. It is well known that medical students often make their specialty choices before they have had an experience in the field or have met a role model (Lowenstein 1979: 99). For the residency program director, the challenge is: how can you know if the resident will be able to "function under difficult conditions" (Bowen and Rudenstein 1992:252) when the resident has never worked under those conditions? If you cannot adequately test performance, then will there not always be some attrition?

Managers and administrators deal with uncertainty in a variety of ways. For one, they tend to choose people like themselves to carry on their work (Hughes 1971, Lorber 1984), falling back on old habits. People feel most confident in assessing the traits and characteristics of people just like them. They are reluctant to "risk untried workers" (Reskin and Roos 1990) and therefore tend to perpetuate the traits and characteristics of the current workforce in their selection of the next generation of workers. As stated by Konrad and Pfeffer (1991) the "past is one of the most pervasive influences of the hiring practices of the present" (ibid: 152). In the absence of some true measure of aptitude, managers use proxy measures of aptitude and three of the most common proxies are "educational attainment, experience and group membership" (Reskin and Roos 1990: 36). As Reskin and Roos noted, "[e]mployers' rankings of groups of potential workers tend to be stable over the short run because stereotypes and biases change slowly" (ibid: 48).

These are the general difficulties facing employers in every occupation. What are the unique challenges facing the program director of a surgical residency program? First, residency program directors must choose their residents from among medical students. These students have already been chosen by a different group of managers—medical school administrators. As we will discuss in greater length below, a good medical student does not necessarily make a good physician (Linn 1987). Students who are good at taking tests and getting good grades do not necessarily become good physicians, but medical school admission is largely based on strong academic performance. But the same challenges that face the residency program director and employers in general also face the medical school administrator. The great challenge is stated well by Chapman (1985):

> "[There is] a need for a method by which medical school admissions committees can determine reliably some features in applicants in their early twenties that will predict certain personality characteristics fifteen or twenty years later, after the applicants have completed all their training and have become members in good standing of the practicing medical profession...The order is a tall one and very possibly either unattainable or attainable only by means which are too complex and time-consuming to be applied to large numbers of applicants." (ibid: 98)

Not only might the medical schools be selecting students using the wrong criterion for medical practice—good test-taking skills—but little in the medical school curriculum teaches the student the skills a medical practitioner needs. As one of our respondents said:

> "...in their didactic medical school curriculum, they're not designed to think...so many of them are treated as prima donnas and given everything on a silver platter. That and the exams are multiple choice. They do not come out really being independent thinkers or intellectuals. Most medical students are not intellectuals." (A16)

One physician argued that the information you get about a student's performance in medical school is "worthless" (A12) in trying to predict his or her performance in the residency program.

Another challenge is that medicine is a licensing occupation. Licensing occupations have a greater weight to bear than non-licensing occupations when they are choosing their applicants (Evans and Lauman 1983) because once the student has completed a certain portion of the training process, they may be eligible for a license to practice the trade. If poor choices are made during admission, the group may have professional liabilities on their hands—individuals who are licensed but unqualified.

And another complicating factor is that the training program for medicine in general and surgery in particular is very long. The time between starting the process and finishing the process spans over a decade in many cases. During the whole time, a number of internal and external factors can threaten an individual's successful completion of training.

In the first part of this chapter, we will look at this complicated process of matriculation and analyze the successes and failures of each step. Most medical students try to get residency positions in a hospital closely affiliated with a good medical school. Eighty percent of the top American medical students from the top American schools train in this type of hospital. Applications to the programs include dean's letters, grade reports from the medical school, national board scores, and other letters of recommendations. Each residency program chooses a subsample of their applicants to interview. After the resident visits a program and meets with a number of staff members, both interviewers and interviewees rank each other. The results of this ranking system are submitted to the National Resident Matching Program (NRMP) which matches programs and residents so that the optimum number of preferences of both programs and residents are met.

We will first address the adequacy of letters of recommendations before we discuss the use of grades and test scores as proxies for potential.

Letters of Recommendation

The common perception among medical educators, and among many educators in higher education settings, is that letters of recommendation are barely worth the paper they are written on because you can only trust the information in letters from people you know.

> "I try to evaluate his recommendations in terms of people I know. People whose opinions I respect and people I realize will tell me things as they exist." (A23)

These educators complain that letters are either outrageously inflated (with everyone being the best thing since sliced bread) or so vague as to be uninformative (King 1988a: 197, Yager 1988:322). Why are letters so inflated? Medical schools are ranked in part by the placement of their students into good residency programs: the more students placed in "top ranked" programs, the higher the rank of the medical school. Therefore it is not in the short-term interest of the medical schools to document their students' shortcomings in letters of recommendation. According to residency directors, letters that state that something is not right are the only trustworthy ones because the student's errors must have been very grave to overcome the norm of writing glowing letters.

Recommenders also expressed trepidation about saying anything negative about a person for fear of legal action:

> "This guy was so contentious and litigious, all my letter could say was he's a nice guy, prepared conferences well, did his work, that was it. I said nothing about his interpersonal skills, nothing about his technical ability or anything like that." (A27)

Another challenge is codifying in some reasonable manner the kind of information that is provided in a letter of recommendation. Mitchell (1987) presents the problem well:

> "...much of the valuable information provided in application folders is difficult to quantify for research or selection purposes. For example, it is difficult to quantify data provided by personal statements, letters of evaluation, and accounts of extracurricular work or research experience...These sources may reflect personal characteristics that account for important differences between students in medical school performance." (ibid: 25)

But although it may be true that letters do provide some very useful information that can distinguish between eventual good and poor performers, that information is not being harvested in the current selection process. As Ross and Leicher (1988) have found, no thorough study is known which positively demonstrates that letters have any predictive value (ibid: 240).

So the first kind of information used by residency programs for choosing their residents is fraught with problems and has little predictive power. Although it is unlikely that a program would look twice at a resident file that had no letters of recommendation, it remains unclear that letters help those choosing the next generation of residents.

Academic Performance

There is a great deal of debate in the literature about the appropriateness of using grades as a measure of "physician aptitude," since many studies have indicated that there is little to no correlation between grades achieved in medical school and on national examinations and future performance as a physician (Adler 1988:93, Albo 1982:119, Borlase 1986:185, Keck 1979:759, Miller 1982: 143, Werner 1979:133, Wingard 1973:313). The lack of this correlation is true both in medicine in general and surgery in particular (Gough 1987: 265, Schueneman 1988) where performance is either not correlated or negatively correlated with previous academic achievement. A review of the literature makes it clear that the search for a correlation is somewhat akin to the search for the Holy Grail. One gets the impression that the belief is that if medical educators conduct the study in enough different ways, they will find some correlation somewhere. The belief that grades are a good predictor are well entrenched in the medical culture:

> "I think that past performance in educational situations would be perhaps the best clue to the motivation of the resident, the intellectual motivation. And I think probably that is the best clue to how they'll do in the residency experience which is, after all, an educational experience." (A21)

As we noted earlier, medical educators do believe that a certain amount of intelligence is required to master the fund of knowledge necessary to practice good medicine, and that intelligence is reflected in national exam test scores and GPAs, even when they also admit that intelligence alone does not assure success. Intelligence is a necessary but not sufficient trait. Women have a higher than average risk for attrition but also tend to get better grades in medical school (Barondess, 1998: 101), an indication that grades alone do not guarantee success. As we have already discussed, both raw intellect as well as an ability to get along and be judged as competent are important. Piel et al (1982) have noted that older students typically have lower GPA and MCAT scores, but typically do better on interview ratings and letters of recommendation. Here, the life skills out perform the academic skills.

Wingard and Williamsom (1973) argue that academic grades cannot indicate the transformation of potential into aptitude and accomplishment (ibid:313) so they will always be an insufficient measure. So why do medical educators focus on grades? Measuring non-cognitive and non-quantifiable traits is even harder and presents a formidable challenge. As Iverson (1996) states, "scores on exams become 'outrageously important' because of the lack of all other information" (ibid: 144). Grades also fail to test the physical traits that are deemed so vital for surgery:

> "...nonverbal, visuo-spatial problem-solving abilities (i.e. the capacity to rapidly analyze and organize perceptions based on multi-sensory information) and the ability to distinguish essential from non-essential detail even when the 'signal-to-noise' ratio is high appears most crucial to superior technique." (Schueneman in Lnagsley 1988: 257)

> "They have to have tissue intuition. Of course there is no way you can assess that in an interview." (A24)

> "Because sometimes it's almost in the way they handle the surgery. It's hard to define, and is perhaps a deliberate, a careful, a respect for the tissue." (N12)

Finding ways to test these complicated physical traits remains a challenge for residency program directors. Medical educators hope that by the time the medical student applies for training, he or she will have had enough exposure to the field to determine if he or she can physically perform the work. As we will discuss in later chapters, this line of reasoning was faulty for a certain proportion of our attrition group. The residents were accepted into programs only to discover that they could not perform surgery because of visual defects, chronic fatigue, and other physical handicaps.

Non-Cognitive Traits

Grades are poor predictors, but even more than that, program directors and senior faculty admit that it is more important for prospective doctors to possess integrity, interpersonal skills and other humanistic qualities than intelligence (AMA 1989:14, Friedman et al, 1987: 888, Griffen 1987). Medical educators also admit, however, that these attributes are much harder to measure than intelligence, perhaps even impossible to measure in a standardized fashion (Chapman 1985:98, Greenburg 1981:39, Haas and Shaffir, 1987). This was one of the main concerns of the neurosurgeons who commissioned the study.

> "You want to see procedures and results that are reliably reproducible. You want the procedures to be accurate, objective and fair. But you are engaged, at the same time, in trying to measure such smoky and intangible human qualities as integrity, humanity, sensitivity, stability, compassion . . . communication skills, interpersonal skills, and sound personal attributes. Those are quite oppositely removed on the scale of the inductive process from the reliably reproducible research results of work in the laboratory. In other words, your task here is to test the untestable." (Piel 1982:215)

Even when educators try to focus on one non-cognitive attribute, they still face obstacles:

> "Interpersonal skills are far more difficult to assess than psychomotor skills. The NBME spent several years on a study which reviewed all methods available but was unable to develop a simple and practical assessment." (Langsley 1986:25)

What are some of the more important traits that program directors are looking for? In one study of surgical residents, certain traits were noted among the pool of "good" performers, residents who were performing well according to program faculty. The good performing residents "saw themselves as better able to relate to others, emotionally more stable, more flexible, meticulous, tractable, and more often described themselves as dependable and aggressive." (Wilson 1985:38) These all relate back to our earlier discussion of what is needed for survival in the program and in the culture. Residents must be able to get along with the others already in the program; they must face the heartache associated with their work; they must be meticulous; and they must demonstrate some of the expected aggressiveness associated with surgical work.

Others, however, report being more interested in a sense of passion and commitment. Recognizing that every residency training program will be challenging, draining, and test the limits of residents' physical endurance, some educators want to see a certain commitment made to the field:

"One of the things I look for is well-reasoned passion. They should be in love with the brain, in love with neurosurgery." (A31)

"The minute they start worrying about how many weekends they have off a month, or anything along those lines, they're automatically crossed off in my mind. It's got to be, at least you have to be ready for it to be total immersion. If you're worrying about whether you're going to be able to get out on your sailboat, or whether you'll have enough quality time with your newborn baby and things like that—which are legitimate desires for any human being—but if you start off being worried about that, you're just not going to make it." (A19)

"...someone who is totally committed. [Resident X] is an extraordinary resident. He has all of the characteristics. Totally gung-ho, totally enthusiastic, accepts every responsibility as a challenge, as an opportunity to do something good for humanity and himself and the program." (A12)

But whether medical educators are measuring honesty and integrity, commitment or personality, they must find ways to measure these traits before and after matriculation.

Note that program directors believe that residents must possess these qualities and traits *prior* to admission. Program faculty do not consider the acquisition of integrity and other humanistic traits a natural part of the professional training/socialization program.

"Now when it comes to an element such as integrity, I will admit that it is a little like being pregnant—you either are or you are not. You either have integrity or you do not have integrity and, as we were saying a little while ago, it may not be possible to remediate someone who lacks integrity." (Trier 1985:107)

"The humanistic doctors had to develop their humanistic inclinations before they ever arrived at medical school. There is almost nothing in medical training that encourages compassion, empathy, and 'care' for patients." (Conrad 1988:329)

"It is probably that most program directors consider the lack of personal integrity and immorality are characteristics that will have been identified earlier in the education of the physician and if not, that they are not amendable to correction." (Cruft 1985:68)

This belief that these values must pre-exist and are not acquired during the training program challenges notions about the process of professional socialization. Socialization is the internalization of the values and attitudes of the profession (Conrad 1988:329, Light 1980:315), while training involves the mastery of skills or knowledge. Our respondents and the authors cited above appear to believe that humanistic traits are dichotomous. These doctors do not acknowledge that situational factors may cause residents and faculty alike to be more or less honest, humanistic or caring. Autobiographical accounts of the residency years almost always include a reference to a moment in time when an otherwise caring resident stops caring due to fatigue, illness, or stress, yet writings on the medical culture suggest that these traits must exist before the student is accepted into the program. Why? Because nothing in the context of medical training helps instill these traits. Medical educators debate whether these non-cognitive traits must exist before the resident joins a training program, or whether the culture of the program can influence, promote, or instill these behaviors (Albo 1976: 117).

But what is the ideal resident profile? Medical educators and those in other fields like the military have begun to argue that there is no ideal personality type since the total organization requires many different complementary styles in order to function (Argetsinger 1999, Bosk 1984). These new proponents of a more diverse trait profile claim that although honesty may be vital, perhaps aggression is not. Some surgeons may have a different temperament and still do their job well. And if honesty is really the most vital trait, honesty does not have a demographic profile. No one has a claim to honesty based on race, gender, age, etc. (Linn 1987: 101). But since personality and hubris seem so central to the culture of residency training program and the very activity of surgery, it is unlikely that this discussion will fade away or be settled soon (Bosk 1997: 13).

How do residency programs institute a purposeful and manageable system for choosing residents that adequately matches the resident's traits and intelligence and with the particular character of a program? Ideally program directors want a system that works better than random-sampling. Program faculty have a hard time defining a good candidate: "I have trouble conveying to you in words exactly what we are looking for." (A29) The people we surveyed, however, did agree that more attention needs to be paid to non-cognitive assessments.

> "I think if you could set up a system in which you can look at the character of the individual much more closely than it is done now. Then I think you'd have a much better way of selecting quality people. In other words, when I look at a person, I think, 'Is this person honest?'" (R30)

> "Then the issue comes up if you are lucky enough to be interviewing a lot of very bright people who come from reasonable schools and have letters of recommendations that you believe from people you know, then as you sit with that person it becomes the gut issue, which is, do I feel comfortable?" (A31)

"I think the selection has to change from the sort of frantic lottery system...I would like something that would allow us to evaluate the personality, the individual, the person as a human being." (R36)

So when faced with the difficult decision of choosing residents based on non-quantifiable traits, the program directors and attendings resort to "gut feelings" and personality when choosing residents. Here is where personal preferences and cultural stereotypes can adversely affect the choice of next year's residents, perpetuating a system in which white males dominate.

Since non-cognitive traits are important, the personal interview becomes the most important vehicle for assessing these qualities since no other information in the application packet, not even the letters of recommendation adequately report on these non-cognitive traits. The interview is considered by some to be the "most important selection tool" (Ross 1988:233), a "critical and valuable component of the selection process" (Komives 1984:425). Medical educators think of the interview as "the best hope for information about personality and character traits" (Langsley 1988: 4).

"The interview offers a unique and useful glimpse of individual student personality and other non-cognitive factors which may be meaningful for successful performance in a given residency." (Gong 1988: 155)

A lot rides on the interview since the interview is the medical educator's one shot at assessing personality, honesty, and camaraderie. However, this system is fraught with troubles of its own.

The Interview Cut

Who gets called in for an interview? The first cut is always made on the basis of academic performance. The best programs keep the very highest performers and the bar gets lowered as you move from the top university settings to the community hospitals. After a resident makes that cut, he or she is typically invited to spend a minimum of one day interviewing with the senior faculty and residents in a program and getting a tour of the facility. Residents typically spend only about 20-30 minutes in each interview. This is a very short amount of time to assess the whole gamut of non-cognitive traits deemed so important by medical educators. The hope is that along the course of a number of interviews with a number of faculty members, the program will get a feel for how the potential candidate might fit into the department.

How successful are interviews as a screening device both in and out of medicine? Gough (1987) reports that "[o]ccupational psychologists have shown that the unstructured interview, i.e. the sort of interview in which we [medical educators] all participate has as much power to predict later performance as does random selection" (ibid: 265). Although the faculty hopes that over the course of a

series of interviews, different faculty members will come away with similar impressions of the same candidate, this has been shown not to be true. The interview has rather low reliability—different interviewers tend to reach different
conclusions about the same candidate (Holdsworth 1987: 267). Different faculty
members have their own different interests and look for different characteristics
in the candidates (Bucher and Stelling 1977: 23). The faculty member interested
in a community outreach program will be looking for different characteristics
and motivations in the candidate than the faculty member in the same department who is driven to publish in the top medical journals. And finally, interviews have low validity—that is, there is a low correlation between interview
ratings and subsequent job performance ratings (Holdsworth 1987: 267).

> "Despite extensive evidence...that the personal interview has limited use as an
> assessment technique, the interview is still viewed as the most important selec-
> tion tool." (Ross and Leicher in Langsley 1988: 233)

Some individuals and some departments will be skilled at interviewing, either
because they have been trained to do so or because of some "talent" for "identifying candidates with the requisite motivation, personal qualities, and intellectual capacity" (Bowen and Rudenstein 1992: 252). Many of our respondents,
however, were unsure about their abilities to pick the right candidate:

> "Well, I've learned to distrust the interview now, as the years have gone on."
> (A18)

> "I don't know how skilled I am as an interviewer and I worry about that a good
> deal." (A17)

One respondent expressed concern about the subjective quality of the interview
rating process (A25). Medical educators should be concerned given the lack of
correlation between interview ratings and subsequent performance.

The interview is also saddled with the burden and power of first impressions
(Crandall 1978: 333). In the absence of a history of interactions with someone,
we look for familiarities, something about the individual we are meeting that
seems familiar and recognizable.

> "...even chance resemblances between the candidate and some former ac-
> quaintance of ours...we tend to respond more favorably toward those whose
> impact we judge positively, this in turn encourages them to respond better to
> us." (Holdsworth 1987: 267)

This feature of the nature of human interactions tends to favor people who are
like the interviewer. Here again we have a situation that will favor white males
since white males currently hold most of the interviewer seats. The candidate
who seems familiar or who has had similar experiences as the interviewer (i.e.

gone to the same medical school, come from the same state, etc.) will have an advantage over the candidate who lacks this common background.

So if the interview is not very good at predicting future performance, what purpose does the interview serve? This question takes us back to our discussion of camaraderie. In one study, respondents rated the applicant's compatibility with the program as the most important variable determined by the interview (Wagoner, Suriano and Stoner in Langsley 1988).

> "The interview offers a unique and useful glimpse of individual student personality and other non-cognitive factors which may be meaningful for successful performance *in a given residency*." (Gong 1988: 155, italics mine)

So it is the interviewer's self-perceived ability to work with a resident, not the resident's potential, that is being judged by the interview. This potential may actually outweigh other factors used in assessing resident potential and desirability.

> "No matter how irrational it may seem, the ten- to thirty-minute interviews that you will have at the residency programs will count for more, in most cases, toward getting you into the program than the total weight of your previous 3 ½ years of medical school." (Iverson 1996: 333)

> "The evaluation system is not a fair one and you may find out that people who were not as strong a student as you will get a better evaluation simply because they got along better with the residents." (Zaslau 1994: 20)

What other functions does the interview serve? Not only is the program shopping for a resident, but the resident is also shopping for a program. "The interview and hospital visit provide valuable information to the applicant about the social milieu of the institution in question, the physical plant, the morale of the housestaff, and the patient mix of the institution (Komives et al., 1984: 426). The resident also gets a chance to get a feel for the program.

The interview also becomes an occasion to test for that all-important sense of dedication, commitment and passion that program directors are seeking. The resident ideally shows the program faculty that he or she has no major obstacles in private life to prevent total immersion in training (Broadhead 1983: 13). It also offers the faculty a chance to convey to the candidate that "there is no room in medicine for people with split loyalties and conflicts of interest, or who are mediocre or satisfied with being anything but the best" (ibid: 72).

Camaraderie

As stated by Iverson (1996) in his residency program guidebook: "No matter how good an applicant is, he or she has to fit with our program's residents and faculty. This is where our opportunity to talk with and interview the applicant comes in...A personality already exists for the group, the residency, the depart-ment and the institution. Will you fit in? Will they be comfortable with you?" (ibid, 368, 400). In addition to assessing non-cognitive traits and characteristics, the interview is considered an important vehicle for assessing a resident's "fit" with the overall program, not just with individual attendings: "[t]he applicant's compatibility with the program was rated as the most important variable deter-mined with the interview (Wagoner et al. 1988:305). Faculty believe that "dif-ferent personality traits allow one type of young person to serve and learn more effectively than others with a given faculty or physician" (Polk 1983:8). Match-ing personality types is another goal of the interview.

Our respondents had these comments about what they try to accomplish dur-ing the interview/screening process:

> "I try to get at is some feel about whether this is the kind of person who will en-joy being around the kind of people that we are." (A24)

> "People are accepted into residency programs because they fit into the program for one reason or another, not because they're really better than someone who was not taken. He may even not be as good a candidate, but was taken because that is the type of person the program wanted, be it personality, or be it back-ground, whatever is more important, whatever plays a greater role." (R37)

In fact, Zaslau (1994) specifically makes the point that people who are weaker academically than others may get a better evaluation simply because they got along better with the residents (ibid: 20). Remember, however, only strong aca-demic performers make the first cut.

In addition to giving the faculty an opportunity to assess a resident's compati-bility with the program, the authors of various residency program guides point out that the interview process gives the resident an equally important chance to assess the people in the program. King (1988) makes the recommendation that residents try to interview as many people as possible to get a sense if they will be able to work well with everyone (ibid: 31). Others talk about the importance of the resident walking away that day with a "gut" feeling about the program (Arnold et al 1985: 27).

> "After an interview day, some programs will just feel right to you, and you may not be able to articulate the reasons for this attraction or sense of appeal. Do not ignore this feeling: in fact, consider it to be one of *critical* importance throughout the ranking process." (Miller and Donowitz 1997: 77)

How successful is the interview in accomplishing the goal of successfully matching personalities? Not very well by most accounts. Recall that most attri-tion from the residency programs in this study was not due to a lack of intellec-tual prowess, but involved personality clashes and unprofessional behavior. The interview format fails to pick up potential personality clashes that arise after the resident joins the program. In a number of studies, the composite interview score did not predict residency performance (Komives 1984:426). The failure of this process to succeed in matching personalities is not surprising "given the relatively brief nature of the interview and the fact that the interview format was not standardized" (ibid). The fact of the matter is that an individual interview rarely lasts for more than 20 minutes, even though the prospective resident interviews with a number of faculty and other members of the department during a visit. Broadhead (1983) makes the claim that what the interview may actually accomplish is the detection of "gross deficiencies" (ibid: 23) in personality and emotional stability, but most people could keep themselves composed through a typical 20-minute interview:

> "The interview process, I'm convinced it is a faulty one. I don't think there is anything more we can do but introduce ourselves and meet them and make them feel that we're not ogres and make sure that they can at least make eye contact and they are not schizophrenic which you hope you can tell in 15 minutes." (A18)

> "Clunker is somebody who I would believe doesn't match the paper that came in with them, either by their performance, or personality, or psychological make-up. But in twenty minutes to a half-hour, which is all I have to talk to them, even people that I think have major deficits on a daily working basis can get their act together for that half-hour....To tell how people really react, you have to have them for a six-month rotation." (A35)

The failure of the interview to pick up the gross deficiencies was demonstrated in our data set. Even for the residents who displayed bizarre behavior once they joined the program (like the resident who exposed himself to a group of nurses three days after joining the program), there had been no indication from the interview reports that the resident would have any problems in the program.

If the interview system as it currently exists has so many problems, could medical educators improve the process? One respondent offered this option:

> "Maybe we'd have to interview people twice, or you'd have to come here for a couple of days to see that you fit us and we fit you. You know, we only take one resident a year, and it's a big decision on their part—you're taking six or seven years of their life. We're talking about six or seven years of relying on that person." (R32)

Departing from the single-day visit would be a radical departure for the medical student shopping for a residency program. Already, many students spend a substantial amount of money traveling to various residency programs around the country. Less wealthy students are constrained in the amount of money they can allot for this travel. And for students trying to enter the most competitive residencies, having to travel more than once to a program, or having to stay for a couple of days, times the 15-30 programs that they intend on applying to would take a minimum of a couple of months of time invested in this process. Instead of spending a portion of the last year of medical school seeking a program, a minimum of an entire semester would have to be devoted to this process.

Another suggestion has been to standardize the interview process so that any medical educator could interview the resident and any program considering the resident could utilize the resulting report. For numerous reasons, this process will not work. The most important reason that the standardized interview will not work is the overarching desire for camaraderie. Programs themselves are not standardized. If the main raison d'être of the interview is the matching of personalities and the maintenance of the camaraderie of the group, than no standardized interview will fill that niche. The "fit" can only be assessed after faculty and residents have had a chance to interact and that all-important "gut" feeling has been examined:

> "What was striking about the business of selecting trainees was the relative vagueness of the criteria used. Staff of each program attempted to choose people who would fulfill their own professional image of their discipline, but they were remarkably unable to clearly specify the bases on which they accepted or rejected a candidate." (Bucher 1977:54)

So, if the interview is not very successful at matching personalities, and if ways to improve the process are either counterproductive or costly, then what positive function does the interview serve? Perhaps it all comes down to giving the faculty members a sense that they have chosen the people with whom they will be working, rather than having a computer or some standardized interviewer choose their residents (Friedman et al 1987: 893). It may also serve as a ritual which allows the faculty to "make a commitment" to the residents who will be joining their programs (Herman et al 1983: 842). By being so personally and intimately involved in choosing next year's cohort, they collectively recognize their obligation to train and to mentor these incoming residents, and no medical educator would deny that the process of clinical teaching is intensely interpersonal. The interview process as it is currently practiced may serve to solidify faculty/resident relationships prior to matriculation. This may be the primary function of the interview. As stated by some of our respondents, during the interview you look to chose people you want to help, that you want to be a mentor for:

> "One of the things I look for in residents is to have guys/gals around that you want to help so personality makes a difference." (A23)

> "But if you want to, and you want to come under my training, I'm going to devote my energy and skills to train you, I want a guy who is fully committed." (A27)

Calls for Reform

Although the whole matriculation process is recognized as a highly flawed system, an imperfect tool for choosing and evaluating prospective candidates, efforts to devise a better system are challenged by the highly subjective nature of assessing non-cognitive traits, matching personalities within programs, and creating a balance of academic and community practitioners. The challenged is multiplied when we consider the sheer number of medical students who pass through the system each year. This subjective assessment of traits and "fit" is also increased by the new "diversity" of the applicant pool (Wagoner 1988:61). People tend to be far more comfortable with and feel connected to people who are much like them. The challenges faced by both the white male program director and the young African-American female, or the young male medical student from India, in trying to assess compatibility in a 20-minute interview is more formidable than the interview between that same white male program director and the young white male medical student.

Calls for reform and standardization also meet resistance from a subset of medical educators who worry that if the system for choosing residents becomes too stringent and codified, the system will weed out the "mavericks" of medicine before they have had a chance to become great physicians. These educators fear that program directors following a new prescribed code for choosing residents will not be willing to take a chance on "troublesome, but often talented" (Mogul 1985:143) residents who "will go on to successful careers" (ibid). This line of argument is interesting when we recall our earlier discussion of "hubris" and its role in enabling surgeons to do what they do everyday. A necessary amount of "hubris" may make the surgical resident troublesome by definition. But among our respondents, medical students who acted like mavericks at the interview were scorned and avoided:

> "Some people come in here and say 'I want to be a neurosurgeon' and are real cocky about it. Immediately that turns me off because even neurosurgeons I know who are cocky are cocky because they have spent a lot of time and have developed a certain fund of knowledge and ability. If they're going to be cocky, it's because they've earned it. But to come in here, applying for a residency and being cocky, I find that totally unacceptable." (A15)

> "I've had some people say that they want to be the next Harvey Cushing...I feel a little uncomfortable having them tell me they want to be the next Harvey Cushing." (A28)

Our respondents generally felt trapped by this system of choosing that in the end gave them no real power to predict who was and who was not going to be a good resident, just like the program faculty from other residency programs (Adler and Gladstein in Langsley, 1988: 93, Werner and Korsch in Shapiro and Lowenstein 1979: 133).

"It's akin to throwing the applications up and we make some prejudiced evaluations on these people based on twenty-minute to half-hour interviews and a review of their transcripts and recommendations, half of which are not trustworthy, or based on the fact...that somebody is afraid to write what really happened, or what they're really like." (A18)

What is the ideal?

"We look for a complete person. We look not just for grades, personality, or
where they're from or how they are going to fit in, but a combination of every
one of those things." (A20)

But the challenge remains—how do you measure a complete person?
Let us end this section with a quote from Tinto (1993) about the endless
search for an ideal screening process:

"Even if one could 'improve the odds' by so screening students, there is good
reason to question the wisdom of doing so. The great danger of screening procedures is that they may lead not only to self-fulfilling prophecies but also to
the constriction of opportunity for late-developing students and/or those individuals whose abilities are not easily captured on formal admission documents.
Screening procedures tend, by their very nature, to heavily weight the past at
the expense of the future. By doing so they may hinder the chances for admission of those persons who are 'late bloomers' or who tend to flourish only after
being admitted to particular types of intellectual and/or social climates. In a
very real sense they may act counter to one of the presumed ends of higher
educational enterprise, namely the discovery and fostering of individual talent.
It might also be added that screening devices can produce, over time, homogeneous student populations, populations whose limited variety may also serve to
constrain rather than promote the attainment of the educational ends of higher
education." (ibid: 161)

Are program directors in surgical residency programs looking to create an army
of homogeneous practitioners, or a group of unique artisans? The answer will
affect what types of reform these educators implement.

Evaluation

Despite all the enumerated problems above, this imperfect system, along with
the NMRP, matches a new host of residents with a whole host of residency programs every year. And once the residents begin their tour in their new program,
a more intimate and regular evaluation begins. In this section we will look at the
process of evaluation in a surgical residency program. What does the process
typically look like? How frequently do faculty formally and informally evaluate
residents? Who on staff is involved in the evaluations? Are standardized forms
used? Are the problems we noted in the process of choosing residents replicated

in the process of evaluation even after the resident has started a program? The following statements made by two of our respondents foreshadow out findings:

"I think it's pretty subjective." (R45)

"It is always determined on a subjective basis...If you wind up on the chairman's shit list, you are going to get fired and not recommended for anything else." (A33)

Guidelines listed in the Directory of Residency Training Programs published by The Accreditation Council for Graduate Medical Education (ACGME) state:

"It is urged that the performance of each house officer be reviewed by the teaching staff each six months and that a documented record of his performance be prepared and retained for review by appropriate accrediting and credentialling bodies." (ACGME 1982-83: 19)

Most of the programs in our survey follow the guidelines established by the ACGME. Only five percent of the surgical programs in our survey did not report using a standardized form when evaluating resident performance, and only four percent did not review their residents a minimum of every six months. In fact, 66% of the programs actually reviewed their residents more than twice a year. The following table shows the distribution.

Table 2.1. How often are residents evaluated?

Time period	Percent
Monthly	26%
Quarterly	40%
Bi-yearly	30%
Yearly	4%

So these surgical programs do a good job in following the ACGME guidelines for frequency of evaluation, but of course, we have not said anything about what is being evaluated.

What is certain from our analysis is that the same traits and characteristics that the program faculty look for during the process of matriculation continue to be sought and evaluated during the residency training. So, program faculty look for both academic prowess and evidence that the resident is an honest and responsible individual. Again, medical educators are faced with the task of evaluating residents on the basis of test scores, clinical performance and "smoky and intangible human qualities" (Piel in Lloyd 1982: 215) like honesty, integrity, humanity, sensitivity, etc. Academic prowess continues to be measured primarily by in-house and national exam scores as well as the resident's management of on-the-spot questions about diagnosis and treatment raised during rounds.

The medical faculty, however, continue to face the difficult task of assessing the general character of their residents.

As noted by Langsley (1986), "interpersonal skills are far more difficult to assess than psychomotor skills. The NBME [National Board of Medical Examiners] spent several years on a study which reviewed all methods available but was unable to develop a simple and practical assessment (ibid: 25)."

One of the ways that medical faculty attempt to cope with this dilemma is by trying to get a sense of the resident as a "whole person." They attempt to assess the resident's general goodness by trying to see him or her in action outside of the confines of hospital behavior.

> "I try to get a feel for them outside the hospital. Are they rounded individuals or just uni-dimensional?" (A14)

In later chapters, we will review in detail cases of how behavior outside the strict confines of the hospital setting influenced program director's thoughts on whether or not a resident should be terminated.

This phenomenon of extending the evaluation beyond the strict confines of the job may be seen as unfair or oppressive, but it is an aspect of our social lives. Think of our national obsession with the personal lives of politicians and other celebrities and the continuing public debate about whether or not their private and public lives can be separated from each other. Especially when trying to assess a non-quantifiable aspect of character, it is understandable that program faculty would seek other examples of behavior to get a complete picture of the resident. As Light points out (1980), we all have a difficult time making any judgments about others beyond what we see as their level of "general goodness" (ibid: 45). And as Tinto (1993) states in his discussion of graduate education in general, "faculty judgments as to student competence within the classroom are necessarily conditioned by social judgments arising from interactions beyond the classroom—the hallway and offices of the department" (ibid: 236). The challenge is assessing any evaluation process is deciphering how much of the evaluation can be based on "manifest characteristics like cognitive knowledge which can be measured, and to what degree are they based on latent ones such as private judgments, feelings and intentions about personal integrity that cannot be measured" (Bosk 1984: 76)? When a significant amount of evaluation is based on private and subjective judgments, then we must be aware for the potential of discrimination and abuse. But we must also recognize that "resident evaluation can never be fully objective because what is being measured can never be fully objectified" (Bosk 1981: 30).

As we have discussed, subjective assessment opens the door for discrimination and the search for behaviors outside the context of the job exacerbates this potential. Many social behaviors which signal honesty and integrity to the program director may be very "class bound." For example, in his residency program guide, Zaslau (1994) recommends that residents write thank-you notes to program directors after visiting a program. He goes on to say that writing a thank-you note:

> "...shows you have some *class* because, after all, it is your chance to thank the director for inviting you to visit his department." (ibid: 48, italics mine)

Those who recognize this social etiquette will win points.

Diverse Faculty

Another challenge for the medical faculty at any program is the diverse interests and habits of the medical faculty members themselves, who have different views on what is good and bad performance, honest and dishonest behavior. The faculty ideally represents a united front when declaring a resident fit or unfit for practice, but the reality behind that evaluation is much more varied. Polk (1983) provides the following description of this process:

> "There are the faculty 'sweethearts' who have never seen a bad resident. Their counterpart is the congenial grouch with a short memory who has never seen a resident 'as good as we were in my day.' Perhaps even more troublesome to the evaluation process is the ambivalent faculty member who provides a string of complimentary written assessments and then, when it comes time to discuss the young person's progress, is extremely malicious. Furthermore, differing personality traits allow one type of young person to serve and learn more effectively than others with a given faculty or physician. These kinds of misunderstandings reflect the complex psychological nature of the process and require continuous interpretation within each department." (ibid: 8)

We have an example from our respondents' experiences:

> "I think he is an unhappy man to start with and sometimes he can take it out on the residents. He is also insecure. There is an element of arbitrariness about him as well. You are never sure how he will react to a problem. Sometimes he can be very hard on a resident." (R41)

What is being evaluated?

> *"An excellent job is expected and doesn't really get any praise at all, and I mean that's from the attendings, from the patients, everyone expects to come in and have a perfect job done." (R29)*

We know that what continues to be evaluated after a resident joins a residency program are the resident's performance on exams, his or her clinical judgment, and his or her character. What we have not asked yet is the correlation of these different measures with eventual performance as a physician. Perkoff (1989), a medical educator speaking to other medical educators, makes the following statement about the process of producing competent physicians:

> "We all have done it for years, we believe we do it well, but we are hard pressed to specify exactly what we do. And we don't know which parts of what we do are critical to the expected outcome, a well-supervised, competent, caring physician." (ibid: 33)

What is important for producing a competent, caring physician? Good test scores? A physician with good clinical judgment? An honest individual? And how do medical educators weigh the value of each one? How many residents rank high on all three? Dr. Perkoff raises this question—what is critical to the expected outcome? And would everyone evaluating even agree on what constitutes a well-supervised, competent, caring physician?

Medical educators are still embroiled in this debate, but a review of some of the findings uncovers some clues about the process. Researchers have found that there is no or little correlation between program faculty's assessment of a resident's character and personality and his or her performance on exam scores, although there is come correlation between non-cognitive traits and clinical judgment:

> "...qualitative, observation-based performance ratings of program directors are not strongly related to the quantifiable performance of a candidate, i.e., exam scores." (Boggs and Dolch in Lloyd 1985: 120)

> "Clinical scores did not correlate with ABSITE or QE scores. Clinical assessment categories (personality, clinical, overall) correlated well within their respective categories. Resident with high personality scores generally received high scores in clinical and overall performance. However, the examination and clinical performance scores did not correlate." (Borlase et al, 1986: 185)

Bosk makes the point that one of the criteria which attendings use to measure a resident's worth is how well they organize and run a service (Bosk 1997b: 25), a task that involves good organizational and people skills that are quite separate from those used in the doctor-patient relationship. These findings suggest that although program faculty wants residents to have academic prowess, clinical judgment, and stellar personalities, in their experience faculty members find that this three-stellar constellation is not the norm. Residents with good personalities are not necessarily good exam takers, although Borlase et al. (1986) suggest that personable residents typically demonstrate good clinical judgment.

These findings challenge once again the great emphasis on grades and exam scores in the selection of medical students. By the time the medical student has obtained a residency post, he or she has typically passed the intelligence hurdle. The question remains, can that resident both absorb and successfully apply medical knowledge?

Who Is Evaluating?

Who evaluates residents in a typical residency program? The answer varies depending on a number of factors: the specialty, the size of the program, the particular mix of the program faculty, and the degree of autonomy enjoyed by the program director, to name a few. Although the ultimate responsibility for evaluation lies with the program director, the program director typically has very little contact with interns and first-year residents in the average residency program. This is in part the result of the very hierarchical system of medical training, especially in the larger programs. More senior residents typically supervise new residents' work (David 1986:81, Anwar 1981: 35). Because program directors are not often involved in the instruction and supervision of new residents, critics of the current system argue that it is inappropriate that their evaluation of resident performance is given so much weight. These same critics claim that a better alternative would be to have a number of peers and superiors involved in evaluation since peers will have a better handle on a given resident's overall performance (Miller 1982, Bosk 1981: 31, Anwar 1981: 37).

What format of evaluation did the programs in our study have? We will present some data on who was involved in evaluating the residents in our study and see if there were any specialty effects among our surgical specialties. In Survey I we asked program directors to identify which of the following staff members were involved in the evaluation process: program directors, attendings, chief residents, nurses and others. From that information, we get the following table:

Table 2.2. Who evaluates residents?

Who is evaluating?	Percent of programs reporting category of person involved in evaluations, all specialties combined
Program Directors	81%
Attendings	99%
Chief Residents	36%
Nurses	6%

In our sample, it was not true that program directors were always involved in evaluation. For 19% of the programs in our sample, the program director was not involved in evaluation. Two of our specialties, neurosurgery and plastic surgery, were significantly more likely to have the program director involved in evaluations than the other three specialties. These two specialties were significantly smaller than the other three specialties, suggesting that program directors from smaller programs would tend to be more involved with the residents.

Ninety-nine percent of our programs reported that the attendings were involved in resident evaluation. There was no significant variation on this trend by specialty. However, only 36% of the programs regularly involved chief residents in resident evaluation although there is evidence that peer evaluation is an important assessment technique(Stanton 1979: 813). The general surgery programs were significantly more likely to have chief residents involved in evaluation and, along with anesthesiology, were more likely to have a larger number of residents in the programs.

And finally, we look at nurse involvement in evaluation. A mere 6% of programs report involving nurses in resident evaluations. As we will discuss below, nurses do get involved, if only informally. There were no specialty effects in this category.

Our data support others' findings that program directors and attending faculty do most of the resident evaluation. Before looking more closely at the role that the program director plays in the evaluation process, we will look at the under-utilization of reports both from nursing and from patients, especially in the assessment of non-quantifiable personality traits and characteristics.

Nursing and Patients

Nurses occupy an ideal spot on the medical faculty for commenting on the humanistic behavior of residents. Alone with residents at the bedside, nurses are in a unique position to assess residents' independent clinical competence and humanistic tendencies when they are not "performing" for attendings and program directors.

> "Since residents spend a great deal of their working time with the nursing staff, and are taught much by and corrected frequently by nurses, evaluation of residents by nurses has been advocated strongly, especially in getting a handle on humanism and other personal factors." (David 1986: 82)

A number of analysts have noted nurses' unique position (Blurton et al, 1985: 650, Linn 1986). In fact Linn noted that "nurses and other non-physician personnel are willing to evaluate the humanistic behavior of physicians and are reliable and valid sources of such information" (ibid: 920). Some of our respondents made comments that support these assertions:

> "Nurses know more about the residents, probably more than the attendings." (R35)

> "I think in general, nurses know a lot about the residents, about the behaviors that other people may not see...their ability to deal with certain situations, writing orders, keeping up with the IV status on patients, those kinds of things." (N12)

In addition to nursing, attendings report that patients are their eyes and ears when they are not rounding with their residents:

> "There are some residents whom people are always complaining about and there are others whom they say nothing but the nicest things about, plus you get a heck of a lot of feedback from nursing about how residents are dealing with patients and families." (A28)

> "I think most of us rely upon second-hand information from our patients, because the residents make their rounds at different times. But we always hear from the patients, and it is very consistent about who's a wonderful doctor and who's not." (A20)

The challenge for programs then is finding ways systematically to involve nursing especially, but perhaps patients as well in the evaluation of resident performance.

Arguments against Program Directors' Evaluations

We have already noted one complaint against the use of program director evaluations. How can program directors give accurate assessments of performance if they are not supervising residents on a day-to-day basis? Because of the many demands on their time (administrative, clinical, teaching), program directors delegate some responsibility for resident supervision to other faculty members. When the department is functioning smoothly, this system works well. When problems occur, the program director may respond by increasing his or her involvement in daily operations, increasing the level of supervision for all residents. This increased supervision may lead to the detection of "problems" that were not considered problems before the director's reign of intense scrutiny began (Bosk 1979):

> "Once a problem gets noted, then he gets all hyper-focussed." (A18)

> "I think that everyone here does a pretty good job, unless a serious mistake is made. That's when people begin to question. If a serious mistake is made, then everybody kinds of steps back, and they look a little closer." (R37)

This "on-again-off-again" kind of process can have grave consequences for residents. If you are unfortunate enough to work during a period of intense scrutiny, you may be faced with a laundry list of small infractions that add up to a poor evaluation. As Anspach (1988) has noted, once a resident falters, he or she will be suspected of incompetence and will be targeted for closer inspection (ibid: 361).

> "I don't know a single resident who hasn't messed up along the way and then you come under the magnifying scope and under the magnifying scope there is no one who can't be faulted. You will continually do something wrong whether it is major or minor as you go along, but if someone keeps tabs on those things, you can be made to look terrible." (A33)

"You can do 98 things right, or 999 things right, it's sort of the accepted thing. Yeah, you put this in at the right time, yeah, he had a skull fracture and you got him to the OR right away. But you screw up once, and that seems to over-shadow everything." (R43)

If you are evaluated when scrutiny is less intense, many of those small infractions may go undetected and your overall performance may be evaluated quite favorably. This "on-again, off-again" evaluation leaves residents feeling frustrated since they are aware that what the medical faculty deems an infraction one day will be overlooked on another day. The residents start to view evaluations as inconsistent and arbitrary:

"It's almost like being a child of alcoholic parents, and there is an inconsistency. Each day you don't know how that parental figure is going to treat you." (R22)

"I see [Dr. X] as a Dr. Jeckle and Mr. Hyde, where you don't know which one is going to approach you. The residents have also talked about that. Where sometimes he just comes in and just lays their asses out, and other times, he's real polite and friendly, and they are just waiting for the other shoe to fall." (N17)

Potluck

The outcome of an evaluation is contingent on a number of factors. We have already cited one factor—the intensity of the level of supervision. A second factor is the number and variety of people involved in the evaluation process. While a diversity of evaluators–peers, support personnel, and the resident's superiors—might provide a "truer" picture, it is also true that the more people involved in evaluation, the harder it is to achieve consensus among all the evaluators. Additionally, attendings, residents and nurses alike recognize that some evaluators are just difficult to please. And again, just as different faculty members will have diverse opinions of what looks good prior to matriculation, so too will they hold differing views after the resident has joined the program (Griner in Langsley 1992, Friedman et al, 1987: 891, Koran 1975). The following quotes from our respondents offer insights into the complexity of the evaluation process where behavior and personalities mix to influence the evaluation. This process protects some residents, while others are left to feel its subjective sting.

"Dr. X can be very hard on you if he doesn't like you. He likes me so he is easier on me although I do a good job for him as well. To a certain extent, if he personally gets along with you, it's good…If an individual is liked, he is not criticized as strenuously as someone who is not." (R41)

"I mean at M&M rounds they are more harsh towards some people and less harsh towards other people which seems to be based on their reputation, irregardless of whether they made the same mistake." (R31)

"Some of it's subjective, it depends on how you talk, smooth things over, you know? The same problem can happen to two different people and somebody stinks and somebody comes out as the wonder boy." (R15)

"I've had people come up and say things like, 'You're too tentative, you've gotta be more aggressive.' Then the next day somebody will come up and say, 'God, you don't need to be that aggressive.'" (R27)

Practice Setting

Studies have found a correlation between residents' evaluations on a particular rotation and the character of the practice setting (Kastner 1986:257):

"Our study suggests that the traits valued by faculty depend on the medical setting: high faculty ratings were assigned on the inpatient service to residents with high [examination] scores, on the intensive care rotations to those who lacked a primary care and psychosocial emphasis, and on the outpatient rotations to those with positive psychosocial orientation." (ibid:263)

The result of the effect of practice setting can mean that residents' "experience of becoming and being competent varies from rotation to rotation in nonlinear, substantial, and at times frightening ways" (Good 1995:145). This can lead the residents to experience some of the negative evaluations as capricious and arbitrary, especially if they had been given a favorable evaluation on a previous rotation.

Expected Mistakes

But no matter what the practice setting or the identity and number of evaluators, faculty expects residents to make mistakes. "According to the definition of competence . . . nearly every surgeon can be expected to be a deviant at some time in some respect" (Welch 1985:127). The art of medical practice requires action before information is complete, so the potential for a wrong decision is ever present. If every resident is expected to make mistakes, how do evaluators judge the inevitable mistakes made by their residents. What differentiates between a serious and minor mistake? According to Bosk, medical educators are concerned about the level of negligence that contributed to the error, not the mistake itself (Bosk 1991). If the resident does everything he or she is supposed to do within the realm of good standard practice and still makes a mistake, that is expected. But if a negligent resident errs because he or she cut corners, failing to provide good care, that mistake is not expected. How does the medical faculty know once an error has been made whether this error in this particular case was part and parcel of medical practice or the result of negligence? The gravity of the mistake is judged by how the resident responds (Bosk 1985: 87):

> "It is not the error itself, it is the response of the resident and the way it is read by his or her subordinates that determines whether or not that resident is going to be blamed..." (ibid)

In order for the resident not to be "blamed" for an error that is a natural consequence of the training process, the resident must quickly recognize the complication, promptly seek appropriate help, and consistently improve performance over successive trials (Bosk 1984:73).

> "I will try to fix it before it gets noticed, or bite the bullet and notify." (R28)

> "I didn't try to bullshit anyone, I just said, 'Sorry, I screwed up." (R45)

The resident who does not recognize the mistake is negligent. The resident who tries to hide his or her mistake is probably trying to hide the shoddy performance that led to the mistake. And the resident who makes the same mistake over and over again does not have what it takes to become a competent physician, to practice medicine employing a good standard of clinical care. The resident who fails to consistently improve typically demonstrates a "pattern" of mistakes during training.

> "...showing continuous progress, it's more important than your absolute level—if you are always getting better, it seems you are improving at a good rate, that is important to them. Demonstrating that whatever they taught you in the past, you don't forget, so you don't make the same mistake twice." (R17)

> "The people who are really good are really good at everything because the way they got to be good is by taking time to master each aspect of what they do and it takes very little time to master things like getting along with patients, or doing phlebotomy correctly and stuff. The people I've seen who are bad screw up repeatedly." (R29)

The medical faculty looks for a resident who will accept responsibility for his or her mistakes because each physician bears a huge amount of responsibility for the lives of their patients. In the recognition and acceptance of the mistake, the faculty hopes that the resident will not forget and not "make the same mistake twice." This links into our discussion from Chapter I of the fiduciary role of the physician. The young doctor who is afraid to face up to that responsibility should not be practicing medicine. He or she will not be able to avoid repeating the same mistakes.

Documenting Mistakes

Although faculty expect mistakes and may not hold a resident responsible for a mistake they deem a natural consequence of the learning process, mistakes still need to be documented so that faculty can catch dreaded patterns and residents can fight arbitrary evaluations based on personality contests. In other studies, authors have found few if any evaluation reports when reviewing resident files, especially reports documenting poor performance (see for example Bosk 1979, Chapter 5). Our study, however, found that only five percent of our 541 programs did not use a standardized form to document performance. We did not, however, see any examples of those forms so we cannot comment on their content or comprehensiveness. The low percent that did not use standardized forms suggests that the majority of surgical residency programs recognize the need for some reporting mechanism.

Good documentation provides a record of the residents' performance. Good documentation is important so residents can have a clear idea of how they are progressing through the program and a sense for how faculty judge that performance. Clear documentation also facilitates the dismissal of poor performers, otherwise residents can challenged dismissal either informally or legally. And it is also important to justify the profession's right to set the educational standards for its members. If the profession as a whole cannot clearly specify the criteria it uses to judge the overall fitness of physicians, how can the general public be confident that the profession is actually producing competent practitioners? The random patient seeking medical care cares more about the proficiency of the doctor rather than his or her ability to get along with the program director.

Feedback

Documentation itself is not enough, however. Adequate feedback to the residents is vital (Albo 1976). As Voytovich points out, any evaluation which is not assimilated by the resident is "of little value" (Voytovich et al, 1986: 66) since the evaluation does not succeed in instructing or altering the resident's behavior. Blurton and Mazzaferri (1986) report on a study of residents that controlled for feedback. They found that "five of the eight residents from whom questionnaire feedback was withheld displayed no improvement, while six of the eight members of the group given such feedback showed significant improvement" (ibid: 182).

Unfortunately, we did not specifically ask our respondents if there is a standard process through which residents get feedback after their evaluations, so we cannot report on general trends and averages. It seemed pretty clear, however, from our subset of interviews that in these surgical residency programs, feedback is rarely provided to residents other than in a very informal manner. We surmised this based on the residents' unfamiliarity with the evaluation process, and because they specifically reported not getting feedback.

What are the dangers of no feedback? Not only do you waste an opportunity to actually instruct the residents that you have been charged to instruct, but you also risk leading along a resident who thought that he or she was performing adequately. This is a disservice to the resident who is investing a great amount of time and energy in an arduous training program:

> "It seems as though this person did not get much feedback until the first day of chief residency and now all of the sudden, out of the blue, her career was threatened and it seems as though everybody from what I've heard that many of the attending staff said that they had reservations about her all along and nobody ever mentioned it when she was out there doing all the footwork and doing all this scut work. Now that it came time for her to be more responsible and do more in the operating room, all of the sudden everybody is not quite confident...She's technically better than a couple of the attendings on the staff." (R36)

This resident not only was deprived of many opportunities to improve her performance, but her entire career was now threatened. As this resident suggests at the end of this quote, he suspected that even this evaluation was arbitrary since he assessed her skills to be even better than some of the attendings on staff. Again, without clear criteria and processes, the whole process will always be vulnerable to claims of arbitrariness, inconsistency, and subjectivity.

There have been calls for reform by medical educators to address this lack of feedback. Some have suggested that residents should be able to read a summary of each evaluation, signing off after it has been read and having an opportunity to respond to the content of the evaluation (Gordon 1987, Robinowitz 1986: 175). This helps to maintain communication between program faculty and residents as well as documenting that feedback has been delivered.

Type of Feedback

Feedback is important for instructing neophytes. The frequency and quality of feedback are important aspects of the process. Surgical faculty members are notorious for yelling at residents. Yelling as a means of instruction is expected as a part of the culture. From the faculty's perspective, reprimands of this sort underscore the gravity of the physician's responsibility. There *is* a lot riding on every decision made by the doctor for his or her patient, and loud, booming corrections make this point.

> "During the last operation, Dalton had found fault with the residents almost continuously, and when a nurse had come into the room to tell him that he was wanted outside for an important telephone call, he had turned his eyes upward toward the ceiling and dramatically implored, '*Someone* keep yelling at them.'" (Millman 1977: 34)

"[Dr. X.] can make things so uncomfortable that it is embarrassing for me to even be there listening to it, hurtful to me to see this happen to a resident and I know that sometimes it is so bad that there are certain nurses who wouldn't want to be in the same room and be part of it...he just gets down right nasty and I notice sometimes, and this is funny, that when we have guests, he behaves even more in this role." (N14)

Many residents believe that since the wider society no longer tolerates this kind of behavior, it should not be tolerated in a residency program.

"But malicious criticism, a malicious approach to attempting to drive home a point just does not have a place in the modern world." (R34)

The problem was that they sometimes saw yelling as a personal attack rather than a justified reprimand.

"Any excessive yelling is bad teaching. If the yelling can be perceived as personally directed rather than just general, or as ballistoid behavior, which some people can't avoid, that's bad." (R28)

What also bothered some residents was the diversity of the faculty in this regard. Residents saw some members as fair and just, and others as unfair. And they saw some faculty members as beyond the pale of acceptable behavior.

"I have no problems when somebody screams at me for a reasonable mistake. Okay, you made a mistake, they kick you in the rear end, and you correct it. That's part of the residency program. I expected that...What bothered me the most was being accused of something unjustly. Or to be yelled at for no reason at all...There were people in the past who would yell at you and would give you a chance to defend yourself. That's fair. They'll sit down and talk with me...But there were other people who would stab you in the back, and not give you a second chance, even talk to you, and would sell you down the river. That bothers me." (R18)

"I've been in other services where I have been beaten before. Many people who are educators in medicine are jerks, and they really do rotten things to people who are in training—they swear at them, they throw instruments at them, they'll make you go stand in a corner if you do something wrong in the operating room. They berate you." (R30)

Another complaint is that sometimes residents find themselves berated for what they deem "small" offenses that did not compromise patient care and did not deserve the kind of attention they got. Faculty tabulate these minor offensives during times of increased scrutiny. When residents find themselves defending these minor infractions, they feel that their own and the attendings' energies are being spent in the wrong places. It also causes confusion since again the residents are faced with the challenge of deciphering what is really important and not important as the standard to judge performance changes from moment-to-moment and person-to-person—a continuing lack of consistency.

> "The only time it bothers me is when some little picayune incident...meanwhile you did the right thing with the patient. And that may result in a report or something and all they focus on is a little nothing, that is inconsequential to patient care. Then, that hits a raw nerve. Because here you are, working hard, doing the job from the patient's point of view, and then you get nailed on some, you know, point that is really not that significant." (R13)

> "You can't defend yourself in those circumstances because they are blown out of proportion. You're not going to get a logical argument out of it, so I just eat it."(R36)

The inconsistent nature of resident evaluation and the diversity of faculty opinions leads the students to discount negative assessments when they begin to develop confidence in their own doctoring skills. Light (1980) found that by the second year of training, residents in psychiatry and internal medicine discounted even blunt criticism of their performance by attributing it to differences in approach, the same difference in approach and focus that they regularly see demonstrated by attendings. Similarly, Bucher (1977) found that "postgraduate trainees actively discounted occasions in which their performance and competence were criticized by both peers and members of the staff" (ibid:11). Discounting is a natural extension of the initiates' training for control--as the resident's self-confidence grows, he or she will inevitably begin to trust his or her own judgment over others, and recognize that there can be a number of valid approaches to patient care and treatment. We would also argue, however, that this discounting is an unintended consequence of the inconsistent aspects of the current system of evaluation. If residents were clearer on the yardstick that was being used to judge their competency, we believe that residents would be less likely to discount faculty assessments.

Among our respondents we found something different than just discounting: the attachment of certain residents to certain attendings. Residents stated that the opinions of the faculty members they respected were important to them. Other attendings could rant and rave about the residents' performance and it did not impact them very much, but if the attending for whom they had high regard either criticized or praised these residents, they took that evaluation to heart.

> "I care whether some people think I'm doing a good job because I respect them and care about them and care about what they think. But I don't feel that way about everyone." (R22)

> "He is a perfectionist and when he says something is really good, you know that it is really good...he's not bullshitting you, it's something you can really

take home. He was telling me what a good job I was doing and that was really nice to hear." (R27)

"But he just has all those qualities that people respect. So if he criticizes you about something, you take it to heart. And you want to figure out what you did wrong or why you did it and how to make it better." (R23)

Ultimate evaluation

We have already enumerated many drawbacks to the current system of evaluation. First of all, program faculty members have the task of choosing next year's cohort of residents within a process that leaves members with little information to go on. Attendings pick students on the basis of test scores that have no correlation with their ultimate performance. They try to assess residents' personality and character from misleading and at times untruthful letters of recommendation. They also try to assess compatibility during a brief and informal interview process that has the validity of random sampling.

Once the resident enters the program, new problems arise. As the resident makes different rotations, different faculty members with different agendas assess their skills, leaving residents to feel as though their competency has more to do with pleasing a particular individual rather than an objective measure of doctoring skills. Additionally, residents notice that the level of scrutiny is inconsistent, and that when levels are high, minor infractions garner major attention. Residents note that evaluation can often be subjective and involve quite a bit of personality, so that during M & M rounds, some residents will be more severely chastised for an error than another resident who made the same error. Since all of these factors result in the resident's viewing the evaluation process as arbitrary and inconsistent, in the end residents find these reports on their skills to be indecipherable. No reliable standard exists to compare one resident with another.

If all this is true, is there no way to say that one resident is better than another, or that a resident is not qualified to operate? Although there are many problems with the current system, both residents and attendings agree that there is an ultimate evaluation, and the outcome of this assessment is the best measure of whether peers consider a fellow practitioner competent. The evaluators must ask themselves the following question: would you let this resident operate on a family member? If the answer is "no," then that resident should not be released from the program onto an unsuspecting public until the program faculty can, without reservation, answer "yes."

"My own chairman's standard was that by the time you get through residency, if I wouldn't let you operate on a family member of mine, you don't finish the residency." (A19)

"The other four faculty members would not submit themselves to a surgical procedure by him. I think that is the best way to judge any surgeon—do his peers trust him to be cutting on them?" (A33)

"There are some physicians that I wouldn't take my family to, or go to." (R22)

We will now look at some general issues around the last topic of this chapter, attrition.

Attrition

As discussed in the introduction, attrition occurs when an individual fails to complete some socialization process, whether it is an attempt to join a group, a profession, or to complete some training program. As Tinto (1993) notes:

> "Institutions of higher education are not unlike other human communities, and the process of educational departure is not substantially different from other processes of leaving which occur among human communities generally. In both instances, departure mirrors the absence of social and intellectual integration into or membership in community life and of the social support such integration provides." (ibid: 204)

The attrition process can be started either by the initiate or by the target community. Either the initiate decides that community membership is not desired or that he or she lacks a "goodness of fit", or the community decides that the initiate does not have the traits and characteristics necessary to assume a role in the community. But where does the fault lie in either of these situations? The trend in attrition studies has been to lay the blame at the feet of the individual "dropout." As Tinto remarks in the case of the college dropout:

> "...dropouts have been frequently portrayed as having a distinct personality profile or lacking in a particularly important attribute needed for college completion. As a consequence, we have been given the mistaken view that student dropouts are different or deviant from the rest of the student population. Such stereotypes are reinforced by a language, a way of thinking about student departure which labels individuals as failures for not having completed their course of study in an institution of higher education." (ibid: 3)

Attrition reveals something about both the institution and the individual. Specifically, a dynamic exists between the individual and his or her community that the scenario above simplifies to the point of misrepresentation. What would lead the initiate to change his or her mind about membership? Is it a failure of the individual or of the community? What leads the community to reject the individual after initially accepting him or her for community involvement? Was the mistake made in the initial selection? In the case of attrition from educational programs, where does the responsibility lie—with the student or with the teacher? When the student fails, is it because the teacher failed to impart the knowledge, or did the student fail to do the work? Could the student have succeeded with a different teacher in a different environment? How can these different scenarios be tested? These are among the multitude of questions that investigators of attrition raise. The answers to the above questions may differ from case to case, but attrition studies typically fail to examine both sides of the coin, the individual and the community. Raising the level of awareness of the dynamic interplay may foster better studies.

In the attrition literature, analysts like to distinguish between "voluntary" and "involuntary" attrition when possible, although the data do not always allow it. Ideally, researchers want to distinguish between people who resign from their positions and those who are terminated. The constant feedback between individual and community can muddy these lines in way that statistics can never adequately address. As Bowen and Rudenstein (1992) caution: "What is 'voluntary' and what is 'involuntary' becomes murky indeed, and it is hard to see what criteria can be relied on to tell anyone where to draw the line" (ibid: 113).

Many researchers have focused on the selection process in order to find ways to reduce attrition. They argue that if we can get better at matching candidates with communities, fewer people will leave. However, in study after study, little evidence supports such an argument (Cope and Hannah 1975: 86). Also, as noted by Tinto (1993), no evidence supports the existence of an "attrition prone" personality. As we have already discussed, there are many uncertainties in matching candidates and communities. Employers face the difficult assessment of potential and achievement, the uncertain correlation of past and future performance, and the unique problem of assessing how someone who has never performed a particular role will perform that role.

> "...success depends in large measure on commitment, stamina, and the capacity to function under difficult conditions—qualities that are difficult to assess, especially in a student who has not yet enrolled." (Bowen and Rudenstein 1992: 252)

Competing life events can also interfere with any socialization process. All these areas of uncertainty limit the reformation of the matching process.

Given all the uncertainties associated with the process, some programs and individual residents will have inevitably made the wrong choice.

> "Well, people who I thought were very dedicated and interested in neurosurgery proved not to be, and vice versa, people who I thought were not going to be particularly good residents turned out to be excellent residents." (A18)

> "Twenty percent. It's a national statistic. It's not reducible. If we continue along with the matching program as it is, a guy or a woman will come in and

say, yea I want to be a neurosurgeon and then say, well this isn't what I wanted
after all." (A17)

Some people will find that group membership does not bring the anticipated
rewards or that certain skills are lacking. In other instances, the initiate discovers
a discrepancy between the job description and his or her job experience (Jacobs
1994: 3). In these cases, attrition is a positive event since it allows people to
pursue other options that might be a better fit for a variety of reasons (Tinto
1993: 143). In fact, Heimbach and Johansen (1986) define about one-third of
resident attrition as "natural" attrition. By this, the authors mean that due to lack
of exposure in medical school to their chosen residency specialty, the residents
had chosen to pursue a particular path with imperfect knowledge and discovered
that the chosen specialty did not actually make them happy (ibid: 13). There are
restrictions on how much exposure any individual student can be given before
making a choice. Increases in exposure to one specialty means less time spent in
another. The desire for specialized exposure as a medical student has to be balanced with the production of a well-rounded doctor familiar with many different
medical and surgical specialties. This inherent tension is not easily resolved.
    Another argument suggests that the problem is not with selection, but with the
socialization process once the resident has joined a program. King (1988), a
neurosurgeon, makes this argument:

    "Are the failures a selection problem? Or are they a problem of graduate medi-
    cal education 'processing' wherein some fine young people—separated from
    their customary supports and unable to establish new ones—do they need more
    from their peers, new families, the faculty and the program than we proffer?"
    (King in Langsley 1988: 33)

King raises the question: How much attrition results from lack of support from
the socializing unit, in this case, the surgical residency program? How many
residents who leave would have been able to stay had they had more support
during the time of transition when they are learning the ropes, the new skills,
adapting to a new environment, and interacting with a new community of people? This question raises issues vitally important in the analysis of the time of
departure, a theme we will cover in later chapters.

Attrition in Higher Education

    From the five specialties covered in this study, we obtained the attrition statis-
tics reported in Table 2.3. These numbers represent the combined rate of resignations and terminations from the programs sampled. This table demonstrates
that the overall average attrition rate was about ten percent, with a fairly high
deviation between programs (notice the standard deviations). This means that

about 1 out of every 10 residents who began a residency program in any of these five specialties left before finishing the tour in the original program.

Table 2.3: Attrition Rates by Specialty

Specialty	Mean	SD
Anesthesiology	7.38%	.0543
General Surgery	15.61%	.1547
Neurosurgery	11.74%	.1427
Orthopedic Surgery	4.37%	.0513
Plastic Surgery	5.18%	.0903
Total	9.61%	.1232

Note that general surgery and neurosurgery reported the highest attrition rates, about 16% for general surgery and 12% for neurosurgery, while plastic surgery and orthopedic surgery enjoyed the lowest rates. The difference between the rates reported by the general surgery and neurosurgery programs compared to all other programs combined was highly significant. In later chapters, we will look at these trends and specialty effects in greater detail.

How does this overall trend in attrition compare to that experienced by other professional groups and institutions of higher learning? These statistics pale in comparison to higher education in general. As Cooke et al (1995) report, 40% of college students do not earn a degree. The risk of attrition varies with the type of college, type of degree pursued, and race and gender, so not every college experiences such a large attrition rate. This substantial rate represents a national average across colleges.

For those who survive the undergraduate training program and continue their studies in graduate schools or professional programs, the numbers are both better and worse. For those lucky enough to get accepted into medical school, the risk of attrition is greatly reduced. Only about one percent of the nation's approximately 65,000 medical students permanently drop out of school. For those who pursue other professional programs like law, the numbers again are quite good—only 5% of these students experience attrition. Students entering masters programs fare poorly, with 42% discontinuing before earning a degree (Scott 1996: 234). Students who pursue PhD programs fare even worse, with 50% dropping out before obtaining a degree (Bowen and Rudenstein 1992). Students pursuing a law or medical degree are protected against attrition.

Although only one percent of medical students leaves their medical school programs, more than one percent leaves their residency training. But these residents do not tend to drop out of medicine altogether. There is a difference between dropping out of a specialty and dropping out of a profession. But how do the attrition rates we report above for our specialties compare with the attrition rates in other specialties? Although the rates can vary depending on how attrition is measured (temporary vs. permanent leaves, transfers vs. permanent withdrawal, etc.), the numbers across specialties seem fairly comparable, with about 10% of residents on average deciding that their first residency program choice was not the right choice (Hook in Lloyd 1982, Klineberg in Lloyd 1985). We cannot, however, compare our analysis of problematic completers outside of these five specialties since this statistic is not typically measured.

Why are these residents leaving their programs? As others have found and we also found in our analysis:

> "...deficiencies generally seem to be in the realm of interpersonal communications and the humanistic traits rather than fund of knowledge." (Klineberg 1985: 48)

Tinto notes that across educational institutions of all types, professional and institutions of general learning, only 15-25% of failure constitutes "academic failure," or an inability to master the academic work. Another proportion fails to master the ethos of the community (Bucher and Stelling 1977: 218). Over and over again, we find a relationship between non-intellectual factors and attrition (Waenecke 1973: 165). In the case of these surgical training programs, evaluators note non-technical shortcomings before technical ones since residents assume surgical responsibility later in the program. Technical weaknesses can only be evaluated later in the tour (A26).

But we are not suggesting that the remainder of those who leave the program are people with difficult personalities and behavioral problems. For example, studies estimate that about 10% of women pursuing educational degrees in "traditional" fields (such as nursing) leave their training programs due to sexual harassment (for example, Gutek and Morash 1982). Studies of women in non-traditional fields (like medicine, law and business) estimate that about 20% leave due to harassment (ibid). Sometimes women perceive the training environment as threatening or dangerous and this motivates the withdrawal. This perception is noted among individuals entering non-traditional fields where "people just like them" are sorely underrepresented. We already know that women and minorities are underrepresented in professional programs and graduate degree programs (Bowen and Rudenstein 1992: 34, 37). Tinto (1993) makes the point that in order to assure successful completion of a program, institutions should insure that sufficient numbers of individuals of varying types and/or dispositions are found so that every individual chosen for the program will find a support group available within the institution (ibid: 124). The structural and financial constraints of doing so, however, can present significant challenges especially in smaller settings. Also, sometimes outside influences cause people to withdrawal from programs such as family or financial crises. These outside influences have historically disproportionately affected women (Bardoness 1981), and the trend apparently remains. In later chapters, we will analyze the reasons residents left their programs or were terminated and see how sexual harassment and/or external forces contributed to the attrition risk for our women residents.

Cost of Attrition

Attrition is costly for the individual as well as for the institution or community. Although few residents in our study left medicine altogether, they bore a huge cost in joining a residency program and beginning training in a labor- and knowledge-intensive specialty such as surgery. Investing in specialized knowledge is costly, especially when we measure time invested (Evans and Lauman 1983: 15). But the costs for the individual are measured in other ways as well. For the young medical professional, the completion of a residency program is the way to achieve full adulthood within the medical profession (Broadhead 1983: 55). Those thwarted in their attempt to complete this rite of transition find themselves in a prolonged professional adolescence. This prolonged adolescence hampers the young medical professional's development of the mastery and self-confidence so vital in the practice of medicine (Bucher and Stelling 1977: 193). In some ways the medical student has put all of his or her eggs into one basket over a course of many, many years. The prize for all that investment is not a prize easily lost.

For the programs, attrition poses other challenges. Not only has some investment been made in the screening and acceptance of residents (think of the interview time, the processing of papers, the tours through the department), but each unexpected withdrawal also causes a labor shortage in the department. Attrition can also effect housestaff morale and esprit de corps. An unexpected resignation or termination can cause other residents in the program to re-examine their own commitments to the specialty. If both the residents who leave and those who stay view the termination or resignation as the fault of the program faculty, or as unjust, it can stir ill feelings between the remaining residents and the program faculty. The harmony of the department can be adversely affected.

Functional Attrition

Up to this point we have been focusing on the costs or negative aspects of attrition, but attrition can have positive effects as well. Attrition can give a resident a chance to pursue another specialty that will make him or her happier. From the program perspective, potential benefits can accrue. For example, department harmony can be restored when a disruptive member of the resident group leaves. A termination can be functional if it maintains standards of performance, provides a contrast that rewards good performance, and protects the group from poor performers. With these functional aspects in mind, should program faculty convince the resident who wants to leave to stay and/or give the resident who is at risk for termination one more chance. No one wants to make the decision to leave or to terminate prematurely, but postponing a withdrawal bears its own costs, both for the individual and for the department. For the good performing resigner, postponing resignation means wasting time that could be spent pursuing another career option. For the poor performer termination, postponing the termination both keeps the resident from pursuing a more appropriate career and exposes his or her patients to substandard medical care and affects group morale.

> "I think it is better to err on the side of getting rid of someone who is questionable than keeping someone who is questionable...Certainly, if I was questionable, I would hope that Dr. X would tell me because I certainly have other career options where I think I would not be questionable, and it's his duty to let me know so that I can pursue them and become a good something." (R29)

Difficult to Terminate

Many faculty members as well as researchers, however, recognize that asking a resident to leave is difficult. Faculty members recognize that these residents have already invested a great deal of time and energy in their education and they are individually reluctant to be the one that wields the axe that will stop the process, or sully a resident's record:

> "I think they find it very hard to terminate a resident. I think it's a blot on the record, or they feel that way." (A13)

> "It must be the hardest thing in the world to trash, collegially, to trash someone's career like that, and yet, that is the responsibility of a program director, to do that." (R29)

> "You can't just fire somebody, it's their livelihood." (A14)

Additionally, this individual has already been screened by numerous individuals and institutions, and has, therefore, a whole history of approval behind him or her. How can this group of attendings, this one institution, now deem this individual unfit? How can they justify this negative assessment, which is contrary to the implied good opinions of others? This need to "justify" the decision to terminate or encourage to leave again underscores the need for good documentation.

> "Remember, you not only have a medical school investment and a licensure process behind this person, plus several years of preliminary training for some specialties. Now we say you ought to be doing something else, you ought to be growing avocados. That is a tough statement to make unless you have good documentation." (Mankin in Lloyd 85: 99)

There are times when a resident should be terminated or encouraged to withdraw, but whose responsibility is it to terminate the resident? Should the faculty agree on the decision, or should an individual member such as the program director be responsible for the final decision?

> "The chairman is really the one obligated to fire the resident. It's on his shoulders to follow the responsibility to do it." (A20)

Some program directors will accept full responsibility for this decision:

> "I'm responsible for what goes on here. If I send a bum neurosurgeon on the world, it's my fault and nobody else's." (A23)

Leaving the termination in the hands of one individual, however, leaves the decision open to the claim that the decision was unfair, due to interpersonal conflicts, subjective, not unanimous. If a resident or faculty member challenges a decision, the termination can cause internal strife and discontent rather than serve the positive function of expelling a disruptive member. In Chapter 5, we will review the different ways the programs in our study handled the termination decision: who was involved, what was the process followed, how was the resident informed, etc.

Some believe that program faculty should compensate residents for their great investment in their medical education by giving them extra chances early in the training process:

> "I think that people ought to be given lots of chances, though, considering what everyone's had to go through to get to the residency program." (A24)

> "We try to support those people, try to remake them, and graduate them , not like at Hospital X where a person is simply terminated once it becomes obvious that the person has faults in their personality." (R31)

Critics contend that programs tend to be much too lenient since it appears that residents must fail in some catastrophic way in order to be terminated.

> "It appears, at this point, that standards set for actual dismissal, at least in the early years of training, are so restrictive that for a resident to be asked to leave a program, he or she must commit literally the equivalent of repeated high crimes and medical misdemeanors." (Anwar 1981: 38)

> "Nobody gets fired for an isolated incident, unless they rape the head nurse or something like that." (A27)

In our analysis, we uncovered examples of seemingly too lenient and too harsh dismissals with most cases falling in-between. We had one case of a resident being terminated for leaving the building without notifying an attending and another resident who was not terminated even after his carelessness contributed to the death of a patient.

And finally, program faculty say it is difficult to terminate a friend. There is a need and desire for camaraderie among the members of the department. In many cases, residents are chosen to join a program because they fit in well and are well liked. Sometimes, faculty members find themselves faced with the prospect of terminating "one of their own"—someone that they liked very much and want to see succeed:

> "He was a nice guy. I knew his wife. I played racquetball with him. We'd go out socially, have parties together, and this was his life and his career, so that was a hard thing to do...And I thought that it was a matter of him getting a little more mature, and that didn't seem to be the case. But I thought, we'd carried this guy along, now in his fourth or fifth year to say suddenly, 'You don't have what it takes.' It's kind of not the right thing to do and maybe what we should do is get him out to do some extra work in other places."(A18)

What are some of the proven or suggested ways of reducing attrition both in and out of the arena of medical education programs? We will review some of the relevant issues below.

Assimilation

Given that many individual joining a new program or a new institution will be unfamiliar with many aspects of their new community, a vital aspect of early entry and training involves gathering a great deal of information on expectations associated with the initiate's new role. Programs that are created in order to help initiates assimilate to their new environments are crucial in reducing attrition (Crandall 1978: 331). By the term "assimilation program" we mean any program that helps the initiate learn about and adopt the characteristics of the group. It is not helpful to expect a newcomer to perform a function if you do not tell that newcomer both 1) what you want done, and 2) how the job is typically done. The information the newcomer receives must give an accurate portrayal of the work setting and the work. As Crandall notes (1978):

> "Work in industrial and military settings has focused in giving prospective newcomers accurate information about the setting they are about to enter, including realistic negative information. This has generally increased job satisfaction and decreased job attrition." (ibid: 333)

But this transfer of knowledge does not occur during formal information seminars alone, although these sessions would qualify as assimilation programs. It also occurs during a variety of informal and formal ceremonies; over a cup of coffee in the lounge; during a cocktail party; during a walk from one department to the next. Numerous vital rites and ceremonies of both a formal and informal nature help the initiate learn about his or her new surroundings (Tinto 1993: 175). The initiate who is excluded for any reason from these rites and ceremonies (from the information seminar to the cup of coffee in the lounge) will be at a greater risk for attrition.

Quality of Interactions

Lack of assimilation programs contributes to attrition, and so does poor interactions between community members and newcomers. This not only affects attrition, but reports of job satisfaction in general:

> "Whether workers experienced high job satisfaction and high morale, or low job satisfaction and low morale seemed to depend less on the work itself (or even on the salary and benefits) than on the satisfying interactions with bosses and co-workers and the feeling of some control over the work." (Garson 1977, in Jacobs 1994)

Tinto (1990) found a similar relationship among college students:

> "…research demonstrates that the degree and quality of personal interaction with other members of the institution are critical elements in the process of student persistence…the absence of sufficient contact with other members of the institution proves to be the single most important predictor of eventual departure even after taking account of the independent effects of background, personality, and academic performance." (ibid)

As we have already discussed in part and will expound upon in later chapters, the quality of interaction affects the degree of camaraderie felt by the members of the group. When members identify with each other and feel loyalty to the group, the likelihood of leaving is reduced (Groopman 1987: 214). The greater the number of perceived differences between members, the harder it will be for them to have quality interactions. When differences between recruits and current members exist, formal forms of interaction must be developed to assure communication and improve interactions. In these cases, institutions must create opportunities for initiates to become more involved with their communities (Cooke 1995: 686).

Goodness of Fit

When the initiate feels qualified for his or her new post, the risk of withdrawal is greatly reduced. Analysts have noted this relationship both in and out of academic settings.

"...the closer the perceived fit between person's perception of himself and of so-called ideal candidate (graduate), the more likely is persistence" (Tinto 1993: 81).

"...a crucial variable in determining the outcome of socialization experiences is the degree of 'fit' between the individual and his immediate socializing environment." (Rootman 1972: 263)

The trick is figuring out what predicts whether or not the newcomer will feel a goodness of fit. We have already suggested that a greater sense of similarity between mentor and mentee will promote these feelings of a fit between the person's perception of him/herself and the ideal candidate. Since most mentors in these programs will be white males, women and minority residents have the greater challenge.

When Problems are Noticed

In this section we discuss the timing of attrition in surgical residency programs. The common trend in this study was that faculty noted problems, whether they be academic, social, personal, or behavioral, quite early in the resident's tour in the department, typically within the first six months.

"Anybody who has been in this department knows almost immediately if a resident has problems. If they aren't resolved, or showing signs of being resolved within three to four months, they are not going to resolve them. And by six months, it's absolute. No one should ever go over six months." (N21)

The fact that decisions about whose performance is problematic are made so early in the resident's tour presents an interesting dilemma for the foreign, racial minority and female residents who face the greatest assimilation challenge in the community of surgical residents. These residents are often excluded from informal knowledge networks and therefore will have a harder time "learning the ropes" of the department and hospital environment. Foreign and racial minority students may also face language barriers that would take more than a few months to overcome. Racial and gender minority residents bear the burden of early identification of problems.

But what are the costs of delaying? If the resident will never be able to be "transformed" into a competent surgeon, the program should let that resident know as soon as possible that he/she has little chance of success. The resident can then minimize the costs that he or she must bear at this early stage of residency training. There is no point in having the resident invest any more time than they have to in pursuing specialized knowledge:

"If you are not 100% sure at the end of the first year, you should cut the strings right there. You are not doing anybody a favor to string him on for three more years and then tell him, 'You're no good.'" (A35)

"I sort of set a policy for us that our attendings, our residents, need to learn early in their careers here whether or not they're staying on. The business of 'let's give him another year, it's too early,' I find that unacceptable. It's unfair to the program and no fair to the individual." (A27)

Problems that should have been noticed

Residency program directors expressed frustration that they end up choosing residents who obviously displayed problems while they were medical students. Program directors are dumbfounded that after countless years of screening and training—arduous undergraduate premedical programs, a long series of national testing, numerous interviews, a grading system, etc.—they still end up choosing residents who are unfit for graduate training.

"There really must be a failure in the educational system because these are not kids off the street. Remember, they have come from our prestigious universities after four years of training in our most prestigious medical schools for four more years of training. So they have been under the scrutiny of academia for a period of eight years and yet we still seem to get them into our programs totally unwarned and the problem seems to have been unrecognized over that period of time. I think that the tragedy is that it gets to that point." (Klinenberg in Lloyd 1985: 96)

A number of our respondents expressed similar views:

"But in medical school, there were some kids in my class who just lacked any judgment whatsoever, and might have bordered on personality disorders and psychopathies and things like that." (R43)

"In medical school, there were a number, two or three classmates, who were addicted to drugs. Thereby, they cut corners and cheated and really did not pay attention to what they were doing. One of them ended up getting thrown out of school, but the other two went on." (R42)

Although we do not have data that can tell us just how prevalent this problem is in many different medical and surgical specialties, we did ask one question on the survey which can suggest how many problems should have been noted that were not noted before. We asked if there was any indication after the resident interviewed that he or she would have any problems meeting the requirements of the program. We got the following responses for our three attrition categories:

Table 2.4.: Indication of potential problems?

	Percent	SD
Resignations (n=555)	6%	0.243
Terminations (n=247)	13%	0.341
Problematic Completers (n=165)	22%	0.414

Six percent of the residents who resigned, compared to 13% of the residents who were terminated and 22% of the residents who problematically completed their training, had some indication that they would have problems meeting the demands of their chosen residency program. What kinds of indications did the program directors note? The following table breaks down the kinds of indications most often cited for the 89 cases for which we had information:

Table 2.5. Indication of problem

Type of problem	Percent
Poor academic preparation	22%
Prior history of problems	19%
Wrong personality	17%
Unsure of specialty choice	13%
Untruthful letters of recommendation	12%
Outside interests/pressures	8%
Physical problems/handicaps	4%
Poor language skills	2%
No indications/total surprise	2%
Other	1%

(n=89)

The most often cited indication was poor academic preparation.

"Deficient in knowledge." (non-white male, termination)

"One interviewer noted that he was deficient in several areas of technical knowledge." (non-white male, termination)

Program faculty consider poor academic preparation a problem that is not easily remedied within the structure of a normal residency training program. Current program schedules cannot accommodate the poor academically prepared resident and bring him or her up-to-speed. The resident who came poorly prepared will have a more difficult time passing in-house and external exams which faculty use to measure proficiency.

The second most cited indication was a prior history of problems. Despite the prior history, the program decided for a variety of reasons to take a chance on the resident. The prior history most often involved a personality conflict with members in a different residency program:

"Had withdrawn from two residency programs prior." (white male, problematic completer)

"Had some problems as an intern, yet department felt that these would resolve." (white female, termination)

Recall that program faculty are fully aware that personality conflicts can happen so the attendings may have decided to take a chance in the hope that the particular mix of the initiate's personality and their own would be better.

The third most cited indication was wrong personality. In some of these cases, it was thought unlikely that the resident would mix well with the program, but the resident matched nevertheless—"really didn't feel that he was going to fit in (white male, problematic completer)." In other cases, the resident was perceived as being too passive or too timid for the kind of work that surgery involved:

"At interview, he was passive, but said he liked the persona of general surgery." (non-white male, resignation)

"His manner and affect were flat. He seemed laid back, lack of intensity. These traits persisted through residency." (white male, problematic completer)

"We knew this individual was somewhat timid, but he seemed to be bright and willing to work hard and learn." (white male, problematic completer)

In other cases, we note the opposite—the resident's personality was too aggressive for the work required.

"Pushy and overly aggressive in interview. His background and previous research made us take a chance on him, hoping he would be worth the effort. It didn't pan out." (white male, termination)

"Seemed demanding, but had good credentials." (non-white female, resignation)

Uncertainty about specialty choice was the fourth most cited indication. Recall that attendings look for a display of passion during the residents' interviews. When this passion and commitment is not displayed, the faculty believe the resident is at risk for leaving.

"He told me he was not sure of his specialty choice and was deciding between anesthesia and psychiatry." (non-white male, resignation)

"He initially considered anesthesia, then chose general surgery, then switched back to anesthesia." (white male, resignation)

Our program faculty also seemed haunted by untruthful or misleading letters of recommendation. In twelve percent of our cases, faculty discovered a dishonest recommendation after the resident had already matched with the program, so program faculty felt obligated to wait it out and hope for the best:

> "Her anatomy instructor indicated how difficult she was to get along with. The Dean's letter whitewashed everything and made us think that she would be a good surgical resident. He lied—she was impossible." (white female, termination)

> "He was accepted after 3 years of general surgery training on the advice of chief of surgery who then noted after the applicant was accepted for plastic surgery training that resident's performance during his last years of general 'slacked off.'" (white male, termination)

Another indication was outside interests or pressures. In these cases, it was obvious to the program faculty that others outside the hospital had some claims to the resident's time and energy.

> "Resident had a lot of debt and a large family." (white male, resignation)

In one case, a resident was a single parent with no one to share childrearing responsibilities. In another case, a white male who was very athletically inclined ended up leaving his residency program because it interfered with his training schedule. In one of our more tragic cases, a white female problematic completer had to give up a year of additional training to support her family since her husband had gone to prison for tax evasion. Studies of attrition across educational and occupational settings have shown that "life load," or how much responsibility people have in their lateral roles, significantly affects attrition (Scott 1996).

Four percent of our cases involved physical handicaps that were severe enough to interfere with training:

> "Resident had a neurological procedure as a child and had a speech defect." (non-white male, termination)

We also have a case of a woman attempting surgery when she was 51 years old—the program faculty doubted that she had the physical stamina to get through the residency program.

And finally, we have the total surprise. In these cases the program directors recounted their total surprise that the resident had any problems at all given his or her stellar application, test scores, background, letters of recommendation, etc.:

> "He was very charming in the interview setting. He had excellent credentials with excellent letters of recommendation; he had been an honor student in

physics as an undergraduate. There was absolutely no indication, even in retro-spect, that we could detect from reviewing his application folder." (white male, termination)

"This young man passed all interviews with flying colors. His medical school letters reflected this also." (white male, resignation)

What would have happened if the program directors had heeded these warn-ing signs and not accepted these residents into their programs? As we have noted, sometimes faculty discovered the indications after the residents had al-ready matched, but in other cases, the warning signs preceded matriculation. The most obvious answer would be that their attrition would have been reduced. But can we state that from our data? No. We unfortunately do not have the other side of the equation, which is how many residents with these same warning signs went on to successfully complete their programs? Experience may inform these program faculty's decisions to accept the resident with the prior problem, or with the aggressive personality, or even the indecisive resident because in the past these gambles have often paid off. What we can note from this analysis is that overall, among the entire pool of problematic residents (resignations, termi-nations, and problematic completers, n=967), in only 11% (104) of these cases did the faculty recognize any indication that the resident would have any prob-lems meeting the demands and challenges of residency training. This low figure underscores some of the problems with the current selection process, which can-not accurately predict which students will and will not complete training. How-ever, we are not suggesting that all the reform lies in the development of a better selection process. Look at the indications that we enumerated. Poor academic preparation needs to be addressed before the resident even comes up for consid-eration. Sometimes prior problems due to personality conflicts will not be re-peated in another environment. Residents' uncertainty about their choice of resi-dency program can be remedied with better exposure during medical school. Foreign students with poor language skills can get extra training prior to the start of the residency program. We do not need to throw out the student with the indi-cation as much as we need to remedy the situation before the training begins, or reorganize the residency programs so that they have the flexibility to allow stu-dents of varying preparation and talent to move at different speeds. But no mat-ter how many reforms are implemented, some surprises will remain.

Potential Liabilities

"If you're not a good doctor, you're a licensed murderer." (R44)

The resident who withdraws from residency training costs the program quite a lot in terms of wasted resources, time, and manpower shortages. But the resident who withdraws also presents a potential cost to the profession as a whole.

Armed with a licensure process behind them, and in some cases, preliminary training for some specialties, the resident who fails out of a residency program can still practice medicine even if his or her instructors were displeased with his or her standard of care (Mankin 1985: 99). The poorly trained and poorly skilled physician poses a risk to the public (Kapp 1981: 560):

"I get extremely angry at this current generation of senior physicians who I think are turning a blind eye as to who is being trained and sent out." (R39)

"The effect of the quality of future patient care from residents who leave to enter practice before completion of training, especially those who are discharged for incompetence and performance difficulties, is incalculable but should be of concern to the profession." (Baldwin et al, 1995: 1124)

The resident who withdraws or who is terminated may end up pursuing additional training, but he or she may also go straight into practice.

"The transient house-staff members, or those poorly matched with their learning environment, without anyone ever intending it, may become orphans in a series if foster homes in medicine and they may drift out to the fringes of the medical system somewhat beyond the control of their medical colleagues." (Mumford 1970:223)

"A lot of these people are practicing in situations where there is no one directly around who is really capable of supervising these people." (A24)

More disturbing than the resident who resigns or who is terminated and therefore does not have the certification of a residency program behind them is the problematic completer who at least on paper has the backing of whatever institution promoted him or her. As stated by some of our respondents, the diploma paints a false picture of the resident's overall proficiency and will lead others outside the program to assume that this resident is competent:

"He has finished a very adequate program, a very well-respected program, then he must be a very good neurosurgeon, otherwise they wouldn't finish him. Which, frankly, should be true. It is the responsibility of the program to filter out people who are not going to be competent neurosurgeons or competent doctors in general and not sanction them to be in neurosurgery." (A14)

"The two guys who graduated from here when I first came on, one of them clearly should not have gone out." (A15)

And another account of a woman who will finish a residency program but who will fall into this same category of certified professional liabilities:

"We are in a hell of a dilemma and believe me, we just don't know what to do. You have to ask yourself, would you let this person operate on a relative of yours in the future and my answer would be absolutely not. Could you recommend this person to somebody in practice? Absolutely not. Could you recommend her to a university service where she didn't have any clinical responsibilities and did research? Probably, but I'm even worried about that. Well, the bottom line, we thought, was that she put in all this time and can't change her career. We'll finish her and see if she won't develop a strong interest in research." (A26)

Are there liabilities roaming about out in the wider society, unsupervised physician who had been poor residents who are wreaking havoc in the medical community? The answer without a doubt is "yes." Our respondents had their own encounters with the liabilities:

"I'm operating on a patient next week who had an operation done by a neurosurgeon who missed the tumor, opened up the guy's head in the wrong place." (R39)

"Probably more like manslaughter...a certain surgeon was operating near the brain, but outside the cranium itself, resecting a tumor, and he got into the intracranial vault where there was a cerebral-spinal fluid leak and he did not call a neurosurgeon. He finished the case in his gallivant style. She did not wake up from the surgery and finally a neurosurgeon was called, but nothing could be done, and then we opened her head up and her brain was just very swollen, and she was brain dead at the time." (R43)

We are all familiar with the most extreme cases of malpractice in this nation because these cases draw the attention of the mass media. In the past few years we have been treated to a number of malpractice nightmares: a physician carving his initials into the belly of a woman (Wong 2000), and a fake doctor performing plastic surgery using animal anesthetics in Florida (Bragg 1999). But it is not the extreme case that interests us here (every profession will have its abhorrent members), but the average experience across the nation and across specialties. What is the risk for the average patient seeking care of encountering a poor performer? We cannot review all the literature on doctors in practice here, so we will review two articles that give some indication of how many liabilities are on the loose.

We have already discussed the challenges that reviewers face when judging physician performance since medicine is considered an art and not a science. Attempts to quantify and standardize performance measures are always challenged by the medical profession since the art of medicine is the application of general science to a unique individual. In one study (Schaffer et al 1988), the staff at an ambulatory center checked the credentials of physicians who were applying for ambulatory-staff privileges. When cross-checking references, they found that 5% (39 physicians) provided false information on their applications.

Twenty-seven of these 39 had falsely reported their residency training, and ten falsely reported being board-certified. That these physicians made these false reports is troubling indeed but does not directly measure their performance.

In another study (Norman at al 1993) conducted by The College of Physicians and Surgeons of Ontario, the authors did make some hard choices on how to measure physician performance. Between 1971 and 1982, 391 randomly selected practices were studied and analyzed on quality of care and patient records. The researchers concluded:

> "...if we follow a sample of 1000 physicians through the process, an initial peer assessment of randomly selected physicians will identify approximately 10%, or 100, as having possibly serious deficiencies. Of these, about half will be self-correctable, and after 6 months, the deficiencies will have been resolved without further intervention. Of the remaining 50, the PREP results imply that about 30% (11/37), or 15 out of 1000, have very serious problems that require mandatory education or removal from practice, and about 10% (5/37) or 5 out of 1000 physicians will require removal from practice." (ibid: 1051)

The average patient in Ontario, then, has about a 1 in 10 chance of encountering a physician with serious deficiencies. These are not very encouraging odds.

Attribution

Where does the fault lie when a resident leaves a program? We have tried to impress that attrition is the result of a dynamic interaction between the community and the individual, so in many cases, the failure lies in the mixture of these elements rather than in one or the other. We have also tried to show the amount of uncertainty involved in matching individuals and communities at many different points in the process. All this uncertainty will inevitable result in poor matches.

If you asked the community or the individual who withdraws where the fault lies, what answer will each group give? Attribution theory predicts that the failing resident and the program faculty will have different explanations for poor performance or lack of perseverance.

> "Attribution theory predicts that accounts of failure depend on who is queried. Presumably, the failing person tends to attribute the failure to situational factors beyond his or her own control while observers tend to attribute failure to dispositional weaknesses . . . people can attribute behaviors to relatively long lasting personality characteristics of individuals . . . or to relatively unusual environmental circumstances... Presumably, most of us are not completely unbiased when it comes to making these causal attributions; i.e., we make them in ways to maximize our self-concept." (Schroeder 1984:149-150)

Prior research on the problem of resident attrition conducted by medical educators has sought to locate the problem almost exclusively in the individual resident (Albo et al. 1976, Cruft 1982, King 1988, Lloyd (ed) 1982, Polk 1983, Veloski et al. 1979), providing a good example of attribution theory. Researchers have paid little attention to the possible effect the structure and organization of medical education, the selection process, and medical practice may have on residents' ability to complete training. Although speaking about physician impairment, Morrow (1985) notes that "[i]mpaired physician programs do not commonly prescribe treatment for the organization of medical work, i.e., do not attempt to alter workloads or otherwise ameliorate structural sources of stress in medical training and practice" (ibid:171). As we saw in Chapter 1, the environment of medical education is objectively difficult, but Morrow's observation suggests that medical educators will resist attempts to reform the structure of these residency training programs since this is not the place where they believe the problem lies.

In the next chapter, we will explore what has often been ignored in the attrition literature—the effects of program structure on attrition rates. We will take a concentrated look at one half of the dynamic process. We will ask, what characteristics of the structure and organization of the residency program are associated with higher and lower attrition rates?

III

The Effect of Program Structure on Resident Attrition

"I think a big part if the success of a residency program is the interaction of residents within and the structure that the programs have. Programs differ greatly in the way they treat residents." (R32)

The resident quoted above tells us that the success of a residency program rests on two things: the interaction of the residents and the structure of the program. In Chapter I, we reviewed many aspects of the culture of the surgical residency programs and the need for camaraderie among the residents. In this chapter, we will take a targeted look at the structure of residency programs to see what relationship there is between certain aspects of program structure and attrition rates. We are asking a similar question to the one posed by Jacobs (1994): how can environmental factors on the job be used to explain job satisfaction and career paths without invoking personality theory (ibid: 67)? While shifting the focus from the individual to the environment, we employ a different sort of personality analysis. Instead of looking at the personality of individual residents, we look at the personality of the program as a whole as it is manifested by its culture and organization. What kind of programs do we have in our sample? Small and intimate, large and impersonal? A "gentleman's" program (R20), an academic powerhouse, a place focussed on research, a place that is devoted to community service? We have a mix of different types of programs among our sample. We will try to decipher which particular mix of residents, which form of evaluation, and which forms of interaction are associated with higher or lower rates of attrition. Is it possible that some formula for successfully reducing attrition lies at the feet of the institution?

Prior Research

As we discussed at the end of the previous chapter, prior research on the problem of resident attrition both in surgical residency programs and other specialties has sought to locate the problem almost exclusively in the individual resident (Albo 1976: 115-121, Klineberg 1985, Leonard and Harris 1980: 57-59). Personal flaws such as lack of integrity or deficient motivation are often cited as the reasons for resignation or termination of residents (Cruft 1982, King 1988). Since the problem is understood as one of "flawed" individuals, proposed solutions have been focused at this level. There have been attempts to develop personality profiles which, when combined with national test scores and in-house exam results, identify both superior and inferior performers (Herman et al, 1983, Keck et al, 1979). There have also been repeated discussions of how to improve the selection process so that programs are assured of accepting only "the best" applicants (Clarke and Wigton 1984, King 1988, Komives et al, 1984, Langsley 1988, Lloyd and Langsley 1986). To date, this focus on the individual has yielded little in terms of more reliable screening or selection mechanisms or reduced attrition. There is a lot of evidence that the structure and organization of institutions is significantly associated with attrition. The size of the program, the amount of financial support given to students, the mix of the student population, all of these institutional characteristics have been shown to be associated with attrition (Bowen and Rudenstein 1992). The community is a key unit of study.

New Direction

The absence of progress yielded by a concentration on individual level variables and the recognition of attrition as a process involving both the individual and the community, suggests a reconceptualization of the problem of attrition is in order. Although a few researchers have suggested that individual program variables impact training outcomes (Bucher and Stelling 1977: 264), very few studies have questioned or systematically examined the effect variations in the structure and organization of a residency program have on a resident's ability to successfully complete program requirements (Anwar et al, 1981, Cousins 1981, Heimbach and Johnson 1986, Light, 1980: 318, Lloyd 1982). In this chapter, we will demonstrate that program structure and organization exert a significant influence on resignations and terminations from surgical training programs.

The data reported here are from Part One of our two-part survey on attrition sent in 1990 to the program directors of all certified programs in anesthesiology, general surgery, neurosurgery, orthopedic surgery and plastic surgery. Part One of the survey collected information about rates in our three outcome categories—

resignations, terminations, and problematic completers—as well as information about hospital characteristics, support systems, and general organization of each program. One hundred thirty-two (29.42%) of the 469 programs in our sample reported that they had experienced no problems during the five-year span covered by the survey—they had no resignations, no terminations, and no problematic completions. A breakdown of these programs by specialty is shown in Table 3.1.

A total of 245 (51.24%) of the programs experienced no resignations, 319 (66.74%) had no terminations, and 293 (61.68%) reported no problematic completers. Since so many programs took on the value of zero or "no problem(s)" for one or all categories of attrition and problematic completion, we used tobit analysis to test for relationships between rates of resignation, termination, and problematic completion and program characteristics (Tobin 1958: 24-36). The remaining observations followed the usual characteristics of a continuous normal variable. Because so many observations were truncated at zero, however, we could not use ordinary least squares regression analysis. Tobit analysis corrects for our inability to observe a problem rate less than zero. The resulting tobit coefficient estimates can be viewed as ordinary least squares regression coefficients corrected for the bias induced by the truncation of the dependent variable. Tobit employs maximum likelihood estimation under the assumption that the attrition and problematic completion rates are truncated normal variables.

Table 3.1. Programs Experiencing No Attrition

Specialty	Percent Reporting No Resignations, Terminations, or Problematic Completers
Anesthesiology	10.00% $_{(n=6)}$
General Surgery	23.45% $_{(n=34)}$
Neurosurgery	33.75% $_{(n=27)}$
Orthopedic Surgery	30.77% $_{(n=36)}$
Plastic Surgery	52.24% $_{(n=35)}$
Total	29.42% $_{(n=132)}$

Separate Categories

Are programs that experience one type of attrition more or less likely to experience other kinds of attrition? Our analysis indicates that the experience of one type of attrition does not necessarily increase other kinds of attrition. There were no strong correlations between the three target outcomes for all five specialties. Correlations are as follows: resignations and terminations, 0.1466; resignations and problematic completions, -0.0511; and terminations and problematic completions,

0.0910 (Table 3.2).

Table 3.2. Correlation of Problem Rates

	Resignations	Terminations	Problematic Completers
Resignations	1.0000		
Terminations	0.1466	1.0000	
Problematic Completers	-0.0511	-0.0910	1.0000

The absence of a stronger correlation between the three target outcomes suggests that each outcome should be discussed separately. In this way, we can assess the contribution of program structure and organization to each outcome category. The overall rate of attrition and problematic completion for the five-year period under study was 14.0%. The overall resignation rate was 6.6%; the termination rate, 3.0%; and the problematic completion rate, 4.5% (Table 3.3).

Table 3.3. Summary of Attrition Rates

Attrition	Number of Programs	Mean	Standard Deviation
Overall	469	0.1404	0.1459
Resignations	480	0.0657	0.0994
Terminations	480	0.0299	0.0592
Problematic Completers	475	0.0446	0.0773

We will first look at how our program characteristics are associated with the different problem categories and then discuss the various findings.

Resignations

Resignations were the most frequent cause of attrition from the programs surveyed. A gross resignation rate, however, overstates the number of residents who voluntarily withdraw from surgical training because it combines those residents who withdrew on their own initiative and those who were coerced into resigning by program directors unhappy with their performance.

Resignations initiated by program directors function as pre-emptive terminations. Using items from Part Two of Survey Two, it was determined that 20% of all resignations in the programs surveyed were made under duress. Treating resignations under duress as terminations rather than as resignations would reduce the overall resignation rate to 5.3% and elevate the termination rate to 4.3%. In the next chapter, we will see what distinguishes between these voluntary and involuntary resignations.

Table 3.4 . Descriptive statistics of sample

Variable	Mean	SD
Is program university affiliated?	0.71	0.46
How many beds in hospital?	826	975
Is program director a male? (1=male)	0.81	0.39
How many years has program director been in job?	8.71	7.19
How important is having information about the following traits, aptitudes and skills prior to admission? (1= not important, 5 = very important)		
Personality	4.33	0.75
Honesty	4.93	0.30
Maturity	4.45	0.65
Ability to handle stress	4.36	0.72
Cognitive knowledge	4.23	0.70
Manual dexterity	3.64	0.88
Clinical judgment	4.24	0.75
Staff relationships	4.29	0.69
Patient relationships	4.46	0.69
Information sent to resident about hospital, department or community prior to matriculation (0=no information, 5=extensive information)	2.24	0.94
Is assistance provided to new residents in the following forms: housing, childcare, education, community resources or spouse employment? (0=none, 5=assistance in all)	2.81	1.64
Are any of the following social activities organized by the department: coffee hours, lunches, dinners, journal clubs, staff parties? (0=no activities, 5=all of the activities)	2.83	1.20
Standard evaluation form used? (1=yes)	0.95	0.22
How often are evaluations conducted? (1=monthly, 2=quarterly, 3=bi-yearly, 4=yearly)	2.79	1.57
How many different categories of people are involved in evaluations: program director, attendings, chief residents, nurses) (4=all categories)	2.22	0.76
Are the following people involved?		
Program director	0.81	0.39
Attendings	0.98	0.11
Chief residents	0.36	0.48
Nurses	0.06	0.24
Do residents evaluate teaching? (1=yes)	0.74	0.44
Are merit raises given? (1=yes)	0.08	0.27
Is moonlighting allowed? (1=yes)	0.41	0.49
If moonlighting allowed, are there restrictions? (1=yes)	0.60	1.20

A variety of program characteristics were tested to see if they exerted any impact on the resignation rate. Table 3.4 describes the variables that appeared on Survey I. The full model, which incorporates the variables showing strong bivariate relationships and interaction terms that control for differing effects by specialty, is shown below. The probability of the full model chi2 is 0.0000. We can see from the full model above that the number of residents in a program effects the resignation rate for three of our specialties: neurosurgery, plastic surgery, and orthopedic surgery. In neurosurgery and orthopedic surgery, for each additional resident, the average resignation rate increases. For neurosurgical programs, that increase is on average by 1.47%, while for orthopedic programs, it is only by 0.3%, holding all other variables constant. Plastic surgery programs, on the other hand, experience an opposite effect. For each additional resident, the resignation rate decreases by 1.9%.

For each additional resident, the resignation rate decreases by 1.9%. The average number of residents in each of these three specialties was 7.58 for neurosurgery, 20.43 for orthopedic surgery, and 9.91 for plastic surgery. The corresponding standard deviations were 3.39, 11.23, and 3.93.

The full model suggests a number of other interesting relationships. There is a significant relationship between the number of social activities a residency program offers and its resignation rate. The more programs offered, the lower the resignation rate. In Survey I, we asked if the department formally organized any of the following social programs: coffee hours, resident lunches, resident dinners, journal clubs, and staff parties. Our variable, number of social activities, was able to take on a range of values from zero to five. The model estimates that for each additional social program offered, the average resignation rate decreases by a rate of 2.1% (p = 0.002), holding all other variables constant. The average number of social activities for the programs surveyed was 2.83 with a standard deviation of 1.20.

We also asked programs directors to rank the importance (1=unimportant, 5=very important) of having information about the resident on a variety of traits, attributes and social skills prior to matriculation. Traits asked about in Survey I included: personality, honesty and integrity, maturity, ability to handle stress, cognitive knowledge, manual dexterity, clinical judgment, staff relationships and patient relationships. Of these, only manual dexterity was shown to have a significant relationship with resignation rates. The higher program directors ranked the importance of having information on a resident's manual dexterity, the lower the average resignation rate (p > .003), holding all other variables constant.

The model also predicts that programs that award raises based on merit experience a higher resignation rate than similar programs that do not award raises on merit. It also predicts that programs that provide information about the hospital and community prior to admission to the program also experience higher average rates of resignation.

And finally, we note that the more people involved in the evaluation process, the higher the resignation rate. Program directors were asked to indicate who in the department was regularly involved in the evaluation process: program director, attending faculty, chief resident, and nurses. Our variable took on a range of values

Table 3.5: Tobit analysis of resignations rates and program structure

	Tobit coefficients
Number of residents in neurosurgery	0.0147**
	(0.0061)
Number of residents in plastic surgery	-0.0188****
	(0.0034)
Number of residents in orthopedic surgery	0.0032**
	(0.0014)
Number of social activities offered by program	-0.2104****
	(0.0069)
Importance of information on manual dexterity	-0.0290****
	(0.0095)
Use of merit raises	0.0606**
	(0.0299)
Number of different evaluators	0.0182*
	(0.0109)
Amount of information provided by hospital	0.0189**
	(0.0088)
Neurosurgery program	-0.1352**
	(0.0537)
Orthopedic surgery program	0.1249****
	(0.0369)
Prob > chi2(10)	0.0000
-LL	22.9347
Sample size	441

* $p < 0.10$; ** $p < 0.05$; *** $p < 0.01$; **** $p < 0.005$

from 0 to 4. We did not ask how many individuals within each category were involved, so our variable has to be interpreted as the number of *categories* of people involved rather than the actual number of people involved. Nevertheless, it results in a significant relationship at $p < 0.10$. The more categories of people involved, the higher the resignation rate. For each additional category, the rate increases on average by 1.8% ($p = 0.096$).

Finally, our full model includes dummy variables for neurosurgery and orthopedic programs that experience on average a lower overall resignation rate than general surgery, anesthesiology and plastic surgery programs combined, holding all other variables constant.

Other structural variables were also tested to assess their direct impact on the resignation rate. No significant difference was noted between university and non-university programs, nor between large and small organizations (measured by overall bed size). Also, there was no significant difference between programs headed by male and female program directors (19% of all programs were headed by a female program director). Although length of tenure of the program director did show a strong bivariate relationship with resignation rate, with each additional year of service decreasing the average resignation rate by 0.66%, this relationship lost its significance when other variables were added to the model. This finding suggests that tenure is an indirect measure of other organizational structures. There were no significant differences in the salary scales between programs and therefore no relationship between salary and the resignation rate.

Terminations

In absolute numbers, there are fewer terminations than resignations. However, since terminated residents have to be forced out of programs, this outcome is often more troublesome to program directors than resignations. Also, since residents who resign may be performing acceptably while residents who are terminated by definition are not, terminations raise larger concerns about attrition.

Here we look at the relationship between a program's organizational structure and its termination rate. The full model, reported below, suggests a number of interesting relationships between organizational structure and termination rates.

In this model, we find that the number of residents is a significant predictor for neurosurgery programs just as it was in the resignation model discussed above. This independent variable even has a similar magnitude and relationship: the more residents in the program, the higher the termination rate.

We also see that a different trait is identified in the termination model: honesty. The more important honesty is ranked by program directors as a screening device prior to admission, the lower the average termination rate, holding all other variables constant ($p < 0.002$).

Just as in our model for resignation rates, the structure of the evaluation process appears to effect programs' rates of termination. When attendings are involved in the process, the average termination rate is lower. Conversely, involving chief residents in the process appears to increase the termination rate in every specialty except orthopedic surgery, where the influence of the chief resident works to further reduce the termination rate.

Table 3.6: Tobit analysis of termination rates and program structure

	Tobit coefficients
Number of residents in neurosurgery	0.0125****
	(0.0033)
Importance of information on honesty	-0.0639****
	(0.02022)
Attending involved in evaluation	-0.1611****
	(0.0524)
Chief resident in involved in evaluation	0.0544****
	(0.0152)
Sharing information about hospital program, neurosurgery programs	-0.1789****
	(0.0385)
Prob > chi2(10)	0.0000
-LL	46.430869
Sample size	469

* $p < 0.10$; ** $p < 0.05$; *** $p < 0.01$; **** $p < 0.005$

And finally, we see a unique effect of sharing information about the hospital with residents prior to matriculation for neurosurgery programs. The neurosurgery programs that share information with their residents have an average termination rate that is 17.9% lower than programs that do not, holding all other variables constant. Nineteen percent of all neurosurgery programs reported not sharing information about the hospital prior to the start of the residents' tour through the department.

Problematic Completers

Problematic completers accounted for about five percent of the overall attrition rate. Two organizational variables were significantly associated with problematic completion. First, the greater stress placed by the program on assessing a resident's mastery of cognitive knowledge prior to admission, the higher the average problematic completion rate. In this model, we also see the reappearance of our evaluator variable: the more different types of people involved in evaluating a resident, the higher the average rate. The probability of the full model chi2 is 0.0193.

Table 3.7: Tobit analysis of problematic completion rates and program structure

	Tobit coefficients
Importance of information about cognitive knowledge	0.0125****
	(0.0033)
Number of evaluators	-0.0639****
	(0.02022)
Prob > chi2(10)	0.0193
-LL	92.050489
Sample size	470

* $p < 0.10$; ** $p < 0.05$; *** $p < 0.01$; **** $p < 0.005$

Discussion

These results demonstrate that certain elements of program structure and organization exert a powerful impact upon the rate of resignation from, termination from, and problematic completion in the residency programs we surveyed. In addition, our survey discovered that 29.42% of all the programs we surveyed experienced no resignations, terminations, or problematic completions during the five-year period under study. What are we to make of these results? What revisions, if any, in current policy and practice do these results suggest? We will address some of the major findings separately.

Size of Programs

In our model of resignation rates, we note that three of our variables are not easily subject to manipulation. These are the variables which control for the number of residents in a program interacted with three of our specialties: neurosurgery, orthopedic surgery and plastic surgery. In neurosurgery and orthopedic programs, bigger programs had larger resignation rates. This finding is upheld in studies of many different educational settings (Bowen and Rudenstein 1992)—in all programs, smaller programs have better completion rates. Unfortunately, most programs would resist reducing their current size in the name of reducing attrition. The larger programs are proud of their size and the patient loads they currently manage. That is the reason why this particular area of possible reform is not subject to much manipulation.

The reason why bigger programs may experience greater resignation rates, holding all other variables constant, is not hard to find. Larger programs are in a better position to absorb the "costs" of resignations than smaller ones where the burdens are spread across fewer individuals. The size effect exerts an influence both on the resident considering resignation and the program director counseling him or her. Residents in smaller programs may feel deeper camaraderie to other residents in the program and to the attending faculty (ibid: 235). Aware of what their resignation will mean to their peers and to patient care, they may find themselves much more hesitant to defect. They have to overcome stronger resistances than do their peers from larger programs. From the program director's perspective, those in smaller programs face larger logistical problems as a consequence of resignation than do those in larger programs. As a result, they may be more inclined to encourage residents to ride out difficult periods and may generally place more obstacles in the path of a resident who thinks about resigning. The longer a resignation is delayed, the greater the sunk cost in becoming a surgeon, the harder resignation becomes. In smaller programs, a little temporizing on the part of program directors may go a long way. Why, however, this effect appears limited to neurosurgery and orthopedic programs, and is actually reversed for plastic surgery programs, suggests that there is some interaction between program size and the nature of the work in these different programs. One influential factor is that plastic surgery residents have already completed a general surgery residency before beginning their plastic surgery tour. These residents already have many market opportunities available before started their specialized surgical training. Market availability very likely influences residents' decisions to stay or leave.

Social Activities and Support

The finding that the presence of social activities is associated with lower resignation rates does point to an important area of possible reform. Implementing coffee hours, resident lunches/dinners, or journal clubs in those departments that currently do not organize these functions, or increasing the quality and use of the programs already in place, may result in lower resignation rates. Our survey asked about the presence of these activities and not the frequency or quality of the function. We have little doubt, however, that better organized and more frequent functions would result in lower attrition. We would hypothesize that social functions would be most important in the first few weeks of the residency programs where they would function as assimilation programs. As Crandall (1978) and others have noted, assimilation programs reduce attrition since they act as introductions to a new environment (ibid: 331). Before informal social networks develop, formal social activities are important ways to help newcomers adapt to new environments and gain the information that they need to succeed in their new positions (Eaton and Beau: 639). Since as we noted earlier that women and minorities are excluded more often from informal networks in white-male dominated work settings, these formal assimilation programs would be even more important for reducing minority and female attrition.

Since there are historical and inherent obstacles to their easy assimilation, women and minorities need these programs to help develop a sense of belonging to the community while simultaneously giving the community a chance to formally welcome these residents (Cooke et al, 1995: 686). Formal networks can also facilitate the eventual formation of informal networks.

Not only do these social functions help residents to adapt to their new environments, they also function as "support structures." Social functions like those suggested above allow residents to "take a break" from the demands of their work. They also function as demonstrative signs of care and concern on the part of the program. Organizing meals, parties, and breaks contributes to the residents' sense that the program cares about their well being, and as some residents noted, these outward signs are often lacking:

> "There are all sorts of family services and social workers to help families deal with all the different types of problems. What we don't have here is someone to help the residents." (R33)

But perhaps most importantly, regularly organized social functions give residents an opportunity to air their doubts and concerns about meeting the challenges of their residency posts with others residents who undoubtedly have some of the same concerns. Everyone can "blow off steam" together over a cup of coffee, especially when out of earshot of attendings and program directors. Finding out that others share their anxieties and frustrations about the job may go a long way in keeping residents from resigning prematurely. Data from Survey II indicated that 58% of all resigners resigned in the first year, and that the majority of these residents were ranked as performing "above average" when they resigned. Program directors were understandably reluctant to see the above average performers go. There remain some, however, in medical education circles as well as in graduate education that believe that the point is to create a stressful environment because it is only in a stressful environment that you can "separate those who have emotional as well as intellectual toughness" (Hall 1998:124) to become great practitioners from those who do not. Convincing the hardcore medical educator that the residency program does not have to re-create "battlefield conditions" (Bosk 1979) in order to produce competent physicians poses challenges of its own.

Skills and Attributes

Another interesting result from our analyses above is that each of our three outcome models identified a different trait, attribute or skill as an important predictor of the outcome (resignation, termination, or problematic completion) that a program could expect to experience. For our model of resignation rates, manual dexterity

was significant. For termination rates, it was honesty. And for our model of problematic completers, it was cognitive knowledge. These traits and skills give us some
insight both on how residents fall into each category and how faculty categorizes the
"problem" residents in their programs. The more importance a program director
ranks manual dexterity, the more likely it appears that some residents in those programs will conclude that they cannot succeed in the chosen surgical specialty or in
that particular program and resign in order to pursue training in another specialty or
program. A greater focus on honesty and integrity, both as a screening device for
new recruits, and, we would argue, as a continuing evaluation device throughout a
resident's tour through certain departments, appears to lead to more frequent detec-
tions of "breaches" of honesty by faculty members and to subsequent termination
procedures. And finally, highly valuing a resident's store of cognitive knowledge in
a program appears on average to result in the identification of a greater number of
problematic completers. A program director's misgivings about a problematic completer's ability to practice without supervision, therefore, may be associated more
with his/her assessment of the resident's general fund of knowledge about the
proper identification and management of surgical problems than with the resident's
technical skill per se. These associations suggest that more focussed research on
how departments categorize their problem residents may yield more insights into the
process of attrition. We will explore these relationships in greater detail in our separate chapters on resignations, terminations and problematic completers.

Number and Type of Evaluators

Finally, we note that the form of the evaluation process exhibits a significant effect in each of our three models. For resignation and problematic completion rates,
we find that the more types of people involved in the evaluation process, the higher
the average rate of resignation and of problematic completion. This relationship
suggests that the more people involved in the process, each of whom may focus on a
different set of traits and attributes for evaluation, the harder it is for the residents to
please everyone. We discussed this phenomenon in some detail in Chapter 2. Residents are quite aware that the faculty can have very diverse views about residents:

"I also learned that different attendings have different perceptions of performance
and things like that, sort of very diverse, actually." (R26)

With more opinions involved, the more likely someone will identify a "problematic" component in the resident's performance. Getting negative feedback about
some aspect of performance from an evaluator may be an impetus for some resignations, even if the program director regards the resident as an "above average" performer. More opinions also appears to lead to the identification of a greater average
number of problematic completers among those fulfill all program requirements,

even if the "problems" are not deemed grave enough to warrant the resident's expulsion from the training program or prevent his or her graduation.

In our termination model, we find that the involvement of an attending(s) is associated with a smaller average rate. The "attending(s)" effect is quite substantial. The average termination rate for programs that involve an attending(s) is 16.1% lower than similar programs that do not. What can explain this relationship? The logic is similar to that employed in our discussion of resignations and terminations above. Although involving many different voices in the evaluation process may increase the likelihood that a problematic component will be identified, it simultaneously increases the likelihood that a resident will garner some faculty support. Termination is difficult to achieve without unanimity, since the absence of unanimity raises questions about fairness, so if the resident has impressed or befriended a faculty member or support personnel during his or her tour through the program, the harder it will be for the department to initiate termination procedures:

> "I think that when you are dealing with ten attendings, there is always one or two who don't feel as strongly, and feel that perhaps we should try to re-educate them." (R31)

> "There have been people who have been saved by their necks by the fact that some attendings have spoken up for them, by the fact that some nurses had the audacity to go to a doctor and say, 'I really think he is better than you think he is because...he has done exemplary things and he basically is an overall good person." (N14)

The involvement of a chief resident(s) increases the average termination rate except in orthopedic programs. We suspect that involving chief residents in evaluations increases the chance that instances of poor performance will not only be brought more regularly to the attention of the program director and/or faculty, but may also be more formally documented. The citing and documentation of poor performance by chief residents may facilitate termination procedures.

Attrition-Free Programs

The finding that close to 30% of all the programs that participated in this survey experienced no resignations, terminations, or problematic completions is intriguing. Some alternative explanations suggest themselves. These programs may either employ better procedures in selecting residents or more skillfully employ the same procedures than those programs that experience adverse outcomes. Alternatively, these programs may more laxly employ standards for evaluating residents. Ideally, however, these programs may be just very good at doing what other programs wish they could do—take a handful of young residents and successfully transform them into competent surgeons. A more detailed study of these programs would be needed to explore these various explanations. We suspect that we would need all of these alternative explanations to describe the programs that experience no attrition.

Despite the existence of attrition-free programs in our sample, we have shown that a considerable proportion of the rate of resignation, termination, and problematic completion is attributable to program organization and structure. The setting of the program is an important piece in the attrition puzzle, and one that has been sorely under-studied. We have suggested ways in which the program structure could be re-organized to reduce attrition. We have also shown how some attrition is the byproduct of the evaluation process rather than an objective measure of a resident's performance.

In the next chapter, we will begin a focussed discussion of our first attrition category, resignations. In Chapter IV, we explore in detail the interaction of program characteristics and resident characteristics as we describe the resignation process.

IV

Resignations

The voluntary leaver from a training program is different from the forced leaver. When we speak of "resignations," we most often think of individuals who decide for themselves that they do not want to stay with a particular occupational group or in a particular position. In many cases the person resigns because the work does not meet his or her expectations, does not bring happiness or fulfillment. The work environment may be less than ideal, stressful, unclean, dangerous, etc. The work itself may be unrewarding or unappreciated. Or the work demands may interfere with the enjoyment of other social roles. For example, the length of an average workday may make the roles of spouse and parent nearly impossible to fulfill. The individual may also decide that he or she does not have the right skills for the job and opt out. The person who resigns does not necessarily have another career option in mind, but he or she has decided to change directions.

As noted earlier, individuals also resign "under duress." Those who are asked to resign, or are for all intents and purposes, forced to resign, are much more like forced leavers than the voluntary and self-directed resigners. In many of these cases, the teachers or evaluators decide that the person-in-training does not have what it takes to complete the program before the individual has come to that same conclusion. In fact, the individual might never have come to that conclusion on his or her own. Instructors suggest and encourage the initiate to pursue another career. This scenario is different, however, from the individual who is forcibly terminated. In the case of the resignation under duress, the individual is offered a "graceful" exit. He or she is given an opportunity to leave under his or her own volition. This voluntary departure gives the appearance that the individual rejected the work, not that the community of professionals rejected him or her. The seed of the decision appears to lie within the person who resigned and makes him or her appear self-aware and self-directed. The fact that this opportunity is presented to the person who resigns under duress suggests a good personal relationship between teacher and student even if barriers to success remain. Twenty-two percent of the resignations in this survey were made under duress.

As noted earlier, the overall risk of resignation from a surgical residency program was approximately seven percent; that is, seven out of every 100 surgical residents resigned from their surgical training programs. This risk varies quite significantly based on the resident's race and gender. For white males, the overall risk is only about six percent. For white females, this figure rises to 16%. For non-white males, the risk stands at 19%, and for non-white females, we calculate the risk as almost 30%. Therefore, white females are 2.7 times more likely to resign than white males, while non-white males are 3.2 times more likely, and non-white females are about 5 times more likely. In this chapter we will look both at the typical resignation, and at the effects of race and gender on the resignation process.

Resignations: A Profile

The residents who resigned were on average self-directed, confident about employment options, and above-average performers. Fifty-eight percent were not married. The average medical school rank of these residents was 61 on a scale of one to 126. Only 12% had trained in international medical schools.

Seventy-one percent of these residents initiated talks about leaving their programs, most often citing the desire for a less stressful specialization as the reason for their dissatisfaction. Fifty-seven percent of the residents left their programs within the first year, with another 29% leaving by the end of the second year. Most of the residents who resigned (94%) discussed their plans to leave with the program director, but six percent were able to secure other residency positions without ever discussing their plans with the head of their program. Residents held on average only three discussions with program faculty before formally resigning, even though program faculty tried to convince about half of these residents to stay. At the time of resignation, the overall performance ranking of 75% of the residents was average or above average. Thirty-four percent were ranked above average, and the performance of 10% was outstanding. The most common reason for leaving the program was to seek a less stressful specialization (44%). The next most often cited reason was marital/family pressures (24%).

Only 54% of the residents sought help in securing a new position once they had decided to leave the program. Program directors were most likely to write letters of recommendation for those residents seeking help. After resigning, residents were most likely to enter a different specialty at another institution. This accounts for the movement of 35% of the residents who resigned. The next most popular move was to enter a different specialty at the same institution. This option was pursued by 19% of the residents.

The residents who resigned did very well in their next appointments. Their performance in their new settings was ranked as above average. Program directors were most likely to hear reports on the residents who moved into another specialty at the same institution.

Why Do Surgical Residents Resign?

Why do some residents decide that surgery is not the life for them, or that training in a particular program does not suit their needs? Part II of the survey asked program directors to note the reason the resident gave for resigning. The data from that response appear in Table 4.1 below. We report in responses accounting for over five percent of the residents:

Table 4.1: Reasons Residents Cited for Resigning

Reason	White Males	White Females	Non-white Males	Non-white Females	Total
Less Stress	46.49%** (139)	46.84%** (37)	32.43% (12)	22.22% (4)	44.34% (192)
Marital/Family Pressures	21.45% (62)	34.18%** (27)	24.32% (9)	29.41%** (5)	24.41% (103)
Faculty Advice: Incompetence	10.53% (30)	7.04% (5)	17.14% (6)	11.76% (2)	10.54% (43)
Belief Firing Imminent	10.03% (29)	5.63% (4)	16.67% (6)	11.76% (2)	9.93% (41)
Economic Pressures	7.32% (21)	5.48% (4)	5.56% (2)	5.88% (1)	6.78% (28)
Other	17.79% (53)	16.22% (12)	21.62% (8)	35.29% (6)	18.54% (79)

* $p < 0.10$, ** $p < 0.05$, *** $p < 0.01$, **** $p < 0.001$

Residents were most likely to cite "desire to seek a less stressful specialty" (44.34%) and "marital/family pressures" (24.41%) as a reason for resigning. Residents were able to cite more than one reason for leaving the program and typically cited 1.2 reasons, with no difference on the total number of reasons based on race and gender. Less than five percent cited any of the remaining reasons for resigning: faculty advice based on dissatisfaction (3.19%), chronic illness (2.46%), substance abuse (1.48%), self-perceived deficiencies in cognitive knowledge (1.47%), in manual dexterity (4.65%), and/or in clinical judgment (4.15%), occupational hazards (3.67%), or a desire to relocate (0.25%).

Desire For a Less Stressful Work Environment and Relationship to Support Programs

A desire for a less stressful work environment was a significant force motivating the greatest percentage of resignations. This result is not surprising given our earlier description of the culture of residency programs. There is unquestionably a lot of stress involved not only in the training schedule but also in the very nature of surgical work. Take the demands of the schedule coupled with a very sick patient base, it is not hard to imagine that a desire for a less stressful work environment would motivate many of the departures.

The desire for less stress links back with our earlier analysis of the relationship between the number of social supports a program has and the program's resignation rate. We found that for every social activity provided by the program, the overall resignation rate decreased by an average of two percent. We argue that the social activities provide not only a much-needed break from work pressures, but also a forum for residents to discuss their anxieties about performing under pressure. Too few programs provide enough activities that can potentially relieve some of the early stress. Some of these activities might be orientation programs, while others may just be for entertainment.

The timing of the resignations underscores the need for formal programs, early in the program, before residents establish informal networks. Most resignations occur quite early in the tour through the program. Residents start thinking about resigning quite early in the training period, with 20% of residents who eventually resign first talking about the possibility within the first six months. Twelve percent of these residents actually resign within that same time period. Another 39% resign by the end of the first year, so just over half of the resignations occurs within the first year. An additional 31% drop out by the end of the second year. There is not much of a honeymoon period. On average, resigners decide quite early that the work environment is too stressful. Unfortunately, they also seem to think that the only response to the stress is to leave the work environment. Those who resign adopt a flight response rather than try to seek support during the stressful first few months.

Table 4.2: When did the resident first talk about the possibility of resigning?

	Total
First six months	20.84%
Second six months	36.93%
Second year	28.70%
Third year	11.52%
Fourth year	1.65%
Fifth year	0.37%

Table 4.3: When did the resident formally resign?

	Total
First six months	12.34%
Second six months	39.38%
Second year	31.03%
Third year	13.43%
Fourth year	3.45%
Fifth year	0.36%

As noted in Table 4.1 above, whites were significantly more likely than non-whites to cite a desire for a less stressful work environment as the reason for resigning. This is because non-whites were significantly more likely than whites to resign under duress. In these cases, the residents wanted to stay in the training program, but were encouraged to leave by the program faculty. The following probit model shows the resident characteristics associated with citing a desire for a less stressful specialization. When our race variable was added to the model with the variable "under duress," our duress variable was insignificant:

Table 4.4. Probit analysis of citing a desire for a less stressful specialty/work environment

	Probit coefficients
Anesthesiology	-1.1032****
	(0.2013)
Ranking on patient relations	-0.3840**
	(0.1504)
Ranking on staff relations	0.4459***
	(0.1419)
Resigning under duress (1=under duress)	-0.5457****
	(0.1653)
Prob > chi2(10)	0.0000
-LL	250.81848
Sample size	402

* $p < 0.10$; ** $p < 0.05$; *** $p < 0.01$; **** $p < 0.005$

The model notes that anesthesiology residents were less likely than the residents in our other surgical fields to cite stress as a reason for resigning. Since many residents who resign because of stress actually enter anesthesiology, this finding supports our analysis that residents consider anesthesiology less stressful than surgery.

The next two variables measure the quality of the residents' interpersonal relationships with patients and with staff members. The first variable indicates that the better the relationship the resident has with his or her patients, the less likely the resident is to cite a desire for less stress as a reason for resigning. An opposite relationship exists for staff relations. The better the relationship with faculty and support staff, the greater the likelihood that the resident will cite this reason. The first of these two variables suggests residents who fail to establish good relationships with patients experience greater stress. On the flip side, the better the resident's relationship with program staff, the more likely he or she is to take his or her concerns to the faculty and seek a release from his or her unhappy situation.

As reflected in many of the interviews with neurosurgery residents, the quality of patient interactions has a profound impact on their experience of their programs. Surgical residents, and neurosurgery residents in particular, deal with some profound trauma. For neurosurgery residents, interaction with patients is often impossible since some of their patients are comatose or unable to communicate. Doctors in general derive some personal and professional satisfaction from appreciative patients—an acknowledgment of the doctors' efforts. One attending described this interaction in this way:

"I think that they, patients I enjoy, have an attitude of appreciation, though not a fawning attitude, but appreciate that there is someone who is trying as best they could." (A21)

Another resident (R36) said that he likes patients who are "grateful" and not "obnoxious." Residents compare these patients to patients who are, as one attending (A13) put it, "ungrateful wretches." It is hard to get this kind of "payment" from the incapacitated patient. Even those who are not incapacitated may still be quite uncomfortable after surgery, in great pain, or greatly fatigued— these conditions hamper the doctor/patient interaction. Also, in many of the large medical centers where these residency programs are found, residents see a lot of poor patients, including some who are homeless, drug addicts, unemployed, mentally deficient, or even sociopaths—people who residents describe as "the pits of society." The following descriptions of "bad" patients illustrate how these encounters exacerbate the stresses of the training program:

"The drunks that come in—I don't think you can be a human being and not be disgusted by those people." (R21)

"...drug abusers, with problems that aren't surgical, but were self-induced..." (A22)

Good patient relations can help relieve stress and bring joy to the resident's work, while poor and even abusive interactions can compound the stress.

The last variable in the model, "under duress," is a dummy variable that indicates the resident was asked to leave by the program faculty. Residents who were asked to resign were less likely to cite a desire for less stress as a reason for resigning.

Lack of Anticipatory Socialization

Some anticipatory socialization occurs before any individual joins an organization or training program. Many medical students have a fairly good idea about the culture of medical training from personal experience or from stories and myths encountered by the pre-med student (Merton 1957, Fox 1989, Hafferty 1991). Although medical students seem to have a good deal of lore under their belts, this appears less true for surgical residents. In their own writings, program directors bemoan the fact that many residents seem to have little to no idea about what they are getting into prior to the start of a residency program despite having done some clinical rotations in their third and fourth years of medical school. Students' exposure to the more esoteric specialties is either quite limited or nonexistent during medical school. This situation exists for three of the surgical specialties in this study. Few students get much exposure to surgical specialties and often make their choice to pursue training in these fields with little practical experience. What evidence do we have that demonstrates this lack of "anticipatory socialization?" The large percent of residents who resigned because of too much stress suggests both that the structure of the residency training programs lacked support programs, and that these residents did not anticipate how much stress was associated with the work. Although they originally thought they would enjoy anesthesiology or surgery, they found that the work did not make them happy. Here are some quotes which help illustrate this point:

"Decided that surgery was not right for him." (white male, general surgery)

"This was a case where the resident had made the decision to enter orthopedics too early, and he perceived it as wrong for him once he got started. He did not like to work long hours and disliked stress." (white male, orthopedic surgery)

"She had performed well, but decided that she did not want to be a surgeon." (white female, general surgery)

We also have a number of examples where the resident could not decide between specialties. His or her experiences in medical school did not help the resident settle on a particular career path. As indicated in Chapter II, program directors usually shy away from the indecisive resident precisely because they are afraid the resident will resign.

"Initially considered anesthesia, then chose general, then switched to anesthesia." (white male, general surgery)

"He told me he was not sure of his career choice and was deciding between anesthesia and psychiatry." (non-white male, anesthesiology)

And a rather extreme case of indecision:

> "He went into Radiology, but he again quit for uncertain reasons even though his performance was acceptable. He previously quit a Family Practice program. He's a 3X quitter!" (white male, general surgery)

In other cases, residents attribute their lack of happiness and enjoyment to a "personality mismatch." The resident does not possess the kind of rugged, decisive personality that we outline in Chapter I. Not fitting the mold, the resident resigns in order to pursue a better "fit" in another specialty setting. These cases represent mistaken anticipatory socialization. The resident underestimated his or her ability to fit the mold.

> "Specialty/personality mismatch." (non-white male, neurosurgery)

> "Personality mismatch with specialty. Began to get interested in Critical Care medicine. New employer agreed that resident had potential future in Critical Care. Resident eventually went into anesthesiology and completed training program." (white male, neurosurgery)

> "Poor personality match." (white male, neurosurgery)

And finally, we have two cases in which the socialization is so tenuous, and the work so unrewarding compared to other life pursuits, the residents left medicine altogether.

> "Wanted to leave medicine altogether. He became a professional golfer." (white male, general surgery)

> "Resident was a triathlete. He couldn't keep up with his training schedule as a surgery resident." (white male, general surgery)

Marital/Family Pressures:

Program directors cited marital/family pressures as the second most common reason for resigning. It will come as a surprise to few readers that women were significantly more likely to cite this reason than their male counterparts, although white female surgical residents were significantly less likely to be married than the male and non-white female surgical residents. We show the breakdown by married status in Table 4.5 below. Non-white females are most likely to be married and to be divorced. Equal percentages of non-white males are married and single, and white males are more likely to be single than married. Probit analysis revealed that white females ($p=0.009$) and non-white females ($p=0.000$) were significantly more likely to be divorced than either white or non-white males.

Table 4.5: Marital status of surgical residents by race and gender.

Race/Gender	Single	Married	Separated	Divorced	Widowed	Total
White Males	59.01 %	40.47%	0.26%	0.26%	0%	100% (n=383)
White Females	64.65%	29.29%	1.01%	4.04%	1.01%	100% (n=99)
Non-white Males	48.98%	48.98%	0%	2.04%	0%	100% (n=49)
Non-white Females	36.36%	50%	0%	13.64%	0%	100% (n=22)
Total	58.23%	39.60%	0.36%	1.63%	0.18%	100% (n=553)

Pearson chi2(12) = 41.2666 Pr = 0.000

The fact that being married carried a greater risk for resigning for marital/family pressures for women is demonstrated in the following probit equation. The dependent variable is a dummy variable for citing marital/family pressures as a reason for resigning. The independent variables are dummy variables for "married" and gender.

Table 4.6. Probit analysis of citing marital/family pressures as a reason for resigning

	Probit coefficients
Gender (1=male)	-0.4378***
	(0.1699)
Marital status (1=married)	0.6436****
	(0.1531)
Overall rank in program	0.3012****
	(0.0777)
Medical school rank	0.0048**
	(0.0021)
Prob > chi2(10)	0.0000
-LL	181.02139
Sample size	364

* $p < 0.10$; ** $p < 0.05$; *** $p < 0.01$; **** $p < 0.005$

We see from this output that both our variable for marital status and our variable for gender are significant. We therefore conclude that the likelihood of citing marital/family pressures is significantly greater for women than for men even after we control for marital status. So among the resigners, women, both married and single, faced a greater risk for resigning for marital/family pressures than their male colleagues.

Looking at some of the comments that were recorded on the reports about residents who resigned for marital/family reasons gives greater insight into the different challenges faced by men and women in these training programs. Both the men and the women in our survey who resigned for family/marital pressures faced problems that challenged their ability to continue training. Residents became pregnant, their spouses become pregnant, they dealt with medical problems, and faced troubles supporting a family on a resident's salary. There were some very real differences, however, in the way residents managed these challenges and in whether or not the program director thought the resolution was admirable or "non-remarkable."

For example, let us look at the descriptions of some white male residents dealing with the birth of their children during residency training:

"The resident married after he began his residency. When their first child was born, he realized that if he continued in surgery, he would not have time for his family. He opted to pursue a field that would not be so demanding." (white male, general surgery)

"The resident and his wife wanted a child. The wife had undergone extensive diagnostic studies. The resident felt that the demands of the orthopedic program were too great and he went into an anesthesiology residency." (white male, orthopedic surgery)

"His infant son was born with life-threatening medical problems. He reassessed his life priorities." (white male, orthopedic surgery)

"This was a case of extreme marital stress. His wife was institutionalized and he had two small children." (white male, neurosurgery)

There were also comments for two white male general surgery residents who had large families to support and who resigned in order to better support their families.

The comments made for the women who were also dealing with pregnancy and childbirth are less comprehensive, detailed, and sympathetic. In three cases, the program director reported simply that the women "resigned because of pregnancy." These statements appear without the same kinds of supporting text that appears for the male residents. For the males, we learn that they are conflicted, faced with a dilemma, reassessing their life priorities. For these women, we learn only that they are pregnant.

In a case of a non-white woman who had had a complicated pregnancy during her training, we hear: "She was a problem resident, very demanding, expected special care. I did not discourage her resignation. Her husband relocated. She had been in and out of our program with a complicated pregnancy. She took time off for childcare, avoided call, etc." The two adjectives that describe this woman in the first sentence are "problem" and "demanding." We do not find language that conveys sympathy for the woman's difficult situation.

Program directors tended to see pregnancy for women as "something simple." The experience of one white female neurosurgery resident is described in these terms: "She simply got married, got pregnant, and felt that she had to join her husband in Texas. She went into Neurology rather than Neurosurgery." Describing this woman's experience of all of these major life events—a marriage, a pregnancy, a transfer, and a career change—as a series of events that "simply" happened to her, ignores the tremendous impact all of these events had on her life. It refuses to acknowledge that a pregnancy, a marriage, a move, and a decision to resign may cause any of these women great personal turmoil. It would not be hard to believe that when these women reassessed their life priorities, the process was difficult and challenging.

The cases discussed above concern residents who resigned because of pregnancy and/or childcare, but we also have instances where resignations occurred because of the demands of a relationship or of a marriage alone. Of the nine cases where relationship pressures lead to the resignation, in only one instance did a man resign. In two other cases, one involving a non-white female, and the other, a white female, program directors simply noted a desire to get married. In the second of these, the program director helped the woman secure a new residency post in the city where her fiancé was located. In other cases, we have more information about the particular demands of the relationship:

> "Her reason for leaving—LOVE AFFAIR" [capitalization in the original] (white female, neurosurgery)

> "Her husband wanted her to resign. She left medicine altogether and became a housewife. She may have gone back into training into a low-key specialty later. The resident was married to a pediatric resident. He would have completed his training a few years before her. This subject was breached during the initial interview. Candidate felt that her husband would be busy with fellowships or other activities in training." (white female, neurosurgery)

> "She married a fellow resident. She felt the demands were excessive. Resigned after eight months—non-remarkable." (white female, anesthesiology)

> "Resident told no one about resigning. She resigned to take care of her new husband." (white female, anesthesiology)

And finally, our one male representative:

> "His explanation for leaving was to marry a woman with two children living in a distant city who wished to stay there [in the distant city]. Although he did not say it, I suspect he was disillusioned about surgery and returned to a field he had already tried." (white male, general surgery)

Note that in the one case where a man was cited as willing to relocate for his fiancée, rather than having the woman move for her husband, his stated intentions were questioned. According to this program director, the true reason for his resignation could not have been his desire to relocate, but rather his disillusionment with surgery.

All of these quotes taken together reflect certain stereotypes about women in the workplace. They seem to support the idea that a woman should relocate for her husband even if this means that a "higher" status, higher paid woman (i.e. our neurosurgery resident above) should relocate for her husband (the pediatrician) who has less status and less pay. It also supports the idea that pregnancy and childbirth are things that happen to women who take this particular life event in stride, not a decision women make with the knowledge that it will impact their life choices. It would be interesting to know whether any of these women mourned the loss of their residency post when they resigned. The comments provided by the program directors suggest not. The absence of richer descriptions of the women's thoughts and feelings surrounding their choice to leave the program—some sense of the conflicts, or a better appreciation of the external demands on their time and energy—suggests that the quality of the interpersonal relationships between these women and the program director was not as good as the same relationship between the program director and the men who resigned. We see this theme played out throughout this study.

These observations do point to a chicken-and-egg dilemma. We could argue that the program directors, knowing that married women are more likely to leave the program because of pregnancy or other family pressures, are less likely to develop closer relationships with them.They may be reluctant to invest many resources, personal or otherwise, in someone who is more likely to leave. However, if these same program directors go into their relationships with these preconceived notions, the process is unlikely to change. Medical educators must consider some creative solutions to this circular problem.

Resignations Under Duress

Forced resignations call into question our usual definition of a resignation as a voluntary act. A resignation under duress occurs when the faculty encourages the initiate to leave the training program. The faculty decides before the student may fully agree that he or she just does not have the proper skills, talents, or character to complete the training program.

By giving the resident a chance to resign before termination proceedings begin, the program faculty gives him or her an opportunity to reject the program rather than be rejected by the program. This ability to "save face," to appear to have initiated this decision, is an important gift for the resident. In his or her subsequent job searches, he or she will appear less like some other program's reject and more like a self-directed person in pursuit of job fulfillment.

> "She was in the middle of a divorce. I didn't want to terminate her because to dismiss her would have been bad for her records. I was happy that she decided that she would resign. In the end, we did the right thing. She got divorced, she looks great, and has put her life together in an excellent ortho program." (white female, orthopedic surgery)

And from the records of a white male orthopedic resident:

> "Resignation allowed him to continue his training in a fresh environment in which he was able to get a new start."

Offering this opportunity not only provides a service for the individual resident/student, but it also saves the program faculty from a costly and arduous termination procedure. We hypothesize that the individual who receives and accepts this offer will on average have a better working and interpersonal relationship with the faculty than individuals receive and reject the offer and are eventually terminated[1].

Using information from Survey II, we noted that 22% of all resignations were made under duress. We consider a resignation "under duress" if the program director cited one of the following reasons for the resignation: (1) resident was told he or she would be fired if he or she did not resign, or (2) program director asked for the resignation.[2] We see from the following table that non-whites were significantly more likely to resign under duress than their white counterparts.

Table 4.7. Resignations Under Duress

Under Duress	White Males	White Females	Non-white Males	Non-white Females	Total
no	80.26%	83.33%	53.06%	72.22%	78.08% (n=424)
yes	19.74%	16.67%	46.94%	27.78%	21.92% (n=119)
Total	100% (n=380)	100% (n=96)	100% (n=49)	100% (n=18)	100% (n=543)

Pearson chi2(3) = 20.8907 Pr = 0.000

Note that about 47% of the non-white males who resigned resigned under duress, and about 28% of non-white females also fell into this category.

Non-whites in this sample came from lower ranked medical schools and a greater proportion of them came from international medical schools. We used the Gorman ranking scheme to rank all the medical schools in our sample. The lower the number, the higher the ranking of the school. All foreign medical schools were ranked in our data set as "126," one lower than the lowest ranked American medical school. Although we do not deny that the quality of the foreign medical schools varies considerably more than is suggested by this blanket ranking, for lack of better information, we relied on this coding. The following

---

[1] We cannot identify among the pool of terminated residents those who were given an opportunity to resign but rejected the offer and were eventually terminated, so we cannot test this hypothesis at this time.
[2] Note in Table 1 that the next most often cited reasons for resigning after "desire for less stressful environment" and "marital/family pressures" are "faculty advice based on incompetence" (10.54%) and "belief firing imminent" (9.93%).

tables show the average ranking of medical schools by race and gender and the
percent of residents in each category that attended a foreign medical school.

Table 4.8: Average Medical School Rank

Race/gender	Average Rank	SD
White Males	57.89	36.30
White Females	59.10	37.84
Non-white Males	68.94	47.28
Non-white Females	90.54	48.42

Non-whites in this sample came from significantly lower ranked medical
schools than their white counterparts.

Table 4.9. Is resident an international medical graduate?

Race/gender	Percent from International Medical Schools
White Males	8.27%
White Females	6.06%
Non-white Males	28.30%
Non-white Females	59.09%
Total	11.76%

Pearson chi2(3) = 69.0905   Pr = 0.000

These data suggest that on average non-whites came to these surgical residency programs with a weaker educational background than the white residents.
Medical educators typically think of residents from international programs as
having a poorer knowledge base. As noted on one non-white male general surgery resident's survey:

> "Resident came from a Mexican school and clearly had deficiencies in medical
> knowledge."

And recorded for an Asian-American male orthopedic resident:

> "Several decisions in 'on-call' status indicated a deficit in fund of knowledge.
> Resident probably sensed that dismissal was a consideration and resigned.
> Resident was an excellent person who fell far behind the academic standards of
> the program."

The lack of a good cognitive knowledge foundation greatly hampers performance in a residency program. Unfortunately, program directors cannot amend
this shortcoming in the current context of medical training. There are too many
demands both of faculty time and on the residents' time for years of basic
knowledge to be "caught up." Surprisingly, however, neither medical school
rank nor attendance at an international medical school is significant when
plugged into the following probit equation that predicts the likelihood of being
forced to resign among the pool of resignations. The absence of these variables
suggests that on average, attendance at lower-ranked medical schools and at

foreign medical schools does not have a direct effect on the likelihood of resigning under duress.

Although we do not see a school effect, we do see some other effects in the probit model in Table 4.10. The first variable indicates that non-whites were significantly more likely than whites to be asked to resign. We also note that residents who were ranked higher than their peers on clinical judgment were less likely to resign under duress. When other individual characteristics, traits, and aptitudes were added to the model along with race, clinical judgment, and resident's apparent dissatisfaction, there were no significant effects. The other variables tested were the residents' ranking on personality, honesty, maturity, ability to manage stress, cognitive knowledge, manual dexterity, staff relationships, and patient relationships. Therefore, forced resigners differ from voluntary resigners only on their ranking on clinical judgment when we control for these other factors.

Table 4.10. Probit analysis of resigning under duress

	Probit coefficients
White (1=white)	-0.6171****
	(0.2199)
Ranking on clinical judgment	-0.5274 ****
	(0.0808)
Perceived dissatisfaction	0.8055 **
	(0.3879)
Prob > chi2(10)	0.0000
-LL	169.03803
Sample size	373

* $p < 0.10$; ** $p < 0.05$; *** $p < 0.01$; **** $p < 0.005$

Program directors were more likely to ask residents to resign if they thought that the resident was incompetent ($p=0.000$), though program directors rarely specified in what respect the resident was incompetent. In about half the cases, program directors ranked incompetent residents as "below average" in matters of clinical judgment. Cross-referencing with the other traits and variables cited above yielded no significant relationships.

This model also indicates that faculty asked "dissatisfied" residents to resign. We could not decipher from the surveys how dissatisfaction was defined and demonstrated. In one case, the program director specified only that the white male general surgery resident had a "lack of interest." Can we assume that the program directors' assessments were accurate in these cases since the residents did resign? Without the resident's voice represented, it is hard to say.

All of these results raise some questions, especially since the race effect remains significant even after controlling for these other factors. What are program faculty measuring when they evaluate clinical judgment? Faculty members within the same institution do not always agree about a course of action, even when presented with the same case. So to what extent was the poor evaluation of clinical judgment in these cases a matter of a faculty members' idiosyncratic taste for doing things in a particular way, and to what extent is it an accurate measure of the resident's competency? In some way, this hard-to-quantify attribute, clinical judgment, may reveal more about the program faculty's general unease about a resident's performance than dissatisfaction with a particular aspect of his or her work. If this is true, then program faculty must work harder to articulate what they seem to have some trouble articulating. This would help make sure that judgments are fair.

The fact that race remains a robust predictor even when we test other traits, aptitudes and characteristics in the model suggests that there is bias involved when asking residents to resign. Non-whites are asked to leave in greater proportions even though it is hard to decipher from this data the substantive ways in which these residents differ from the voluntary resigners. A preconception that the non-white will perform below par may affect the evaluation process. Program directors may believe that a resignation under duress is better than termination for residents of color, but this explanation also fails to identify the way these residents failed as compared to the voluntary resigners.

Unfortunately, the comments that accompanied this subsample of residents who resigned under duress do not give much insight into these lingering questions. Here are some of the comments:

> For a non-white male, general surgery resident, we learn that he displayed "emotional instability" which is never classified or defined.

> In another case involving a white male, plastic surgery resident, we learn only that there was a "rumor that he had cheated in his exams."

> Another white male, general surgery resident had a "personality disorder."

For two other cases, the reason the faculty requested the resident's resignation is much more clear. One white male plastic surgery resident had falsified physical examinations and quit before the termination proceedings began. A non-white male neurosurgery resident left the hospital without notification. This act was deemed so reprehensible by that particular program's faculty that the resident was immediately given the option of either resigning or being terminated. The resident chose to resign. In two out of seven examples, however, we do have a clear picture of the resident's behavior (see also, Bosk 1979). The lingering vague uneasiness needs to be better expressed.

The Physical Bar

Although a relatively small percent of residents left their programs because they could not meet the physical demands of the work, we want to take a closer look at this phenomenon since it illustrates our earlier themes of anticipatory socialization and the arduousness of the residency program. It also demonstrates the different physical challenges faced by the medical student as compared to the medical resident, and the different physical demands associated with different medical specialties.

All tolled in our sample, resignations for "physical" reasons account for only about nine percent of the resignations. Physical constraints include chronic illness, substance abuse, and problems with manual dexterity. We are not including pregnancy in this section since we discussed it in our analysis of marital/family pressures. Its absence does not indicate that we do not consider pregnancy and childbirth a physical challenge, only that we are considering more enduring physical impairments or conditions in this section.

The same physical problems that precipitated the resignation did not deter some residents from pursuing surgical training in the first place.

"Suffered from narcolepsy." (white male, general surgery)

"Resident had a tremor in one hand. He switched to radiology." (white male, general surgery)

"This resident had a real problem with manual dexterity due to a visual defect." (non-white male, general surgery)

These conditions apparently existed before the resident began training. These conditions would surely be handicaps for the surgeon. At one level, it is reassuring to know that these residents decided to pursue another medical career.

Other conditions became apparent after training began:

"Poor eye-hand coordination. Resident would drill 2 cortexes of bone, place a screw, and be unable to get screw in far side of bone 85% of the time." (white male, orthopedic surgery)

"Resident suffered from a back condition and this condition influenced his training to some extent. It was the Chairman's feeling that his condition would make his training in anesthesiology a very difficult one and advised resident to re-evaluate his career choice." (white male, anesthesiology)

We should note that these residents apparently did not have enough exposure to the demands of their chosen specialties during medical school to adequately assess their physical ability to do the job. We also raise the question of whether these residents received adequate advising in medical school. This lack of exposure speaks to the frustration of many program directors that residents come ill prepared for the work. The physical demands placed on medical students, even the medical student in clinical rotations, often do not adequately mirror the physical demands placed on residents.

In two other cases, program directors reported that the residents had "personal health problems." We do not have information on the nature of those health problems so we do not know whether their health problems were related to the schedule and pressure of the residency training program. In another case we know that the resident's health problems were associated with his obesity.

Another case involving a 51 year-old woman reminds us again of the physically arduous nature of these training programs. The young physician-in-training tolerates many conditions that the older physician finds hard or even unbearable—sleeplessness, general fatigue, poor eating habits, lack of exercise—pressures tolerated more easily by the young body than the old.

> "Resident felt that she had made an error in trying to switch from psychiatry at age 51 and pursue anesthesiology. She did not have the stamina for the work and study involved. We doubted her having the stamina for the residency, but she insisted and had a distinguished career as a teacher." (white female, anesthesiology)

We also have six cases of residents who resigned because of substance abuse. As cited earlier, physicians as an occupational group are more prone to drug and alcohol abuse than the general population and mental health researchers attribute this finding to the stresses and strains associated with medical work. The physical effects of drug dependency are extraordinarily debilitating. The drug-addicted resident, who has already invested so much time, energy, and finances in a medical career, now finds himself or herself addicted to the medicines over which he or she sought mastery.

> "Resident was recognized as a drug abuser. He was referred to a treatment center and subsequently returned under a contract for monitoring. After one month, he voluntarily resigned." (white male, anesthesiology)

> "Substance abuse—received therapy, but never returned." (white male, anesthesiology)

Even other medical professionals could not help these residents overcome their drug dependency.

Of the six residents who resigned because of drug abuse, one switched to another program, two pursued no additional training, one left medicine altogether, and the last two fell through the cracks. Program directors had no additional information about these residents once they left their programs. We will pick up this discussion on the fate of drug abusers again in our chapters on the terminated residents and the problematic completers.

The fact that residents with pre-existing physical problems still attempted to pursue training in a surgical field can be understood as a reflection of the culture of medical education, from undergraduate pre-med programs through medical school. These individuals have been pushing the envelope, working against all odds for years, denying their own physical limitations in order to succeed as an undergraduate, succeed as a medical student, and succeed as a resident. Physicians lead lives that they would never prescribe for their own patients. They deny their own needs for sleep, exercise, food and rest in some sense as a challenge to the very diseases and malfunctions that they spend their lives trying to cure. Physicians' self-sacrifice and denial exemplifies the tenacity of the human spirit, but also take their toll. The toll the self-sacrificing, boundary pushing physician pays is dramatically portrayed by the fate of the young drug-abuser.

Now that we have covered some of the reasons residents resign, we will look at the process. What steps are taken by the resident who wants to or is asked to resign? How do these residents compare with the residents who stay in the program? And how does the resident's race and gender impact this process?

"I'm Thinking About Resigning"

Communication between faculty and residents can be formal or informal. Discussions about plans and performance can occur during rounds or in a formal review session. We tried to assess how information was usually transferred between attendings and their underlings. Some of our questions specifically addressed this issue while other inferences were made from comments that appeared on the survey and from interviews. In this section we will specifically address the question: with whom did the resident speak about his or her plans to resign?

Table 4.11. With Whom Did the Resident Discuss His or Her Plans to Resign?

Program Director	93.49%
Attending	41.44%
Chief Resident	13.40%
Notified Program in Writing	13.64%

The majority of resignations take a formal path. As this table shows, residents were significantly more likely to talk with the program director than with any of the other program staff (p=0.000). We can understand this finding in the context of the hierarchical organization of the program and the timing of the decision. Recall that residents decide to resign fairly early on, perhaps before they have established good working relationships with attendings or with chief residents. Therefore, the more formal route of interaction is probably the more obvious one taken.

Residents have an average of only 3.5 discussions with the program director, attending or chief resident before they finalize their plans. The paucity of discussions suggests that for the most part, these residents were fairly determined to leave the program. Their decisions were probably fairly firm before they even approached the program director. This description certainly applies more to the voluntary resigner than the resident who resigned under duress who had an average of 4.4 discussions with his or her program faculty before resigning—a significant difference (p=0.003).

No race or gender category was more likely to speak with any of the program faculty over any other program faculty. For example, white males were not more likely than white females to speak directly with the program director.

Program Director's Response

We asked the program directors the following question: When the resident first informed you that he or she was thinking about resigning, what was your response? Table 4.12 shows the results. We note from this table that non-whites are more likely to be asked to leave by the program director when the conversation about possible resignation takes place. The full model, which predicts the likelihood of being encouraged to leave by the program director, follows Table 4.12.

Table 4.12. Program Director's Response to Resident's Intent to Resign

Race/Gender	Encouraged to leave	Encouraged to stay	Suggested a leave of absence
White males	45.53% (n=117)	51.36% (n=132)	3.11% (n=8)
White females	48.48% (n=32)	46.97% (n=31)	4.55% (n=3)
Non-white males	75.00% (n=27)	22.22% (n=8)	2.78% (n=1)
Non-white females	60.00% (n=6)	40.00% (n=4)	0% (n=0)
Total	49.32% (n=182)	47.43% (n=175)	3.25% (n=12)

As Table 4.12 above demonstrates, about 50% of the residents who either express an interest in resigning or have been asked to resign are encouraged to leave by the program director. The first relationship demonstrated in the model is between specialty and the likelihood of being encouraged to leave. Residents in anesthesiology are less likely to be encouraged to leave than residents in the other specialties covered by this survey. We also note that our race variable appears again. Whites are less likely than non-whites to be encouraged to leave. Also note that the higher a resident was ranked on his or her manual dexterity, the less likely was the program director to encourage the resident to leave. This model also suggests that if the resident cited a desire for a less stressful work environment or family marital pressures as a reason for resigning, the program director was less likely to encourage the resident to leave. And finally, if the reason the resident cited for his or her resignation was a belief that firing was imminent, the program director was more likely to encourage the resident to leave.

Table 4.13. Probit analysis of being encouraged to leave

	Probit coefficients
Anesthesiology	-0.5136 **
	(0.2233)
White (1=white)	-0.5867 **
	(0.2934)
Ranking on manual dexterity	-0.3739 ****
	(0.1054)
Desire for less stressful specialty/environment	-0.3916 **
	(0.1773)
Marital/family pressures	-0.7857 ****
	(0.2116)
Belief firing was imminent	0.9107 ***
	(0.3387)
Prob > chi2(10)	0.0000
-LL	154.45068
Sample size	268

* $p < 0.10$; ** $p < 0.05$; *** $p < 0.01$; **** $p < 0.005$

The probit model is informative not only because of the variables that appear, but because of the absence of other variables we predicted would have affected the likelihood. For example, when we added the variable that distinguishes between resignations made under duress and those that were voluntary, the variable "duress" was insignificant. We also note the absence of any ranking variable other than manual dexterity. When added to the model, the residents' overall ranking was not significant, nor was these residents' ranking on any other trait, aptitude or characteristic other than manual dexterity. We again have an unfortunate race effect that remains significant even when we control for particular shortcomings in other definable aspects of performance.

Although program directors are less likely to encourage those residents who wish to seek less stressful work environments or who are overwhelmed by marital or family pressures to resign, they are unlikely to suggest either a leave of absence or some modification in the program as a way to address these residents' problems.

Now we look at the factors associated with being encouraged to stay. If we flip the analysis on its head, we find that many of the variables that were associated with the likelihood of being asked to leave are also associated with being asked to stay. We do, however, note a few differences. In our model predicting the likelihood of being asked to stay we find that "belief firing imminent" drops out and two new variables are added: the specialty neurosurgery and the resident's overall ranking compared to his or her peers.

Table 4.14. Probit analysis of being encouraged to stay

	Probit coefficients
Anesthesiology	0.8053 ****
	(0.2242)
Neurosurgery	0.6809 **
	(0.2944)
White (1=white)	0.8578****
	(0.3018)
Desire for less stressful specialty/environment	0.4770 ***
	(0.1767)
Marital/family pressures	0.8002 ****
	(0.2055)
Overall ranking in program	0.4581 ****
	(0.0901)
Prob > chi2(10)	0.0000
-LL	155.32267
Sample size	281

$* p < 0.10; ** p < 0.05; *** p < 0.01; **** p < 0.005$

Program directors in neurosurgical residency programs are more likely to encourage their potential resigners to stay. Note that in the previous chapter we found a relationship between program size and a reduction in attrition. The neurosurgery effect we find here may be an indirect measure of program size. It may also be true that program directors in neurosurgery, acutely aware of the particular stresses associated with neurosurgical work, are more likely to encourage their potential resigners to ride out the initial as well as subsequent periods of stress. The following quote from a neurosurgical resident sums this sentiment up nicely:

> "There are times you say to yourself, 'What am I doing this for? I'm getting out of this. Does it make sense?' I remember my chief saying, 'If you don't think about quitting once a week, something is wrong. It happens to all of us.' But you move on and the next day you are a little more sane." (R18)

In this analysis, we find that a resident's overall ranking as compared to his or her peers rather than the identification of a particular trait or characteristic is associated with being asked to stay. Unfortunately, however, even when we control for overall ranking, our race variable remains significant. Being non-white significantly decreases one's chance of being asked to stay.

Ranking in the Program

In two cases above, we noted an absence of a stronger association between a resident's ranking on a variety of traits, aptitudes and characteristics and his or her risk of resigning under duress and of being encouraged to leave once plans to resign were announced. The race effect remained significant even when ranking measures were added to our models. Recall that for resignations made under duress, residents' ranking on clinical judgment was negatively associated with the risk of this event. Recall also that the only aptitude that was associated with a resident being encouraged to leave the program was manual dexterity. Again we noted a negative association. The higher the resident was ranked on this trait, the less likely his or her risk of being asked to leave. The race effect, however, remained significant in this model even when manual dexterity was included. What do we make of these results? In this section, we will take a closer look at how the residents who resigned compared on a variety of traits and characteristics based on their race and gender. [3]

Resigners as a group were performing slightly above average as compared to their peers at the time of their resignation. This helps explain why program directors actually encouraged about 47% of these residents to stay. The table above indicates that non-white males were ranked significantly lower than their white colleagues and lower than the non-white female residents on three traits, aptitudes and characteristics. Specifically, the non-white males were ranked lower on manual dexterity, clinical judgment, and patient relationships. Non-white males and non-white females both were ranked lower than their white colleagues on ability to handle stress and on cognitive knowledge.

Recall that residents who were asked to resign ranked lower on clinical judgment. But even when we controlled for clinical judgment in our model predicting forced resignations, our race effect was still significant. This finding suggests that the relationship between race and clinical judgment in this table does not adequately explain the relationship between race and resignations under duress that we discussed above. Likewise, residents who were encouraged to leave were ranked lower on manual dexterity, and we find that non-white males are ranked lower than the other race and gender categories on this aptitude. Again, however, both race and ranking on manual dexterity were significant in our model predicting likelihood of being asked to leave, so this relationship does not sufficiently explain the trend. Both non-white males and non-white females were ranked significantly lower than their white colleagues were on their ability

---

[3] In the original survey, program directors were asked to rank the resident in relation to his or her peers on the traits, aptitudes and characteristic included in the table above. Respondents used the following scale to rank the residents: 1=unaccpetable, 2=below average, 3=average, 4=above average, and 5=outstanding.

to handle stress. This result raises the obvious question: how do program directors assess residents' ability to handle stress? We would hypothesize that different race and gender groups have different ways of dealing with and expressing stress.

Table 4.15. Ranking of Aptitudes, Traits and Characteristics by Race and Gender: Averages and Standard Deviations

	White Males (n=361)	White Females (n=91)	Non-white Males (n=47)	Non-white Females (n=17)
Personality	3.5764	3.7065	3.4167	3.7059
	(0.9203)	(0.8961)	(0.8208)	(0.9852)
Honesty	3.8284	3.8587	3.6667	3.8333
	(0.9290)	(1.0001)	(0.9964)	(0.9235)
Maturity	3.3646	3.4673	3.2292	3.3889
	(1.0427)	(1.0425)	(0.9507)	(1.0922)
Ability to Handle Stress	3.2568	3.2088	2.7708***	2.8333*
	(0.9858)	(1.0803)	(0.9280)	(1.1504)
Cognitive Knowledge	3.5121	3.5761	2.9792****	2.7778****
	(0.9605)	(1.0080)	(1.0415)	(1.0033)
Manual Dexterity	3.3548	3.4130	3.0213***	3.1667
	(0.8612)	(0.8467)	(0.8467)	(0.7859)
Clinical Judgment	3.3666	3.4348	2.8333****	3.0556
	(0.9475)	(0.9642)	(1.0383)	(0.8726)
Staff Relationships	3.5296	3.5652	3.2917	3.5000
	(1.0156)	(0.9978)	(0.8495)	(0.9235)
Patient Relationships	3.6450	3.7391	3.3333**	3.7222
	(0.9066)	(0.9593)	(0.9302)	(0.8264)
Total	3.5115	3.5531	3.1843	3.3464
	(0.7761)	(0.7557)	(0.7002)	(0.8406)

* $p < 0.10$, ** $p < 0.05$, *** $p < 0.01$, **** $p < 0.001$

We can recall Zborowski's (1969) classic study on the expression of pain (surely a source of stress) in a hospital setting. He found that social factors impacted on people's experience and expression of pain. While the Jewish and Italian patients that he studied openly and emotionally expressed their experience of pain and discomfort, the "Old American" (white, native-born, Protestants) patients did not publicly cry out but rather bore their discomfort stoically. So, too, we might suspect that white residents and non-white residents possess different means of coping with and expressing the stress of residency training. The model of effective coping within the medical training culture mimics that of the Protestant patient—a stoic, detached management. Residents who raise their voices in protest or who break down and cry are considered by program faculty to be "not handling the situation well." Program faculty do not entertain the possibility that a "good cry" might be just the thing to release stress and enable the resident to get back to work. Although we do not have enough descriptive data to test our prediction that there are differences in the way non-whites and whites manage or express stress, we do know that crying episodes, outbursts of any kind among junior staff, and any behavior that smacks of being "all emotional" are correlated with being ranked low on ability to handle stress. Among the resigners, these behaviors are not necessarily associated with poor patient care but rather suggest to the program faculty that the resident is having trouble handling the workload.

We also note that non-whites ranked significantly lower than whites in cognitive knowledge. We wanted to test to see if non-white residents' ranking on cognitive knowledge was associated with their coming from lower ranked medical schools to start, or if the effect remained even after controlling for rank of medical school. To test this effect, we ran an ordered probit predicting the residents' ranking on cognitive knowledge controlling for both race and medical school rank.

Table 4.16. Ordered Probit: predicting score on cognitive knowledge controlling for race and medical school rank

	Probit coefficients
Rank of medical school	-0.0046 ****
	(0.0012)
White (1 = white)	0.6277 ****
	(0.1448)
Prob > chi2(10)	0.0000
-LL	683.34673
Sample size	504

* p < 0.10; ** p < 0.05; *** p < 0.01; **** p < 0.005

The possible values for medical school rank ranged from "1" (top school) to "126" (international medical school). This model suggests that the "lower" ranked medical schools are associated with an increased risk of being ranked lower on cognitive knowledge. We also note, however, that again our race variable remains significant even after we control for the quality of the medical school. Being white increases the likelihood that the resident will be ranked higher on cognitive knowledge even after controlling for the quality of the medical school. We can explain this lingering effect of race in two ways. It may be true that even within a medical school setting, non-whites still fall behind their white counterparts. Certainly there is evidence that non-whites typically enter the medical school setting more educationally disadvantaged than white students (Tinto 1993). This finding may be showing that non-white medical students are graduating their medical school still disadvantaged. White and non-white students are not graduating equally prepared, even from the same institution. The other possible explanation is that program directors operate with a lingering bias and assume a poorer cognitive base despite the ranking of the resident's medical school. We unfortunately do not have enough information in this survey to support or refute either of these hypotheses. The finding does suggest, however, that further research into this phenomenon is warranted.

White women and both male and female racial minorities face a greater risk of resigning from the surgical residency programs in our study than do their white male colleagues. Our analyses thus far have demonstrated that these groups still face a greater risk even when we control for a variety of intermediate factors. The fact that gender and race remain significant suggests that race and gender affects the process of resident evaluation in ways that are not easily captured by our list of traits and characteristics. These findings call for a review of the measures and processes that are used to determine the retention of the resident who is overall an above-average performer. The fact that there were no significant differences between men and women, or whites and non-whites on many of the traits, aptitudes, and characteristics suggests that talent is being wasted. That waste may begin at the medical school level when minority students are not brought up to speed with their white classmates. It may also occur in a program environment where race negatively biases evaluations.

Securing a New Position

White males were less likely than the other race and gender categories to seek help from the program director in either deciding upon or securing a new position. Only 51% of white males sought help versus 61% of the other residents (p=0.044). The significance of this difference will be considered when we examine the positions that the residents ended up taking after leaving their current programs. White males did not suffer as a result of not seeking help.

We asked program directors to specify what kinds of help were offered to the resigning residents. The breakdown of help and the frequency it was given is noted in the table below. There were no differences between the forms of help offered to any of our race and gender categories. As noted above, program directors were most likely to offer letters of reference to residents seeking new positions. Directors wrote letters for a whopping 86% of residents who sought help (n=305). There was no correlation between residents' ranking or reason cited for leaving and the likelihood of having a letter written, nor was there a correlation between being encouraged to leave or to stay and getting a letter.

Next to letters of reference, program directors were most likely to counsel residents who resigned about programs in other fields. Program directors were more likely to talk with residents about career options in other fields when the resident cited a desire for a less stressful work environment as a reason for resigning and when the resident was ranked higher on clinical judgment.

Table 4.17. Help Offered to Resigning Residents

Help Offered	Percent of Residents Offered Help
Counseling about programs in same field	18.26%
Counseling about programs in other fields	48.02%
Calls of reference to aid in placement	45.06%
Letters of reference	85.57%
Counseling about non-medical careers	2.16%
Referral to professional help	5.19%

Program directors made calls of references for 45% of the residents who sought career and placement help. We found no differences based on race, gender, rank, reason cited for leaving, etc., between the residents for whom calls of reference were made and were not made. Finding no evidence of discrimination in this realm is encouraging since we would argue that calls of reference go a longer way in securing better job opportunities than letters of reference which are held in suspicion by most medical faculty (see Chapter 2). The two variables that were associated with the likelihood that a call of reference would be made were the resident's medical school rank and whether or not the resident had talked to at least one attending about his or her plans to resign. In both cases, the association was positive. The higher the resident's medical school's rank, the greater the likelihood that a call of reference would be made. This finding suggests a certain "strength of potential" or halo effect behind the resigning resident. The other variable, discussion with an attending, suggests that the resident was able to garner the support of at least one faculty member who may have been the impetus behind the call of reference. Even within a short period in the program, the resident may have found a mentor of sorts who was willing to help the resident secure a new post.

Program directors counseled just over 18% of the residents about pursuing training in a similar program at another institution. Directors were more likely to recommend this option to the residents who cited marital/family pressures as a reason for resigning. We cannot decipher from our data whether the program directors were suggesting that the resident move to a program which was "less intense" than his or her current program (a bit of downward mobility within the same specialty) since we do not have this ranking information. It may also be that this recommendation substitutes for a leave of absence—residents are being advised to enter a similar program once their marital/family pressures and demands subside.

Program directors were more likely to send the residents who suffered either from some chronic illness or substance abuse to professional help. In most cases, the form of the help came in counseling and a psychiatric assessment. In the case of substance abusers, many of these residents entered rehabilitation programs, but as noted in our section on physical limitation, they were unable to overcome their addictions and subsequently resigned from their programs. Just under two percent of all the residents who resigned were substance abusers. And about two-and-a-half percent of the resigners suffered from some form of chronic illness.

All the residents received about two different forms of help from program faculty, whether that help was a letter and a call, a counseling session and a letter, a call and a referral, etc. No one race or gender category received any more help on average than any other group, although we cannot comment on the quality of the help given.

The Residents' New Position

Table 4.18 below shows where the residents who resigned went after leaving their programs. There are some striking race and gender trends evident in this table even though help securing new positions was offered to all race and gender groups. Non-white women appear more likely to enter a similar program at another institution than the other race and gender category.

Table 4.18. What did the resident do after resigning?

	White males	White females	Non-white males	Non-white females	Total
Entered a similar program at another institution.	16.79%	17.53%	17.65%	31.82%	17.58% (n=99)
Entered a different specialty at the same institution.	21.63%	17.53%	7.84%	4.55%	19.01% (n=107)
Entered a different specialty at the another institution.	36.13%	35.05%	35.29%	18.18%	35.17% (n=198)
Took a position that required no additional training.	18.07%	17.53%	21.57%	9.09%	17.94% (n=101)
Left medicine altogether.	1.27%	2.06%	0%	0%	1.24% (n=7)
No information	6.11%	10.31%	17.65%	36.36%	9.06% (n=51)
Total	n=393	n=97	n=51	n=22	100% (n=563)

Pearson chi2(15) = 40.8701   Pr = 0.000

The other trend is that whites appear significantly more likely than non-whites to enter another specialty at the same institution. Since so many non-white females enter a similar program, we subsequently notice fewer non-white women entering a different specialty. And finally we note that program directors were less likely to have information about the next job position of their non-white resigners than of their white resigners. Let us look at these categories in greater detail.

Similar Program at Another Institution

What factors predict whether a resident who resigns goes into a similar program at another institution? About 18% of all resigners went into a similar program at another institution, but for non-white females, this percentage is higher, about 32%. This difference, however, is not statistically significant, partially because we only have seven non-white women in this category. The variables that predicted whether or not a resident chose this option were the resident's level of maturity, desire for a less stressful work environment, and medical school rank. The greater the resident's maturity as assessed by the program director, the less likely he or she was to seek a position in another similar residency program. We may suppose that program directors considered not seeking a similar situation a sign of maturity. Likewise, if a resident was seeking a less stressful work environment, he or she was significantly less likely to seek a position in a similar residency program. And finally, the rank of the resident's medical school was inversely related to the likelihood that he or she would seek a similar position.

We expected that at least a significant portion of the residents who chose this option would have also expressed a desire to relocate or a need to move for a personal reason, such as the work transfer of a spouse, but neither of these responses was correlated with this variable. We did not capture in this survey residents who resigned because of personality conflicts. We suspect that some of these residents transferred to another similar program because they were experiencing personality conflicts with faculty members. By resigning, some of these residents probably were not rejecting the work per se, but particular colleagues. The fact that a significant bivariate relationship exists between the quality of staff relations and the likelihood of choosing this career option suggests that this hypothesis may be correct. The poorer the quality of staff relations, the greater the likelihood of transferring to a similar program ($p=0.001$).

Entered a Different Specialty at the Same Institution

There is a significant bivariate relationship between race and the likelihood of transferring to another specialty within the same institution with whites more likely to have this option ($p=0.004$). This difference drops out, however, when we control for a resident's perceived ability to handle stress. We hypothesize, therefore, that the race effect works through this other variable, "ability to handle stress." Recall that there was a difference by race on resident's average ranking on ability to handle stress with non-whites being ranked lower than whites on this ability. Without more information on how "stress management" skills are assessed, we cannot rule out the existence of discrimination in this case.

We can argue, however, that for the resident who is resigning, this career move has advantages over other options. Although the resident still faces the challenge of joining a new program, he or she does not have to move from his or her current residence, nor does the resident have to learn the particular layout of a new hospital system, or the layout of a new neighborhood. We view this move as less costly in many ways for the resident providing that the resident's interpersonal relationships with the faculty and staff in the original program were good.

The only other variable that differentiates the residents who chose this career option and those who do not are "calls of reference." Recall, however, that there was not a difference based on race between the residents for whom calls of reference were placed and those for whom calls were not made. This result does show the relative power, however, of a call of reference versus a letter of reference.

Entered a Different Specialty at Another Institution

Residents who chose to move to another specialty at another institution were significantly more likely than residents who chose other paths to have cited a desire for a less stressful work environment as a reason for resigning (p=0.001). Choosing to move to another institution may be an indication that these residents found both the work environment of the residency program and the general environment of the medical center to be stressful. They were also less likely to have cited a "belief that firing was imminent" as a reason for their resignation, as indicated in the full probit model (p=0.000). They were, however, more likely to have been African-American (p=0.014). Residents leaving programs in anesthesiology were the least likely to chose this practice option. Residents from anesthesiology programs were more likely to either transfer into a similar program or take a position that required no additional training.

Took a Position that Required No Additional Training

About 18% of all resigners took a position that required no additional training. The residents who took these positions were on average older (p=0.010) and had cited economic hardships as a reason for resigning (p=0.008). Faced with both age and monetary constraints, these residents needed to find employment rather than new educational opportunities. They were ranked lower than their peers on "personality" by their program directors (p=0.024) and were less likely to seek help from the program director in identifying and securing a new position (p=0.022). It is possible in these cases that the giving up of educational pursuits affected the program director's assessment of the residents' personality. Relinquishing the chance for more educational training was very likely frowned upon by the program directors, whose own identity is grounded in medical education. These residents, burdened by other life concerns, must have appeared unmotivated.

> "Age 38 with children. Resident was concerned about financial impact of residency program on his family."

And a more extreme example of similar pressures:

> "Resident was in deep personal debt. He and current wife were sleeping in his car in the parking lot. Wife was pregnant and then miscarried. Teen-age child

from a previous marriage sought him out. Hospital gave him an interest-free loan for direct repayment of debt. Resident paid back some of the loan and then disappeared." (white male, orthopedic surgery)

No Information

We see from the Table 4.18 above that program directors were less likely to have information about the subsequent plans of non-white females and non-white males than their white colleagues. While program directors did not have information on a total of about nine percent of the residents who resigned from their programs, this percentage was about 18% of "no information" among the pool of non-white males and 36% among the pool of non-white females.

The race effect remains even after we control for the residents' ranking on a variety of traits, aptitudes and characteristics. The only variable other than being a non-white male or a non-white female that is significantly associated with the "no information" variable is the variable "sought help." If a resident did not seek help from the program director in finding and securing a new position, the program directly was significantly less likely to have information about where the resident landed after leaving his or her program. That the program directors had less information about the plans of non-whites even after controlling for whether or not the resident sought the program director's help suggests that the overall quality of interaction between program directors and non-whites was less good. We can hypothesize that within the brief time that the non-white resigner was in the program, that resident had a harder time developing the kind of relationship with the program director that would have facilitated continued contact.

Life After Resignation: Inquiries and Reports

In addition to asking about the placement of the resident after resignation, we also asked a number of questions about the residents' performance in their new practice settings. We wanted to test if the change in venue and work had indeed helped improve performance and satisfy needs. We wanted some way to see if the problems these residents experienced in the one program setting followed them from one work setting to another or not. In the cases of resignations under duress, we also worried that because of poor documentation and lack of follow-up reports, troubled residents would move from one residency program to the next with few checks being made on their past performance. We know that in the name of professional courtesy, and even in some case, gag rules, program directors provide limited information with other program directors about a resident's tour.

The first question we asked was: did the resident's subsequent employer ever ask to discuss the conditions under which the resident resigned? We were curious to see how often other program directors and employers, surely aware that not all leaves are voluntary, make those follow-up reference checks. We note two significant findings. Subsequent employers made follow-up calls on only

22% of all resignations. The remainder of the residents landed employ-
ment/educational opportunities without any reference calls being made to their
last employers. Some of the reference calls could have been made to attending
faculty so that the program director was just unaware that a call had been placed,
but it is still a very low percent.

**Table 4.19. Did the resident's subsequent employer ever ask to discuss the condi-
tions under which the resident resigned, controlling for race and gender.**

Discuss	White Male	White Female	Non-white Male	Non-white Female	Total
No	78.89%	77.01%	75.00%	76.19%	78.10%
	(n=284)	(n=67)	(n=36)	(n=16)	(n=403)
Yes	21.11%	22.99%	25.00%	23.81%	21.90%
	(n=76)	(n=20)	(n=12)	(n=5)	(n=113)
Total	100%	100%	100%	100%	100%
	(n=360)	(n=87)	(n=48)	(n=21)	(n=516)

Pearson chi2(3) = 0.5057 Pr = 0.918

   The second finding is that there is no race and gender effect in predicting
whether a subsequent employer will inquire about the conditions under which a
resident resigned. We suspected that given that more non-whites transferred to
other institutions, more inquiries would have been noted for non-whites than for
whites, but the facts do not support this suspicion.

   What factors are associated with the likelihood that a discussion will take
place? The full probit model appears in Table 4.20 below. The first variable,
"duress," notes that if a resident resigned under duress, the chance that the next
employer will seek a discussion with the program director increases. We do not
know the reason for this association. It seems that the subsequent employer finds
out through some form of communication that the resignation was not entirely
voluntary. We also note that inquiries are more likely to be made if the resident
resigns for marital/family pressures.

   Our next two variables contrast. Discussions result from calls of reference and
are less likely to occur when program directors provide letters of recommendation. During a call of reference, it is natural that the discussion we are testing for
occurs, while when a letter of reference is in hand, the next employer apparently
relies on the information within the letter to substitute for a follow-up call. We
found this result both surprising and understandable. Even though program directors repeatedly bemoan the inadequacy of letters of recommendation in giving accurate and reliable assessments of residents' potential, they are already
under great time constraints and may find it difficult to follow through with calls
of references in many cases.

   The final factor associated with a discussion taking place is the dummy variable which denotes the field of neurosurgery. Perhaps because any fall from
neurosurgery is viewed as a fall from grace, the subsequent employer is more
likely to make that call and follow up on the resident to make sure that there
were no serious problems that prompted the resignation.

If subsequent employers asked program directors to clarify the conditions under which the resident resigned, program directors reported feeling obligated to talk to the subsequent employer in about 90% of the cases. They felt most obligated to talk when the resident resigned either due to overall incompetence or when the resident believed that he or she would have been fired had they not resigned. Few program directors actually explained why they felt or did not feel obligated to discuss the conditions under which the resident resigned even though an explanation was requested in the original question.[4] We have no information to explain why the few program directors who were asked but who did not feel obligated felt the way they did. In two cases where program directors did not feel this obligation, the residents resigned based on faculty advice due to incompetence. That the program director did not share information on these two incompetent residents is disturbing.

In the few cases where program directors explained their answers, the directors cited either an obligation to be truthful with other medical directors, or a personal obligation ("I knew the guy who hired the resident, so I had to talk to him.") as a reason for discussing the conditions.

Reports

Of the 573 residents in our survey who did resign, program directors reported having follow-up reports on 255 (44.50%) of them. We might surmise that the program directors would be less likely to hear follow-up reports on the non-white residents since they were less likely to know the post-residency plans of this group. Surprisingly, however, there is no significant difference in the proportion of residents heard about when we control for race and gender. So, if race and gender are not associated with the likelihood of hearing a report, what variables are associated? The full probit model is shown below. In a simple bivariate analysis, we found that the higher the resident's overall rank, the greater the likelihood that the program director would hear a report once the resident resigned. We were curious to see how that broke down by individual traits, aptitudes and characteristics. We find that three traits are associated with hearing reports: personality, maturity and ability to handle stress. The higher the program director ranked the resident on personality, the greater the likelihood that a report was heard. Being ranked high on personality was probably associated with developing good working relationships even during a brief stint with the residency program. These residents were probably more likely to keep in touch with the program director or with other residents even after resigning.

---

[4] The original questions were as follows:

21. Did the resident's subsequent employer(s) ever ask you to discuss the conditions under which the resident resigned?

22. If the employer(s) did make such a request, did you feel obligated to discuss the resident's resignation with him or her? Please briefly explain your answer.

The next variable, maturity, is more puzzling. Being more mature decreased the likelihood that the program director heard any reports. This result suggests that the mature resident was more independent and broke ties more completely with his or her former colleagues once he or she resigned. Our next variable indicates that the higher the program director ranked the resident on his or her ability to handle stress, the greater the chance of hearing a report.

Table 4.20. Probit analysis: predicting discussion between new employer and former program director.

	Probit coefficients
Resigning under duress (1=duress)	0.6554 ****
	(0.2198)
Marital/family pressures	0.7568 ****
	(0.2232)
Call of reference made	0.4480**
	(0.2003)
Letter of reference written	-0.5449**
	(0.2449)
Neurosurgery	0.7725**
	(0.3043)
Prob > chi2(10)	0.0000
-LL	109.39771
Sample size	204

* p < 0.10; ** p < 0.05; *** p < 0.01; **** p < 0.005

Table 4.21. Have you heard follow-up reports on the resident controlling for race and gender.

Heard a Report?	White Males	White Females	Non-White Males	Non-White Females	Total
no	53.52%	58.59%	59.26%	68.18%	55.50%
	(n=213)	(n=58)	(n=32)	(n=15)	(n=318)
yes	46.48%	41.41%	40.74%	31.82%	44.50%
	(n=185)	(n=41)	(n=22)	(n=7)	(n=255)
Total	100%	100%	100%	100%	100%
	(n=398)	(n=99)	(n=54)	(n=22)	(n=537)

We also find that if the resident had sought the program director's assistance in finding and securing a new educational or employment opportunity, the greater the chance of hearing a report. The resident may have either reported directly back to the program director, or the program director, knowing the placement of the resigned resident, may have made his or her own inquiries.

If the subsequent employer made a request to discuss the conditions under which the resident resigned, the program director had a better chance of hearing a report. The discussion itself may have been the occasion when the program director heard a follow-up.

Table 4.22. Probit analysis of hearing a follow-up report on resigning residents

	Probit coefficients
Ranking on personality[5]	0.3190 ***
	(0.1018)
Ranking on maturity	-0.3329 ***
	(0.1001)
Ranking on ability to handle stress	0.2715 ***
	(0.0921)
Resident sought help with new position	0.3993 ***
	(0.1277)
Employer wanted to discuss conditions under which resident left former program	0.4936***
	(0.1611)
Resident went into a different specialty at same institution	1.0044****
	(0.1758)
Resident went into similar program at another institution	0.3756 **
	(0.1648)
Prob > chi2(10)	0.0000
-LL	276.37025
Sample size	475

* p < 0.10; ** p < 0.05; *** p < 0.01; **** p < 0.005

And finally we see that there is an association between the practice setting and the chance of hearing a report. If the resident chose to switch into another residency program in the same institution, or chose to switch programs but remain in the same specialty, the program director was more likely to hear a report. It would be much easier to hear reports from colleagues at the same institution about the resident who remained at the medical center, and follow-up reports for those within the same specialty are likely to be shared at professional meetings and through the professional pipeline.

This analysis raises the obvious question: Who falls through the cracks? There is no difference between the residents for whom we have reports and those for whom we do not based on their average ranking on cognitive knowledge, manual dexterity, or clinical knowledge once we control for such other traits as personality, maturity, and ability to handle stress. This finding suggests

---

[5] Recall, ranking on scale 5-point scale with 1= not important to 5 = very important

that the quality of interpersonal traits and characteristics are more important than technical skills in determining whether continued contact and reports are made. It would be disheartening to find that the residents who fall through the informational network are the worst performers who have been released onto an unsuspecting public. We shall see if the same finding holds true for our terminated residents.

Post-Residency Performance

The resigners performed well in their next educational or job positions. Subsequent employers reported these residents as performing between average and above average (average ranking was 3.72 with 3=average and 4=above average). Although when we control for race and gender in a probit equation, non-white females were ranked significantly lower than their colleagues, when it was added to the full model below, race and gender were no longer significant.

Residents who resigned from programs in anesthesiology tended to be ranked lower than residents who resigned from any of our other four specialties. Why this is so may be related to the job choices that most of the residents who left anesthesiology made. Recall from our earlier analysis than residents from anesthesiology programs were more likely to transfer into similar programs at other institutions (a move that tends to be frowned upon by the faculty) or take positions that required no additional training. The prejudice against these choices may result in the lower average ranking.

The next variable, clinical judgment, indicates that there is a correlation between the residents' ranking on clinical judgment during his or her tour of duty in the previous program and his or her overall ranking in the subsequent program/position. The higher the program director had ranked the resident on clinical judgment, the higher his or her overall rank in the next situation. This correlation suggests that even though this evaluative category, clinical judgement, has many problems associated with its accurate measurement, it serves as a core part of the overall evaluation. This finding also suggests that there may be some standard within the residency program culture by which faculty assess this aptitude. We also find a similar and even stronger effect of the residents' previous ranking on patient relationships. The higher the program director had ranked the resident on patient relationships, the higher the resident's overall ranking in the next position. We also note a relationship between the timing of the resignation and the post-resignation overall ranking. The later the resident resigned, the higher his or her subsequent overall ranking. We did not expect this relationship since residents who resigned later were more likely to have resigned under duress. However, residents who resigned later were also more likely to have talked to the program director a greater number of times and they were also more likely to have been ranked higher on honesty than residents who resigned earlier.

These residents' higher overall ranking may indicate that the resignation, although perhaps under duress, was the best move for the resident. Having not flourished in his or her previous situation, the resident apparently made the right choice in the next position and found a better match. All in all, resignation was a good choice for the majority of resigners, demonstrated by their good performance in their next position.

Table 4.23. Ordered probit predicting overall ranking of resident who reigned in next educational or job placement.

	Probit coefficients
Anesthesiology	-0.7801 ****
	(0.2096)
Ranking on clinical judgment	0.3047 ****
	(0.0944)
Ranking on patient relationships	0.6072 ****
	(0.1020)
Timing of resignation	0.1559 **
	(0.0745)
Resident went into a different specialty at same institution	0.4130***
	(0.1584)
Prob > chi2(10)	0.0000
-LL	267.58874
Sample size	247

* p < 0.10; ** p < 0.05; *** p < 0.01; **** p < 0.005

Summary

Our analyses suggest that many of the residents who resigned underestimated the stress associated with surgical work, or overestimated their ability to handle the stress. Although many of these residents did have some exposure to their chosen specialties during medical school, it is very likely that the residents who entered programs in neurosurgery, orthopedic surgery and plastic surgery had much more limited exposure to the day-to-day stressors than the residents in anesthesiology or general surgery. Stress levels appear to be inversely associated in part with the quality of doctor-patient interactions since among our pool of resigners, those who left because of too much stress typically had poor patient relationships. This finding also underscores the paucity of options to deal with stress within the current structure of residency programs such as family leaves and shared positions.

A good number of residents also left due to marital or family pressures. These pressures included marriage, divorce, pregnancy, and relocation. We found that women were much more likely to resign for these reasons than their male counterparts, even after we controlled for marital status. We also found a qualitative difference in the level of sympathy expressed by the program directors for the

woman who resigns for these reasons than for the male resident facing the same
major life events. Program directors apparently knew more about the particular
marital/family troubles facing the male residents than the female residents. Descriptions of the challenges faced by the male residents were much "thicker" in
detail than the comparable comments made for the women. This finding suggests that the quality of interpersonal relationships between program directors
and their female residents is on average poorer.

Non-whites were much more likely than whites to resign under duress. Although we had expected that this would be explained by the greater proportion
of international medical graduates among our pool of non-white residents, this
finding did not hold in our model. What we did find was an association between
residents' ranking on clinical judgment and the likelihood of being asked to resign. We also noted that program directors were more likely to ask residents
they thought were dissatisfied with surgical work to resign. While the assessment of both clinical judgment and dissatisfaction are problematic, the race effect remains even after we control for these other factors. Simply being non-
white increases the likelihood that the resident will be asked to resign.

Residents tend to discuss their plans to resign with program directors. We
assume this trend is the result of both a formal reporting structure and the lack of
better developed relationships with other program staff. Residents typically
think about resigning very early in their tour through the department. We hypothesize that friendships may not yet exist between residents, attendings and
other staff members when the resident first thinks about leaving. This may help
explain the heavy reliance on formal routes of communication.

Once the program director has been informed, he or she responds to the resident's request by either encouraging the resident to leave, encouraging the resident to stay, or suggesting a leave of absence. Leaves of absence were suggested
in less than four percent of the cases. Program directors did try, however, to
convince about half of the residents to stay. They were more likely to ask white
residents and residents whose overall ranking was high to stay. They were also
more likely to ask residents who cited a desire for less stress and/or mari-
tal/family pressures as a reason for resigning to stay. Risks for being asked to
leave included being a racial minority and low rank on manual dexterity.

Non-white males fared least well in an overall ranking of traits, aptitudes and
characteristics. Although program directors ranked non-white males slightly
above average overall, they ranked non-white males significantly below their
peers on manual dexterity, clinical judgement and patient relations. Both non-
white males and non-white females scored lower on ability to handle stress and
cognitive knowledge. The difference in cognitive knowledge remains even after
we control for rank of medical school. We also suggest that differences in the
ways non-whites and whites express and manage stress may help explain why
non-whites scored lower on this trait. It remains true, however, that being non-
white increases the resident's risk of resigning under duress and/or being encouraged to leave even after we control for ranking.

Program directors offered a variety of help to the resigning residents in their search for new posts. The most common form of help came in the form of letters of reference. Next came the call of reference. The kind of help offered did not vary by race or gender. Program directors counseled residents who had cited a desire for less stress as a reason for resigning about residency positions in another specialty. They counseled residents who had cited marital/family pressure about positions in similar programs. They referred residents suffering from substance abuse and chronic illness to professional help.

Most resigners (35%) transferred to another program and another institution. About 18% of residents chose each of the following options: transferred to a similar program at another institution, entered a different specialty at the same institution, or took a position that required no additional training. Whites had a significant edge at landing positions within the same institution. The race effect appears to work through differences in how whites and non-whites scored on their ability to handle stress. That program directors were less likely to know the plans of non-whites suggest that they had poorer relationships with non-white residents. The residents who take positions without additional training tend to be older and to cite economic pressures as a reason for resigning.

Program directors tended to hear follow-up reports on residents who scored higher on personality and ability to handle stress. There were no significant differences on the basis of clinical judgment, manual dexterity or cognitive knowledge between the residents for whom reports were heard or not heard. They were also more likely to hear reports on the residents who either stayed within the same field of surgery or who had stayed within the same institution.

On average, the residents who resigned appear to have made a reasonable choice by resigning. Their above-average post-residency performance reflects the appropriateness of their choice. Although the resignation may have been costly for the programs, the residents who resign from these surgical programs do not appear to be liabilities for the medical profession as a whole. They are not typically bad or untalented physicians, but physicians who reassessed the appropriateness of their original choice, or who, with the help of some constructive criticism, decided that surgery was not the right choice for them

Discussion

Resignations constitutes the largest percent of the attrition statistics. For medical education reformers interested in reducing attrition, reducing the number of resignations will have the greatest impact on overall attrition rates. Resignations are costly both for individuals who must change paths and for program that must scramble to replace lost employees.

The culture and organization of medical education at the residency level helps inform all the data enumerated above and provides insight into the resignation experience. We find evidence that many of the residents who resigned from these surgical residency programs did not have adequate information about the stressors associated with their chosen specialties prior to making their choices.

More and better information and exposure before residents choose their specialty in medical school could conceivably reduce attrition since residents could make more informed choices. How medical educators can provide better practical exposure to various specialties while not sacrificing a broad breath of coverage represents a formidable challenge within the confines of a four-year medical school experience.

For reformers seeking to reduce attrition, challenges exist which result from the timing of the residency program. Residents across specialties are at an age in their wider social and physical development when non-professional life events like marriage, childbearing, and the aging of their parents will undoubtedly demand some of their attention. Unless programs can provide some flexibility in the training program to provide time off to deal with outside demands, some residents will be lost to competing priorities. Of course, some medical educators might consider this attrition a natural weeding out of those residents less committed to the profession. Those who hold this view will resist changing the current structure. But the data notes that program directors rank resigning residents as above average performers. Flexible programs that keep good performers on track may well be worth the extra effort for these programs, especially since more and more women now comprise the medical school population. Eventually, medical educators might find that they can no longer feed their appetite for white males and circumstances will force these educators to make revisions in the organization of the training programs that address the needs and concerns of their female workforce.

We also have evidence that race and gender affect the process of evaluation and post-resignation job placement in ways that are not explained by reference to the traits, aptitudes and characteristics medical faculty consider necessary for good doctoring. Women are more likely to leave because of marital and family pressures although as a group they are less likely to be married. We also presented evidence that female residents have poorer relationships with program faculty.

Even when controlling for a variety of skills, non-white residents continued to experience a greater risk for resigning under duress. Program directors tended to encourage non-whites to leave when the resident and program director first talked about a possible resignation. In these two instances, program directors appear negatively influenced by these residents' race when assessing their fitness for surgery. Since whiteness and maleness have characterized the field of surgery over the past century and have only recently been challenged by the influx of racial minorities and women into the field, the traditional idiom of surgical work biases evaluations in ways that are costly for the individual residents and for the programs. However, biased evaluations are not only costly, they are also unjust.

The measures and processes that program faculty use to evaluate residents need to be reviewed. If medical education reformers want to reduce attrition and make sure that the process of evaluation is fair and just, these data point to areas of reform. Greater flexibility in the organization of the residency program could give all residents an ability to deal with outside life events without sacrificing their career choice. And medical educators sensitized to the ways that their judgments about individual residents are affected by racial prejudice could decrease the resignation rate for racial minorities in fields like surgery.

V

Terminations

Evaluators terminate employees when they conclude that whatever problems the worker has are irremediable within the normal work setting. The problems the worker has may be varied. The worker may not have the proper skills, or display the proper work ethic. The worker may be terminated after a single incident or after a series of offenses. In any case, the evaluator deems the worker incompetent, dangerous, or disruptive to the work environment.

In the case of a resignation, the seed of the decision to leave usually lies within the individual worker. In the case of a termination, the decision to expel the worker originates in the boss or evaluator. The community into which he or she had sought membership rejects the terminated worker.

Another aspect of a termination is that the employer has to force the worker out of his or her position. In some cases, the employer terminates the worker because the employer had to scale back the work force, but often we think of a worker being terminated for poor performance. We found no cases of scale-back terminations in our data set.

In residency programs across specialties, program directors often give poor performers an opportunity to resign before termination proceedings begin. We described this process in the previous chapter as resigning under duress. Letting the poor performing resident resign instead of being terminated permits face-saving: the decision appears to come from the resident rather than from the program faculty. We assume that many of the terminated residents in our sample were given this option but either failed to recognize the warning signs or chose to ignore the signs, which points to another aspect of terminations in surgical residency programs. Having to force a resident to leave suggests that the resident and the evaluator did not agree about the quality of the work being done or the fit between the resident and the community. While the program faculty's assessment was that the resident was not qualified, in many cases the resident thought he or she was qualified. In this chapter we will explore some reasons why this difference in perspective can exist given what we already know about the culture and organization of surgical residency programs.

About three out of every one hundred residents who began their surgical residency training were fired before completing their programs. Just as we found for resignations, however, this rate varies based on the resident's race and gender. While the overall risk was three percent, the risk for white males was about two percent. The risk for white females, however, was five percent, for non-white males it was 20%, and for non-white females, it was 23%. Therefore white females were 2.5 times more likely to be terminated than white males, while non-white males were 8.74 times more likely, and non-white females were 9.87 times more likely. In this chapter we will look at the typical termination and at the effects of race and gender on the termination process.

Terminations: A Profile

Comments from the program directors indicated that terminated residents were typically distraught when they were informed that their performance fell below acceptable levels. When first confronted with the program's dissatisfaction with their performance, 26% of the residents denied that there was any problem at all. About 41% of the terminated residents were married, with 26% of them having graduated from foreign medical schools (this compares with 12% of the resigners being international medical graduates). The average medical school rank for these residents was 71 out of a scale of one to 126.

Program directors initiated about seventy-eight percent of the talks about termination, attendings initiated 13%, and residents initiated about four percent. When confronted by their poor evaluations, residents typically attributed their poor performance to a stressful work environment, personality conflicts with staff members, and marital/family pressures. Program faculty noted problems typically within the first six months of training (41%), with another significant chunk identified in the second six months (26%). Therefore, program faculty identified 67% of the problem residents within the first year. Program directors spoke to 97% of the terminated residents about their performance, but gave written notification to only 40%. Program directors ranked terminated residents lowest on clinical judgment, on their ability to handle stress, and on their staff relationships when compared to our other two outcome categories.

The decision to terminate lagged a bit behind the actual recognition of problems. In only 16% of cases did program faculty decide to terminate in the first six months. They decided on another 34% in the second year. In 95% of all terminations, faculty discussed the decision to terminate, and in 74% of cases, a formal vote was taken. Hospital attorneys were rarely involved (17%), and rarely (14%) did residents threaten to take legal action. We cannot determine from our data the order of these two events: the threat of legal action or the involvement of an attorney.

Despite performing poorly, program directors gave 68% of terminated residents help securing new positions. Program directors tried to steer these residents into other fields of medicine. In five percent of our cases, program directors tried to convince residents to leave medicine altogether. After termination, 27% went into a similar program at another institution. Another 27% went into a different specialty at another institution. Twenty percent took a position that required no additional training. Only 29% of subsequent employers asked program directors why the resident had been terminated. Program directors reported that terminated residents were still performing below average in their next educational/employment setting.

Only 11% of the terminated residents had not been selected through the normal application process. Women residents were significantly less likely to be chosen through the normal application process which reflects the match statistics for women that we cited in the introduction. Program directors reported an indication prior to matriculation that there might be problems in only 13% of cases. Also, 13% of terminated residents had done a clinical externship with their program so the faculty had already been able to observe the resident prior to accepting him or her into their ranks.

What is A Problem Resident?

Unlike our resigners who were performing above average at the time of their resignations, terminated residents were performing below average and continued to perform below average in their next work setting. What are the signs of a below-average performer? We will review what surgical attendings and fellow residents describe as the warning signs. Recall that most attrition result not from a lack of intelligence, but because of non-cognitive factors—outside life events, behavioral problems, personality clashes, etc. Among our total sample, only 25% of the people who left their programs left because of academic or physical difficulties. But among our pool of terminated residents, 62% were ranked as below average on technical skills and cognitive knowledge, and 25% were deemed poorly prepared even before beginning their programs.

> "Most of the mistakes I've seen made, most of the little errors that I've seen made in the last three years, have been made because people just didn't know their stuff." (R29)

Despite a long and arduous educational program, some residents still do not know their stuff.

Another early warning sign is a pattern of mistakes. Although mistakes are expected, the faculty is loath to see a resident who does not learn from past mistakes. Patterns of mistakes are typically noted early in the tour:

"But it is the monotonous litany, repetition of never quite being on target, never quite doing what he is supposed to be doing." (A29)

"Even a bad resident is smart enough to disguise their ignorance in front of me. We don't always pick it up the first ten or twelve times." (A24)

Although the first ten or twelve times may go unnoticed, the pattern and repetition of mistakes does become apparent and program faculty label the resident a poor performer.

Another early warning sign is a lack of passion and zeal for surgical work. Recall that program faculty were eager to see this passion displayed during the interview. Program faculty believe that passion and zeal can carry the residents through sleepless nights, failed cases, the trial and tribulations of the residency program. If the passion is not there in the first couple of months, attendings cannot imagine how the resident will make it through the next four-to-six years:

"Most of the time it wasn't that they weren't bright enough, it was just for whatever reason they'd become burned out, disinterested in the problems that were going on. I think that is the best way to describe it, lack of interest." (R16)

"I was having some ambivalent feelings and I let that show on more than one occasion." (R28)

And we come back to our old standard: camaraderie among the residents. A lack of social skills in dealing with his or her peers is another warning sign for attendings:

"There are residents who are relatively intelligent and yet have such problems with their interpersonal skills that nobody can stand their guts...there are residents who over the years just seem to aggravate everybody in the hospital." (A28)

"He doesn't smooth anybody over, he angers people. He makes people feel that he doesn't respect them. He can be completely competent but if he gets people pissed off at him, if he doesn't have anybody to support him in the end, he's gonna sink because nobody is gonna stand by him. People could help him out, but they won't and you got to work with people." (A36)

Relations among peers is important, but attendings admit that sometimes problems are due to personality clashes with faculty:

"Sometimes there are personality conflicts and you think that perhaps another one of the attendings is reacting based on that...you have to be careful in order to be fair." (A28)

"I thought that he had a personality disorder, the others didn't. We compromised and sent him to a psychiatrist. The psychiatrist said he thought the guy was pretty straight...Well now a couple of years have gone by and the problem is he and I have a personality clash—there is clearly bad blood between us...I can't put my finger on his personality flaw." (A29)

Personal clashes between members of a department do not necessarily determine who is and who is not a competent physician. Since so much of resident evaluation, especially of non-cognitive traits, are subjective by nature, medical educators must be very self-conscious of how their personal feelings, either positive or negative, influence their evaluations.

Residents also appear to get tripped up by the stress associated with their residency positions. According to the doctors we interviewed, troubled residents find it hard to cope with the stress.

"He was very touchy, unpleasant, very insecure guy who couldn't, was always dealing with people by flying off the handle, even the most minor sort of questioning. I think he felt threatened by anybody who even asked him a question, particularly a nurse. He was an incredibly rude and disruptive force." (A28)

"He was very distant and could not deal...he was very cold and impersonal and really delivered a lot of unfeeling things to people. He was sometimes cruel in interactions with faculty, residents and nurses. He was having a lot of personal, family-type strains that made life very difficult for him, but things got to a point where he was really undermining the care that patients were getting...The person decided to change fields...he realized that there were fields that were less taxing both emotionally and physically as far as the work aspect." (R27)

And the extreme example of a resident who really could not handle stress:

"He would get into shouting matches with nurses, he would abuse them, at least verbally. He once squirted blood down the front of a nurse's uniform from a syringe. The nurses claimed that he had pulled a long line catheter out of a patient without first cutting the sutures and I found that unacceptable, wanton cruelty to a patient no matter how awake the patient was. That basically showed a disrespect for his co-workers and a disrespect for his patients at times of personal stress...I might add that he scored highest of any resident on the written boards at his level. It had nothing to do with intelligence." (A31)

According to these same doctors, the worst problem is dishonesty. When asked what they meant by dishonesty, program directors responded:

"I mean, I think the bad resident is the guy who is dishonest, who evaluates patients superficially and attempts to give you a report based on a haphazard exam." (A18)

"I mean dishonesty in the sense that they will try to bluff their way through things they don't know. Like when they are taking care of a patient and there is say a lab value that they should have checked but didn't. Rather than saying,

'Gee, I should have done this, and I just didn't think of it,' they'll come up with
a million different excuses or they will make up a lab value and subsequently
go and check it. They may get away with it, but only for a while." (R45)

The dishonest resident is also the resident who thinks he or she knows more or
can do more than he or she can, who is being dishonest with himself or herself
about their level of skill:

"The most dangerous kind is the person who thinks he can do it and can't.
They're very dangerous gunslingers who end up rapidly taking the wrong action, which is probably the worst thing of all." (A24)

"I think the worst residents are dishonest. The next worse are the impulsive
smug group—primarily people who overestimate their own intelligence...I
think the biggest problem with not being honest, not only with others but with
themselves, is not admitting there is stuff they don't know." (A29)

The challenge of evaluating a residents' honesty/dishonesty and the concomitant
need for residents to know their limitations is such an important issue that we
devote an entire chapter (Chapter VII) to its analysis. Dishonesty in this context
means a myriad of things: lying, failing to take responsibility, cutting corners,
blaming others for poor performance, not admitting your own ignorance.

What insight do we gain from this description of problems and warning signs?
We can compare our survey results against this list of typical problems. Below,
we will be able to see which of these problems seemed most prevalent among
our group of terminated residents. We will tally these categories and see if there
are differences in the way residents were treated based on the type of problem
they presented as well as on their race and gender. Before we begin that analysis, however, we will look at when program faculty first noticed problems.

When Are Problems Noticed?

Program faculty note problems quite early in a resident's tour through a department, and often the kinds of problems they note, such as a lack of cognitive
knowledge, are not remediable within the normal context of a residency program. Program faculty identified 41% of the terminated residents within the first
six months of training. There was no difference based on race or gender in the
risk of being identified early. The only statistically significant relationship between when program faculty first noted a problem and the kind of problem that
residents displayed involved stress. Program faculty identified residents unable
to handle the stress of the workload earlier rather than later. If the resident's
problem was the result of a stressful work environment, program faculty were
significantly more likely to make changes in the resident's program, hopefully in
order to reduce some of the stress. Program faculty adopted this modification,
however, in only 30% of all cases where stress was identified as the root of the

resident's substandard performance. Program faculty did not specify the type of modification made, but given the arduous schedule that residents work and the seeming inflexibility of that educational/work schedule, the modification did not prevent these residents' eventual termination.

Table 5.1. When did program faculty become aware of poor performance?

Time period	Frequency	Percent	Cumulative Percent
First six months	99	40.57%	40.57%
Second six months	62	25.41%	65.98%
Second year	60	24.59%	90.57%
Third year	16	6.56%	97.13%
Fourth year	4	1.64%	98.77%
Fifth year	3	1.23%	100.00%
Total	244	100.00%	

The Problems: What were the Problems that Terminated Residents Presented?

In Survey II, we asked program directors: Can you describe any critical incidents that would give an indication of the difficulties the resident had? Of our 289 observations, we got information about critical incidents for 158 (54%) of the terminated residents. We will compare the descriptions of the troubles these residents had against the list of problems from above. Recall that we obtained this list from the interviews with the program directors, attendings, nurses and residents from five neurosurgery programs. The actual descriptions below come from cases of residents who were terminated from programs in anesthesiology, general surgery, neurosurgery, orthopedic surgery and plastic surgery. There is both overlap and deviations from the list we provide above.

Before we begin the analysis, we need to ask whether the residents for whom we have descriptions of critical incidents are different from the residents for whom we have no descriptions. There are three characteristics that separate these two groups. We are significantly more likely to have descriptions for white residents and married residents and less likely to have descriptions for residents terminated from general surgery programs. We need to keep these distinctions in mind as we conduct our analysis.

We will present the description of critical incidents in the order of their magnitude—what problems were most prevalent among the terminated residents? Table 5.2 shows the distribution of problems as reported by program directors. Of course, a number of the residents displayed more than one problem, but for the sake of our analysis, we categorized the problems by the resident's main problem according to the program director. We will look at each of these categories separately, looking at the descriptions of the critical incidents, and test for any race and gender effects in these categorizations.

Table 5.2. Problems	% Cases
Inappropriate behavior	**19%**
Poorly prepared/physical problems	**14%**
Substance abuse	**14%**
Failure to progress during training	**13%**
Personal conflicts with staff	**8%**
Poor fit with the residency staff	**8%**
Made a grave mistake in patient care	**6%**
Lost passion or interest in specialty	**5%**
Defensive response to teaching	**4%**
Dishonest	**4%**
Distracted by outside interests/events	**3%**
Could not follow orders	**2%**

n=158

Inappropriate Behavior

The largest category captures a variety of behaviors that are considered inappropriate in the context of the residency program. It includes such behaviors as leaving your assigned post, unconventional behaviors, and bizarre behaviors associated with mental illness. In all these cases, it was not a technical error in the surgical theater or the ordering of wrong medications that indicated that the resident should be terminated. The strange behavior indicated that the resident did not have what it takes to become a competent physician. The resident who leaves the building without permission did not take his or her fiduciary responsibility seriously, did not recognize why this is unacceptable behavior for a physician who has been entrusted with the lives and welfare of patients. The unconventional resident may or may not have a mental illness, but the faculty found it challenging to evaluate these residents' moral fiber. And the bizarre performers were incapable of providing medical care since, according to a professional assessment, they needed some care themselves.

Here are some descriptions of residents who shirked their duties:

"Leaving the intensive care unit where she was assigned. Not reporting to operating room for scheduled surgery, not responding to telephone calls while on duty." (non-white female, general surgery)

"Was on call for emergencies as a resident and phones in to ask the chairman to arrange coverage since he was picking up his airplane 800 miles away and was caught in bad weather." (white male, orthopedic surgery)

"She did not respond to repeated telephone calls from a recently discharged patient. She left the hospital without signing out midday." (non-white female, neurosurgery)

In these cases, the residents failed to sufficiently recognize and fulfill their obligations to their patients and fellow staff members. They failed to recognize the gravity of leaving their posts unfulfilled even though as residents, they may not have had the final authority over the patients in their care.

The next set of descriptions describes residents whose behavior was unconventional enough to cause concern:

"Inappropriate behavior, dress, comment." (white female, general surgery)

"Asked patient under his care in the ICU for a job for his girlfriend, other abuses of power relationships, misrepresenting patient data. Did not recognize inappropriateness of unethical behavior." (white male, general surgery)

"Signed another resident's name when checking out library books…beeper always dead or malfunctioning." (white male, orthopedic surgery)

All of these residents' behaviors made the medical faculty uneasy about whether or not these residents had the right traits and characteristics to assume all the responsibilities associated with surgical care. Asking patients for favors abuses the doctor's privileged position, and signing out books under another resident's name suggests that the resident is reluctant to accept responsibility (even for something as simple as a library book).

And finally, we have the bizarre performer—the resident whose behavior was so troubling that the medical faculty thought the resident needed psychiatric care:

"Self-hypnotized himself while he was assisting at surgery. Addicted to gambling." (white male, orthopedic surgery)

"'Out of touch with reality' often used to describe his behavior. Offered to divorce his wife whom he considered the basis of his problems…Wanted him to seek psychiatric counseling." (non-white male, neurosurgery)

"He displayed bizarre behavior. Within the first weeks, he wore a lab coat without undergarments and exposed himself to the nurses. Fired within one month." (white male, neurosurgery)

In these cases, program directors expressed amazement that the resident had gotten as far as the residency program before these behaviors had been noticed and/or addressed by undergraduate faculty, medical school faculty, etc.

There were no race or gender effects under this category. No race or gender group was more or less likely than the other race or gender groups to display inappropriate or bizarre behavior.

Poorly Prepared/Physical Problems

Poorly prepared residents comprised the next largest category. These residents could not handle the rigors of the residency training because they had a weak fund of knowledge, trouble passing examinations, or had a physical problem that made a career in surgery impossible. Here are some descriptions from this group of residents:

> "Trouble passing examinations." (white male, general surgery)

> "Weak fund of knowledge and resident knew it." (non-white female, general surgery)

> "Inability to satisfactorily perform on in-house exam at level which would indicate any possibility of passing the general surgery boards." (white male, general surgery)

> "Poor performance in ABSITE, department exams, and only average on oral exams. No problems clinically, problems primarily related to test-taking." (white male, general surgery)

Many of the quotes specifically refer to the resident's deficiencies associated with test-taking. Recall our earlier discussion of the lack of correlation between test-taking and eventual performance as a physician. So why were the program faculty so concerned about the resident's test-taking capabilities? The RRC (Residency Review Commission) ranks residency programs in part on how many residents from that program pass various in-house examinations and perform on national exams and board exams. Keeping a bad test-taker among the residency pool risks certification. The use of standardized tests as a ranking device disproportionately hurts bad test-takers. Interestingly enough, the majority of poor test-takers cited a lack of manual dexterity as the reason for their poor performance, instead of a lack of cognitive knowledge or problems passing exams. These residents appear to have thought that a lack of surgical skills rather than their poor test scores resulted in their poor evaluations.

Some residents had physical handicaps that could not be overcome:

> "Difficulty with psychomotor skills, surgical procedures. Did not progress during 3rd year to the level necessary for patient management." (white male, general surgery)

> "Resident was legally blind in one eye and therefore had depth perception problems which caused major difficulties in the operating room. It was the opinion of the staff that this problem would prevent her from a surgical career. She was defensive, not realizing that she had a problem and was determined to stay in general surgery." (white female, general surgery)

Again, it often surprised program faculty that these physical conditions, especially along the lines of being legally blind in one eye, did not discourage the pursuit of a surgical career or prevent matriculation.

We found no race or gender effects for this category (keeping in mind that we have an under-representation of non-whites in our description category to start). We had suspected that non-whites would have been significantly over-represented given that they were significantly more likely to come from lower-ranked medical schools. We thought that coming from lower-ranked schools would translate into poor test-taking. Our analysis did not confirm this suspicion.

Substance Abuse

Substance abuse defines our next major category of problems among the terminated residents. Recall from Chapter I that physicians are more prone to suicide, alcoholism and drug addiction than the rest of the population (Gerber 1983: 45, Konner 1987: 28, Ruddick 1985: 211, Vaillant 1979: 372). While about four percent of the residents in this study reported having a drug or alcohol addiction, the drug and alcohol abusers were significantly more likely to be among the pool of terminated residents (65%) than among the problematic completers (23%) or the resignations (12%).

What does our average substance abuser look like among the terminated residents? The substance abuser is not more likely to come from a poorly ranked medical school. He or she is also not distinguished by race and/or gender. Also, the abuser is not more likely to be from one specialty over another although we tend to think of residents in anesthesia having the most trouble with drug addiction. This finding suggests that the surgical residents and anesthesiology residents have equal access to the drugs most often abused.

Program faculty do not notice the drug and alcohol abuser sooner than other problem residents. Program faculty are also not more likely to make changes in the resident's program to accommodate the addiction even though some of our respondents reported sending the addicted resident to a rehabilitation program. Program directors consider the substance abuser to be less honest, less mature, and less able to handle stress than his or her peers. The substance abuser does not differ from his or her peers on the basis of cognitive knowledge, manual dexterity, clinical judgment or staff and patient relationships. During the termination process, program directors are less likely to give help to the substance abusers in the form of counseling or letters of reference. The program director is significantly more likely to refer the substance abuser to professional help.

The normal context of the residency program is obviously ill-equipped to handle drug-addicted residents, but the tragedy of losing a medical/surgical career, the loss of so many years of training and study, and even life itself, suggests that more needs to be done to help the victims of that same long and arduous process. Here are descriptions of some of these residents:

> "Resident was found using drugs in bathroom on one of the nursing units." (non-white male, general surgery)

"Finally admitted drug abuse problem for 2 years, overdosed in hospital."
(white male, general surgery)

"Devious, lying, non-responsive. She admitted to drug use but was not initially
responsive to treatment. Tardy, long-sleeves, Band-Aids on arms, multiple absences. One year delay while she was in a local drug treatment program in psychiatry department." (non-white female, anesthesiology)

"Performance was satisfactory. Drug abuse was the problem. Found uncon-
scious with syringe in bathroom in OR suite. Some suspicion previously. Was
hospitalized for 30 days in substance abuse rehabilitation program." (white
male, anesthesiology)

And the residents whose problems with addiction were so severe that they lost
their lives:

"Inappropriate behavior toward a patient in the ER and inebriated on one occasion. Drug abuse, went into drug treatment program. Resident subsequently
died about one year later. Said to have been caused by an 'overwhelming viral
infection.' We knew that there had been a drug problem. Very sad case." (white
male, plastic surgery)

"Living in Thoracic Surgery on-call room. Faculty smelled alcohol on his
breath. He was late for rounds, failed to respond to nursing calls. Resident
committed suicide—drug overdose a year later." (white male, general surgery)

"Substance abuse—now deceased." (white female, anesthesiology)

Most of these descriptions lack a sense of sympathy or tragedy in their reporting.
We had thicker and richer detail in program directors' descriptions of residents'
family problems than we have of residents' drug addictions. In only one case
above do we hear that this case was a "very sad case." There is also a dearth of
explanation of the addiction—why did the residents use drugs. We note from an
earlier analysis that residents reporting substance abuse were also more likely to
report marital/family pressures, yet we learn nothing about other stresses and
strains in these residents' lives from the descriptions above. In only one case do
we learn that the resident's emotional problems stem from the death of a close
friend:

"Problem was abuse of nitrous oxide. Counseling and therapy begun promptly.
This occurred in the 7th month of training. He entered the medical association
division program immediately which included 4 weeks in-house therapy at
treatment center. Then, in 9th month, returned to residency but gave self a near
fatal does of narcotics in 12th month. Also found to be a heavy alcohol user.
Emotional problems, death of a close friend." (white male, anesthesiology)

Failure to Progress

Failure to progress, although related to poor preparation, was distinct from poor preparation. In these cases, the resident's failure to make progress in the residency program took program faculty by surprise—"nothing in the resident's records would have indicated that there would have been any problems." These residents failed to demonstrate a building of skills over the course of the program, even very early in the program. Program faculty interpreted this failure as a sign that these particular residents could not become competent surgeons:

> "Failure to show progressive acquisition of surgical knowledge and skills." (white male, general surgery)

> "Resident at 3rd and 4th year level could not begin even a very familiar operation without supervision." (white female, general surgery)

> "He just did not progress in his ability to understand clinical problems. He was offered the opportunity to repeat his internship but refused." (white male, general surgery)

Failure to progress did not vary by race or gender. We have no way of knowing whether or not these residents would have eventually progressed had they been given or taken the opportunity to repeat a year of training. We do not know how many residents in the same situation take the program faculty up on their offer to repeat an internship or spend additional years at the junior level who then go on to become competent physicians. We believe from our study of residency programs that this modification is not common. We do have some examples, however, in which the resident's refusal to repeat a year helped decide his or her termination. We want to underscore that residents' lack of progress surprised program faculty demonstrating the inadequacy of paper applications in predicting actual performance.

Personality Conflicts

Program directors recognized that personality conflicts were critical in determining the decision to terminate the resident. The personality conflicts seemed irremediable within the normal context of the residency training program. The resident represented a disruptive force in the department, constantly bickering and arguing with members of the staff. Directors reported that the only way to solve the problem was to remove the resident from the department. We unfortunately do not know in how many of these cases program directors initially gave the resident an opportunity to resign.

> "She felt that she had some personality conflicts with some residents and attendings." (white female, general surgery)

"He could not work with other residents or nurses. He got into verbal fights with nurses and other residents." (white male, general surgery)

"She had poor interactions with peers, faculty and patients." (white female, general surgery)

"Had several fights with his attending staff." (white male, general surgery)

We would hypothesize that if both the resident and the faculty agreed that there were personality conflicts, the resident would be anxious to leave the department. But perhaps the costs associated with moving to a new position were greater in this case for the resident than staying in an unfriendly environment until forced out. Whites were more likely than non-whites to fall into this category. Given our earlier discussions of the culture of surgery in which whites would be more prone to fit, this is an unexpected result. We will examine this phenomenon in greater detail when we discuss the reasons residents gave for their poor performance below.

Poor Fit

Closely related to our discussion of personality conflicts is the "poor fit" phenomenon. In these cases, program directors felt that the resident just did not fit within the program. This recalls our discussion of the need for camaraderie and the culture of the program. Unlike residents who had personality conflicts, these residents did not have interpersonal problems, but stood out like sore thumbs either due to lack of belonging or to language and culture barriers. Here are some descriptions of residents in this category:

"Cultural differences were the cause of problems…repeated communication difficulties." (non-white male, general surgery)

"Inability to relate to team concepts. Ironically went into military medicine." (white male, general surgery)

"Very poor grasp of English." (non-white male, general surgery)

Testing for race and gender effects in this case yields expected results. Program faculty were significantly more likely to describe non-whites than whites as a poor fit with the program.

Grave Mistake

In six percent of the critical incidents described we find a description of a grave mistake. In these instances, the resident severely jeopardized a patient's welfare, or in one case, actually caused a patient's death. Although not one of the top categories, the fact that program faculty failed to adequately supervise the resident's actions suggests that the program must assume some responsibility:

"Resident denied problems...wrong dose of medication resulting in patient's death, inadequate knowledge, poor technically." (white male, general surgery)

"Many lapses in safety, i.e. no flow of oxygen during induction, IV not functioning and no fluid bolus given during administration of spinal. Cannot be trusted to deliver consistently safe anesthesia. Inadequate responses to change in patient's status." (white female, anesthesiology)

"This house officer left an anesthetized patient unattended in the operating room on two occasions. I was not made aware of the first incident until after the 2nd one had occurred several weeks later. A staff anesthesiologist was in the room the first time, but the resident did not inform him that she was leaving for several minutes. She just assumed that he would take care of the patient. The staff person was at the foot of the table checking suction bottles for blood loss when the resident left the room. The second time, no other anesthesia personnel were in the room." (white female, anesthesiology)

When lives are at stake, program faculty cannot tolerate these lapses in care. But is the right response termination? What becomes of these residents who are terminated because of their grave incompetence?

Only one resident who fell into this category took a position after termination that required no additional training. Half of these residents transferred into another residency program (different specialty) at another institution, and the remainder entered a similar program at another institution. Only one resident entered a potentially unsupervised position. We are aware that only by a very fine line did more of our residents avoid this category. Surely the potential for the drug abusing and the poorly prepared physician to cause grave harm to patients is great, but it appears that there was enough coverage and supervision in the majority of cases where there was this potential that harm was avoided. When testing for a race or gender effect we find that not a single non-white was cited as having made a grave mistake in patient care, but the difference was not statistically significant.

Lost Passion

Program faculty terminated some residents because of an apparent lack of interest in surgery. We do not know if these residents had considered resigning. It could be that from the resident's perspective, he or she was riding out a difficult period of adjustment, while from the faculty's perspective, the resident did not possess the necessary level of commitment. It could also be that these residents suffered from the "wrong personality"—failing to display a surgical personality.

> "Interested in a more medical life." (white female, general surgery)

> "Indicated that his interest in general surgery had waned." (white male, general surgery)

> "Lack of interest in clinical care. Became disenchanted with WORK." (white male, orthopedic surgery)

We cannot decipher from the information we have where the truth of the matter lies—had the resident really lost interest, or did the faculty misinterpret the residents' actions? Did a quiet personality get interpreted as a lack of passion? What this category does emphasize, however, is the faculty's desire to see passion demonstrated among the resident pool and the consequences that can occur when faculty note a lack of passion. We again have a situation in which no non-whites fell into this category, but the difference was not statistically significant since such a small percent of terminated residents lacked passion.

Dishonest and Defensive

The next two categories are related. In eight percent of our cases, program directors deemed residents dishonest (the worst problem according to the attendings we interviewed above) or so defensive about critical evaluations that program faculty could not instruct these residents. In some cases defensiveness was considered dishonest since the resident failed to be honest with himself or herself about his or her level of competency.

> "She wrote up the history and physical examination of a patient that she had not interviewed or examined. It took us a while to find out that she frequently lied." (white female, neurosurgery)

> "Made-up a pre-operative evaluation on a patient she had not interviewed." (white female, anesthesiology)

These examples illustrate cases where the resident could have harmed a patient but a grave mistake was avoided.

Dishonest behavior includes making excuses, blaming others for poor performance, or challenging the faculty's assessment:

> "Excuse-making, blaming others, denial, tardiness, failure to return to clinical duty after educational activity, conflict with co-workers, etc." (white male, anesthesiology)

"Denial, unresponsive to patient care requirements, denied performance was poor." (non-white male, general surgery)

"Did not accept negative evaluations. Was angry and bitter." (non-white male, general surgery)

Among terminated residents, program faculty were less likely to label white males as defensive. Given our discussion of the culture of surgical residency programs, women's and racial minorities' stance might be defensive right from the start. Program faculty were significantly more likely to label white females as dishonest in this sample of descriptions. We will see if that label holds in the analysis of the whole pool of terminated residents.

Closely related to the defensive category is the "could not follow orders" category. Although program faculty did not specifically label these residents defensive, the residents seemed pathologically unable to do as the senior staff told them—whether this was due to excessive independence, a lack of team concept, or misunderstanding we cannot decipher from the descriptions.

Outside Interests/Events

About three percent of the residents about whom we have comments seemed excessively distracted by outside events. These events were other interests (hobbies, business pursuits, etc.), or crises that were occurring in his or her life:

"Too many outside interests, often left work early leaving patients unseen." (white male, general surgery)

"Break-up of engagement initiated by his fiancée in first six months was devastating and he never seemed to regain his initial interest although he was allowed to complete his second year." (white male, general surgery)

For these residents, these events occurred at an unfortunate time in their training period. According to program faculty, these residents were so effected by these events that they were unable to work. These residents were not offered leaves of absences or modifications in their programs, suggesting that overall performance or perceived potential was not good enough to prompt these kinds of flexible arrangements.

Can These Problems be Avoided?

In light of what we know about the process of matriculation and evaluation, and about the culture of surgery, we pose the question: could the problems the program directors listed have been avoided? The answer certainly is both "yes and no." For the residents displaying inappropriate behaviors, surely some other evaluators had noted some of the more bizarre behaviors prior to matriculation in the residency program. Better and more honest communication between medical educators is certainly needed. The responsibility for detection cannot lie with the program faculty since these behaviors are difficult to detect in a 30-minute interview. Whether anyone could have predicted the performance of the residents who left their posts is questionable—these residents had not been in positions of such responsibility before, so prediction remains inaccurate.

What about our poorly prepared residents? Our analysis certainly suggests that programs terminated some of these residents because the programs wanted good test-takers, not because the resident was incompetent. Programs need to reassess their over-reliance on the scores as a measure of competency. Some of these residents were most certainly unduly punished for being poor test-takers.

How can programs control the prevalence of substance abusers? Some modifications in the ways programs are organized could help reduce stress levels among residents and hopefully their subsequent substance abuse. But no matter how many theoretical or actual modifications we make, medicine will always remain a stressful occupation since it deals with the reality of life and death, human suffering, and all the meanings associated with those states of being. Physicians will also always have ready access to a variety of drugs. The problem will never disappear.

For the group who failed to progress, what could be done? These residents obviously had progressed at other points in their medical education, otherwise they could have not made it as far as a residency post. Understanding why the resident failed to progress in this particular setting is key in addressing the problem. If the resident is a late-bloomer, than perhaps we need greater flexibility to aid some of these residents. If the failure was due to a lack of interest, then perhaps a transfer to another specialty is the best treatment.

Personality conflicts and poor fit raise the age-old challenge of matching individuals and institutions. The current process of matriculation obviously cannot overcome every obstacle, and personality clashes appear to be an inherent part of some human interactions. The poor fit category seems more amenable to intervention. Residents' language skills need to be brought up-to-speed before they begin their tour. Additionally, formal assimilation programs must be instituted to help the residents who come from different cultural backgrounds than the average surgical resident (white male) get accustomed to their new setting.

How about our dishonest and defensive resident? For the defensive residents, some of the recommendations we make above apply here. The descriptions and the fact that white women and both male and female racial minorities are more likely to act defensively suggest that relationships between these residents and program faculty starts off as combative or strained. Programs that address the tension that inevitably exists between white male faculty members and female and racial minority residents are crucial so that these residents do not feel from the start that they have more to prove than their white male counterparts.

No matter what steps programs take, we suspect that there will always be residents who lose their passion or who become sidetracked by outside events.

We are beings who must inevitably make choices with imperfect information. Imperfect information leads us to occasionally make mistakes. We also simultaneously fulfill many different and at times conflicting social roles. Life demands that some roles take priority over other roles even if only in the short-term.

What Reasons Do Residents Give for Poor Performance?

In Survey II, we asked program directors to identify the reasons the residents gave for their poor performance (Table 5.3). We have already reviewed the critical incidents that the program directors described, but now we can see whether program directors/faculty were in agreement with residents regarding the source or nature of the poor performance.

For the 158 residents for whom we had information about critical incidents, we compared the reason (description) of poor performance provided by the program director with the reason identified by the resident in cases where these were comparable. For example, if the program director identified the resident's problem as a grave mistake, but the resident identified the problem as a personality clash, this was recorded as a mismatch. If the program director identified the problem as poor preparation and the resident cited a self-perceived lack of cognitive knowledge, this counted as a match. In many cases, program directors gave more than one descriptive problem and more than one resident's reason. In these instances, if there was a match on any citation, we counted it as a match. We could make this comparison for 104 (66%) of our 158 cases where we have descriptions. Despite our lenient criteria for matching, in only 38% of these cases did the faculty and the resident agree on the source of the poor performance. This finding suggests that perceptions are skewed depending on who is doing the observing. Because these categories are not mutually exclusive, program directors were able to identify any or all of the above as the reason for the resident's poor performance. We did find some significant associations between citing one reason and another. We detail those associations in Table 5.4 below.

Less than five percent of the residents cited any of the following reasons: belief firing was imminent, chronic illness, cognitive knowledge, or wanted to relocate. Program directors reported that some residents offered more than one reason and on average cited 1.4 reasons.

Table 5.4 tells us that certain reasons tended either to be cited together or not cited together. Residents experiencing marital/family pressures were significantly more likely to cite economic pressures and substance abuse than residents not experiencing marital/family pressures. Residents who experienced the residency program as a stressful work environment were more likely to report simultaneously experiencing marital/family pressures.

Table 5.3 shows that the most common reason given for poor performance by terminated residents were stressful work environment (40%), personality conflicts (35%), marital/family pressures (26%), and self-perceived problems with manual dexterity (16%). We will examine these different categories separately and examine the race and gender effects associated with the citation of personality conflicts.

Table 5.3. Reasons Residents Cited for Poor Performance

Reason	White Males	White Females	Non-White Males	Non-White Females	Total	By Race: Chi2 Prob.	By Gender: Chi2 Prob.
Stressful Work Environment	37% (n=41)	47% (n=10)	37% (n=14)	46% (n=7)	39% (n=72)	0.886	0.294
Marital/Family Pressures	26% (n=26)	22% (n=5)	27% (n=10)	21% (n=3)	25% (n=44)	0.928	0.572
Personality Conflicts	42% (n=45)	38% (n=8)	16% (n=6)	21% (n=3)	35% (n=62)	0.004***	0.618
Substance Abuse	10% (n=10)	9% (n=2)	5% (n=2)	0% (n=0)	8% (n=14)	0.177	0.515
Self-perceived incompetence:							
Manual Dexterity	15% (n=15)	4% (n=1)	22% (n=8)	20% (n=3)	15% (n=27)	0.177	0.348
Clinical Judgment	9% (n=9)	4% (n=1)	11% (n=4)	6% (n=1)	8% (n=15)	0.780	0.401
Occupational Hazards	9% (n=9)	0% (n=0)	11% (n=4)	0% (n=0)	7% (n=13)	0.946	0.053*

* p < 0.10, ** p < 0.05, *** p < 0.01, **** p < 0.001

Stressful Work Environment

Like resigners, terminated residents most often cited a stressful work environment to explain their poor performance. We expected this to be the case in light of our earlier analysis of the culture of residency programs and the very demanding work schedule of the average surgical resident.

Unlike our analysis of residents who resigned, however, we do not see a race effect. Whites were not more likely than non-whites to cite a stressful work environment as a reason for their poor performance. From Table 5.5 below, we note three significant associations with the likelihood of citing a stressful work environment as a reason for poor performance: the resident's ranking on honesty, his or his ranking on ability to handle stress, and the specialty of plastic surgery. The higher a resident scored on honesty, the greater the likelihood of citing a stressful work environment as a reason for poor performance. This finding suggests that the faculty find this reasoning to be honest—an accurate portrayal of the work environment. However, a match between faculty perception and resident perception was not greater for those who cited a stressful work environment compared to other reasons.

Table 5.4. Reasons Given for Poor Performance and Correlated Reasons

Reason	Correlated Reasons *(reasons in italics were negatively correlated)*
Stressful Work Environment	Marital/Family Pressures
Marital/Family Pressures	Economic Pressures, Substance Abuse
Personality Conflicts	*Self-perceived Manual Dexterity*
Belief Firing Imminent	Self-perceived Manual Dexterity
Chronic Illness	
Substance Abuse	Marital/Family Pressures
Self-perceived incompetence:	
Cognitive Knowledge	
Manual Dexterity	*Marital/Family Pressures, Personality Conflicts*, Self-perceived Clinical Judgement
Clinical Judgment	Self-perceived Manual Dexterity
Occupational Hazards	Stressful Work Environment, Belief Firing Imminent, Self-perceived Clinical Judgement

Residents who scored high on their ability to handle stress were significantly less likely to cite this reason as contributing to their poor performance. Of course, we have a cause-and-effect dilemma here. We cannot decipher from the survey whether citing stress as a cause of poor performance lead program faculty to rank a resident lower on his or her ability to handle stress, or whether program faculty noted problems handling stress before the resident gave his or her reasoning. We do need to be aware in this instance that the stress variable does contain a gender effect. Program faculty ranked men significantly higher than females in their ability to handle stress ($p = 0.007$). When both ability to handle stress and gender are added to the model, gender becomes insignificant. Some of the comments made about the women residents appear below:

"Unhappy, cried often, homesick, lonely." (white female, general surgery)

"Unable to function under stress, insecure." (non-white female, general surgery)

"All emotional." (white female, general surgery)

The final variable in this model suggests that residents in plastic surgery programs were significantly more likely than residents in any of our other specialties (anesthesiology, general surgery, neurosurgery or orthopedic surgery) to
identify the stressful work environment as a cause of their poor performance.
We had not suspected that the plastic surgery programs would outrank neurosurgery as a stressful surgical specialty. Addressing this finding would require a
more detailed analysis of the structure and culture of plastic surgery programs
than we currently have available.

**Table 5.5. Likelihood of citing a stressful work environment as a reason for poor
performance.**

	Probit coefficients
Ranking on honesty	0.2401 ****
	(0.0843)
Ranking on ability to handle stress	-0.5916 ****
	(0.1066)
Plastic surgery	0.8434**
	(0.3732)
Prob > chi2(10)	0.0000
-LL	124.67773
Sample size	243

* $p < 0.10$; ** $p < 0.05$; *** $p < 0.01$; **** $p < 0.005$

Personality Conflicts

Thirty-five percent of the terminated residents cited personality conflict as a
reason for poor performance. These residents claimed that interpersonal conflicts resulted in poor evaluations, meaning that the poor evaluation was more a
result of subjective ill will than an accurate portrayal of their abilities. Given
what we have already discussed about the role of subjective assessments in resident evaluation, it would be wrong to dismiss these residents' claims merely as
diversion tactics. Even faculty members agree that sometimes bad feelings result
in poor evaluations that are not accurate reflection of a resident's abilities.

What variables were associated with the likelihood of citing personality conflicts? The following table shows the associations. The first variable in the table
below shows that if an attending confronted the resident about his or her poor
performance, the resident was significantly more likely to report his or her problems as involving a personality clash. The interaction with the attending would
have been separate from any interactions with the program director. Residents
may be reluctant to accept criticism from attendings other than the program director. The next variable shows that the better a resident's relations with staff

members at the institution, the less likely he or she is to cite personality conflicts as a cause of poor performance. This seems to lend credence to the resident's claim that personality clashes were indeed part of the cause. And finally we see that residents in orthopedic surgery were significantly more likely to cite this reason than residents in any of the other specialties combined. As for our earlier finding about plastic surgery, a more detailed analysis of the culture of orthopedic surgery would be needed to address this finding.

Table 5.6. Likelihood of citing personality conflicts

	Probit coefficients
Attending confronted resident (1 = yes)	0.6743 ***
	(0.2429)
Ranking on staff relationships	-0.6816****
	(0.1134)
Orthopedic surgery	0.6714**
	(0.2790)
Prob > chi2(10)	0.0000
-LL	99.140731
Sample size	220

* p < 0.10; ** p < 0.05; *** p < 0.01; **** p < 0.005

The association between the quality of staff relationships and the likelihood of citing personality conflicts as a reason suggests that the resident's assessment was accurate. Can we use the data to decipher how many of these residents were the victims of personality clashes rather than inept physicians? The first thing we can check is the degree to which faculty and residents agreed about personality conflicts being at the root of poor performance. In only 31% of cases where residents cited personality conflicts did program faculty agree that this was a true problem. This compares to a 40% match rate for citing other reasons for poor performance. This 10% difference was not statistically significant—residents citing personality conflicts were not more likely to disagree with their program faculty regarding the nature of their problem. But the difference in opinion where differences do exists is telling. We present some cases for elucidation. In these cases, we present the faculty description of the resident's problem, keeping in mind that the resident attributed his or her poor performance to personality conflicts:

> "Failure to check integrity of anesthetic circuitry, inability to ventilate patients and not recognize failure of adequate ventilation, failure to discuss patient management plan with faculty, inability to insert intravenous catheters, unaware of progress of operation." (white male, anesthesiology)

"Confused, performed invasive procedures on patients without adequate indication." (white male, general surgery)

"Leaving the intensive care unit where she was assigned, not reporting to operating room for scheduled surgery, not responding to telephone calls while on duty." (non-white female, general surgery)

"Wrong dose of medication resulting in patient's death, inadequate knowledge, poor technically." (white male, general surgery)

We did not present these cases to argue that the faculty was obviously right and the resident was deflecting responsibility. These examples, however, raise some doubts about the validity of the residents' perceptions. In these instances, faculty express concern over technical or judgment matters, not about social behavior, while the resident argues that the evaluation is being affected by personality conflicts. The finding above, then, of the association between citing personality clashes and poor staff relationships may be a cause-and-effect confusion. Perhaps the poor staff relations come after the resident has tried to blame others for his or her performance. Or the faculty may use technical faults as a deflection for what are basically personality clashes.

We cannot conclude from our data how many residents truly suffered from poor interactions, although we could surmise that in the 31% of cases where faculty and residents agreed, strained personal relations surely contributed to the resident's problems. We should also be aware, however, that sometimes the "personality" explanation can be used by both residents and attendings to try to deflect negative assessments.

As noted earlier, white residents cited personality conflicts more often than non-white residents as a source of their poor performance. We believe that cultural familiarity helps explain this finding. Whites and American-born residents may be more likely to recognize the subjective aspects of resident evaluation, and therefore also more likely to see their poor evaluation as subjective bias. Foreign residents were significantly less likely than American-born residents to cite this reason. As other researchers have noted, residents' self-confidence could lead them to discount poor evaluations as personal quirks. White residents, more familiar than non-whites and foreigners with the middle-class structure and culture of the residency program, may be more likely to feel self-confident.

Marital/Family Pressures

Program faculty look for total commitment from their residents prior to admission and during the interview. But many residents are married by the time they arrive at the door of the surgical residency program and many of these residents find that maintaining their relationship with their spouse and/or children is difficult if not impossible. Among our three problem categories, 36% of residents who resigned, 39% of the terminated residents and 48% of our problematic completers were married. These numbers are a far cry from the days when residents were only accepted into programs if they were not married.

Who were the residents most likely to cite marital/family pressures as a reason for their poor performance? The married residents. No other variables were significantly associated with the likelihood of citing this reason—not race, not gender, not specialty. During the interview/admissions process, program faculty did not consider the resident's marital status as an indication that he or she would have problems.

What were the problems married residents presented? Overwhelmingly, program faculty claimed that the residents who had marital/family pressures were distracted, unavailable, or unaccountable.

"Helping wife start a business for periods of unsatisfactory performance." (white male, general)

"Failure to appear for scheduled duty." (white male, general)

"Resident unavailable for on-duty assignments, disappeared afternoons." (white male, plastic surgery)

"Often times, left hospital at wife's request and was not able to be found." (white male, general surgery)

Unless revisions are made in the residency program schedule, including flex time, family matters will continue to challenge residents' ability to meet all the demands of their workplace. The medical student/medical-surgical resident already delays many significant life events in the name of his or her education. It hardly seems reasonable to require that residents remain unmarried during their residency tour, although this demand was made by program directors in the past.

Self-Perceived Manual Dexterity

Poor manual skills describe our last category. Residents who cited this reason were significantly more likely to be ranked higher in honesty and lower on cognitive knowledge. The first of these findings suggests that program faculty see this reason as an honest recognition of a personal shortcoming, much like they saw a stressful work environment as an honest assessment of the workplace. However, while the resident cites his or her problem as a lack of manual dexterity, the program faculty see it more as a failure in cognitive knowledge. In the faculty's eyes, the problem is not that the resident cannot manage surgical instruments, it is that he or she does not know what to do when they have the instrument in hand. In the majority of cases above where we discussed residents faculty thought were poorly prepared for their residency positions, the resident claimed his or her problems were due to poor manual dexterity and not poor preparation. In fact these residents were significantly less likely to match the program director in the assessment of the resident's problem compared to all other cited problems. So although the resident accepts responsibility, the resident recognizes the wrong problem.

Why would residents cite a lack of manual dexterity? It may be that within the surgical culture, program faculty remark on "clumsiness" in the surgical theater in the most direct and emotional way, thereby drawing the resident's attention most directly to this shortcoming. It may also be an attribution defense—by identifying a shortcoming limited to manual dexterity, the resident can stay in medicine and pursue another medical specialty. A self-perceived lack of cognitive knowledge would restrict the resident's post-surgical choices.

We have found that residents and faculty agree on the cause of problems in only about 40% of cases. Agreement levels vary by the nature of the cause in three cases. When the problem is drug and alcohol abuse, faculty and residents are in agreement 75% of the time. When the resident cites the problem as manual dexterity, faculty tend to see the problem as cognitive knowledge, so agreement falls to 14%. When the resident identifies the problem as clinical judgment, agreement is the highest, with an 86% agreement rate. For the three top reasons that residents give for their problems—a stressful work environment, martial/family pressures, and personality conflicts—the agreement rate hovers around 40%. In the majority of cases, residents and faculty hold very different opinions on the cause of poor performance in residency programs.

Presenting the Poor Evaluation

How do faculty inform residents of their poor performance? The survey asked: What attempts were made by you and your staff to confront the resident directly about his/her poor performance? The possible responses included, 1) program director spoke with resident, 2) another senior faculty spoke with the resident, 3) chief resident spoke with resident, 4) the program director notified the resident in writing, and 5) change the resident's program to allow greater supervision. These categories were not mutually exclusive—more than one attempt could be reported. The summary of this information appears below.

In almost every case, the program director confronted the resident about his/her poor performance, and the likelihood of other attempts declines as we go down the table. We know the likelihood of each of these attempts, but how many different efforts did faculty make to communicate with the problem resident and did these attempts vary at all by race and gender?

In two percent of cases, no attempts at all were taken to communicate with the resident. This means that four residents in this sample were given no feedback on their poor performance before being terminated. In another 26% of cases, only one kind of contact was made with the resident. This measure represents the form of communication, not how many times. We cannot be sure in these cases where only one kind of contact was tried whether other contacts would have been more successful in altering the behavior or improving the performance of the resident in question. In six percent of cases, all measures were taken to make the resident fully aware that his or her performance fell below par.

Table 5.7. Attempts to confront the resident about his/her poor performance.

Attempt	Percent
Program director spoke to resident	97%
Senior faculty spoke to resident	67%
Chief resident spoke to resident	35%
Resident notified in writing	40%
Greater supervision	18%

Table 5.8. Number of attempts made to communicate with resident about poor performance.

Number of attempts	Frequency	Percent	Cumulative percent
0	4	2.07%	2.07%
1	50	25.91%	27.98%
2	53	27.46%	55.44%
3	47	24.35%	79.79%
4	27	13.99%	93.78%
5	12	6.22%	100.00%
Total	193	100.00%	

Do these different attempts vary by race and gender? We do find some significant effects. Program directors were significantly less likely to speak with non-white females than with any other race and gender category (p=0.003). Both non-white males and non-white females were significantly less likely to be contacted by a senior faculty member (p=0.027). And chief residents were significantly more likely to talk to white males than any other race and gender group. There were no differences based on race and gender on whether or not the resident was notified in writing, but we should note that in only 40% of cases did program faculty inform residents in writing, drawing into question whether faculty adequately informed the majority of residents about their misgivings.

These findings point to two recurring trends. As we found with our resignations, interactions are less likely to occur between non-whites and faculty members among the group of terminated residents. We also find that faculty-resident communication is based on conversation rather than written correspondence. Since we already know that relations between whites and non-whites, and between men and women, are strained within this culture, we question whether the non-white male and female residents were adequately informed of their poor performance. Just as we recommended that formal social gatherings be implemented to facilitate relationships between people unlike each other, so too should formal evaluation processes be instituted.

We asked program directors: Approximately how many times did you and members of your staff speak with the resident about his or her poor performance before he or she was terminated? On average, residents spoke with someone from the department six times. This number was significantly lower for non-whites as compared to whites—again a race effect. The number was also lower for general surgery residents.

How Did the Resident Respond?

In Chapter VII, we provide an in-depth analysis of residents' response to poor evaluations. We will give only some summary statistics here. The program directors responded with brief qualitative responses that we categorized as appropriate or inappropriate responses. We explain the details of this categorization in Chapter VII. According to this dichotomous distinction, terminated residents responded in the following fashion: according to the faculty, fifty-six of residents responded inappropriately to negative evaluations. These residents denied that there was a problem or refused to accept responsibility. Program faculty considered denial the worse offense—34% of the residents denied that there was a problem. We found no race or gender effects associated with denial. White females were the least likely to respond inappropriately, but the difference was not statistically significant. The fact that such a large percent of residents did not respond appropriately underscores our previous comments on the difference of opinion between faculty and residents on both the nature of the problem and its severity. It also demonstrates a large proportion of the residents were either unwilling to give a "good" response to correction, or did not know what constituted a "good" response in this work environment.

Ranking on Character Traits, Aptitudes and Social Skills

We have descriptions of the types of problems these residents had and we also have their ranking on various traits, aptitudes and skills. The list of traits include personality, honesty, maturity, ability to handle stress, cognitive knowledge, manual dexterity, clinical judgment, staff relationships and patient relationships. On average, the terminated resident ranked below average on all these traits and characteristics as compared to their peers, suggesting that the variety of problems the residents presented were not merely behavioral or technical, but a combination of the two. Table 5.9 shows what percent of residents among the terminated residents fell below average on these various measures. Terminated residents suffered most from poor clinical judgment, an inability to handle stress, poor fund of knowledge, and poor staff relationships—a mixture of technical, personal, and interpersonal skills. Skills and attributes that were correlated with one another include the personal traits (personality, honesty, maturity, ability to handle stress, staff and patient relationships) and the cognitive/technical traits (cognitive knowledge, manual dexterity and clinical judgment).

Table 5.9. Percent of Terminated Residents
Ranked "Below Average" on the Following
Traits, Aptitudes and Characteristics.

Personality	34%
Honesty	34%
Maturity	43%
Ability to Handle Stress	51%
Cognitive Knowledge	47%
Manual Dexterity	37%
Clinical Judgment	60%
Staff Relationships	47%
Patient Relationships	33%

Although attrition is typically due to interpersonal and behavioral problems, we find among the terminated residents a greater concern with cognitive knowledge and technical prowess than with behavioral problems per se, even though behavioral problems accounted for 19% of the critical incidents we described above. Program faculty rated a total of 39% of the residents in this sample below average on personal skills (those correlated above), while they rated 62% below average on cognitive/technical skills. The bottom line in these cases appears to be poor surgical skills.

Race and gender appear to have influenced the program faculty's ranking of residents on these various attributes. Program directors ranked white women significantly lower than all other race and gender categories on their ability to handle stress (recall our earlier discussion of women as "all emotional"). They also ranked white women lower on their staff relationships.

The Termination Process

Most terminations took place during the resident's second year in the program (34%). The second largest percent of terminations occurred in the second six months of the first year (28%). In 95% of cases, the program director discussed the decision to terminate with program faculty, and in 74% of the cases, the department faculty took a formal vote. There was little delay between the vote and the actual termination of the resident in the majority of cases.

In about 17% of cases, a hospital attorney was involved in the termination process. The attorney was significantly more likely to be involved in cases where the program director decided to terminate a white male or female suggesting that faculty are more fearful of white residents taking legal action against the hospital. White residents were more likely to threaten legal action, so the faculty's fear appears to have an empirical base.

Finding a New Position

We asked program directors if they helped residents secure new positions after the termination. The program directors provided help to about 68% of the terminated residents. They were significantly more likely to help male than female residents even after controlling for rank.

The following table shows the different kinds of help that were offered to the terminated resident and the percent of residents that were given help.

Table 5.10. Forms of Help Given

Form of help	Percent
Counseling about programs in same field	34%
Counseling about programs in other fields	60%
Calls of reference to aid in placement	34%
Letters of reference	79%
Counseling about non-medical careers	5%
Referral to professional help	20%

Program directors counseled the majority of residents about programs in other fields. Given that program directors ranked a large proportion of residents below average on technical skills, only 34% of the residents received any counseling about programs in the same field. There was no association, however, between ranking on any of the traits, skills and attributes and the likelihood that the program director would counsel a resident about programs in the same field. There was no association between the reason for poor performance and counseling about programs in the same field. We had anticipated that residents who cited personality conflicts might have been more likely to receive this counseling if program faculty agreed that this was a problem, but although the effect was in the expected direction, it was not significant. There were also no race or gender effects.

Program directors placed calls of reference to aid in placement for only 34% of the residents. This compares with a rate of 45% among the resigners. For whom was the program director most likely to make those calls? For white residents. The racial difference was significantly different, with only 19% of non-white terminated residents having calls made for them compared to 40% of white residents. We tested the relationship between overall rank and the likelihood that a call of reference would be made. When we plug race and overall rank into the model, race is significantly associated with the likelihood of having a call made while overall rank is not. Even among the poorest of performers, we find evidence of racial bias.

Seventy-nine percent of residents left their programs with letters of recommendation, a large percent given that these resident's performance fell below average. We do not have any information on the content of those letters, but this finding appears to add to the argument that medical faculty are wary of letters of recommendation. We noted no race or gender effects. We also found no evidence of race or gender effects for the final two categories—counseling about non-medical careers and referral to professional help. Note here, however, the much larger percent of residents referred to professional help as compared to the pool of resigners (20% vs. 5%).

What did the Resident Do?

Program directors reported what the resident did after leaving his or her surgical residency program. Note the relatively large percent of "no information" available, 18% compared to nine percent among the pool of resigners.

Table 5.11.

What did the resident do?	Percent
Entered a similar program at another institution	27% (n=18)
Entered a different specialty at same institution	6% (n=19)
Entered a different specialty at another institution	27% (n=35)
Took a position that required no additional training	20% (n=18)
Left medicine altogether	3% (n=1)
No information	18% (n=9)

A larger percent of terminated residents entered a similar program at another institution than we found among the pool of resigners (27% vs. 18%). This suggests that a larger percent of the residents felt that their problems were program specific instead of specialty specific. These residents appear to have been more likely to think that they could handle the work in another environment with another mixture of faculty and staff. We found no race or gender effects associated with falling into this category. We also did not find other effects such as ranking on traits, skills and characteristics or reasons given for poor performance. The only variables associated with an increased likelihood of pursuing this option were medical school rank and having been counseled about this option by the program director. The more prestigious the resident's medical school, the more likely he or she pursued this option.

The next group of residents entered a different specialty at the same institution. We expected that fewer terminated residents would be able to pursue this option as compared to the resigning residents, given that their average performance fell below average while the resigning residents' performance was above average. While only six percent of terminated residents secured a new post within the same institution, 19% of resigners secured this option. Only one variable was significantly associated with the likelihood of staying within the same institution—personality. The higher program faculty rated the resident on overall personality, the greater the resident's chance of staying within the same institution. We found no race or gender effects in this case, or rank effects. The higher performing terminated residents were not more likely to stay.

Another 27% of the terminated residents secured a new residency post at another institution. The residents who chose this option differed from residents who chose other options in two significant ways. First, they were more likely to be surgical as opposed to anesthesiology residents, and second, program faculty ranked these residents significantly higher on interpersonal traits and characteristics, in particular, on staff relationships. Program faculty may have rated these residents higher on staff relationships precisely because these residents accepted the judgment of program faculty and got out of surgery and into another medical field.

Twenty percent of the terminated residents took a position that required no additional training. The majority of these residents joined emergency room departments at community hospitals. That so many of these residents pursued no additional training is more troubling than the fact that a similar percent of resigning residents chose the same option (18%) since, again, program faculty felt that the resigning residents were performing above average at the time of their resignation. The terminated residents were not. Program faculty ranked the terminated residents who took jobs lower overall than residents who pursued any of the other post-residency positions. These residents were also more likely to be married, a factor that may have pressured them into jobs rather than additional educational positions. They were also more likely to have threatened legal action against the hospital that dismissed them, which may have limited their ability to pursue other residency posts—perhaps the threat of legal action got them blackballed. And these residents were more likely to have come to the residency position outside the official match program.

Given the sunk years of investment in a medical career, we were not surprised that only one of the residents left medicine altogether.

And finally, we have the residents for whom program faculty had no information about their post-residency positions. We find that the percent of residents who fell into this category was greater among the pool of terminated residents (18%) than among the resigning residents (9%). These residents were also significantly more likely to be non-white than white, adding to the picture of poorer communication between program faculty and non-white residents.

Subsequent Employment

We asked program directors a variety of questions about the residents' post-residency positions, including performance in new post and communication between the residents' new employers and the program director. We were interested to see how much information the program director shared with the new employer about the reason for termination.

We were surprised to find that subsequent employers sought information about the terminated resident in only 29% of cases. This low percent suggests that new employers relied on letters of recommendation rather than seek any additional information from the program director. The likelihood of seeking information was associated with only one practice setting—different specialty within the same institution. The new employer in the same institution was significantly more likely to contact the former program director than any other new employer at any other setting. The ease with which inquiries could be made within the same organization may account for this difference.

Although rarely asked, most program directors (79%) stated that they would gladly share information about the resident with any new employer who asked. This was true no matter under what conditions the resident was terminated—whether it was because of an inability to handle stress, marital/family problems, technical problems, or substance abuse.

Reports

Program faculty heard follow-up reports on approximately 45% of the residents who resigned. In the case of our terminated residents, program faculty heard reports on about 39% of the residents—not a big difference between these two groups. On average, the terminated residents about whom reports were heard were still performing slightly below average in their new post. The residents who entered a different specialty at another institution showed significant improvement in their overall ranking. This improvement suggests that the change in specialty was a good choice.

Program directors were significantly less likely to hear follow-up reports on non-white residents, since they were significantly less likely to know what these residents did after being terminated. There was a significant association between a resident's overall ranking in the former residency program and his or her ranking in the new setting, suggesting that at least for the residents about whom reports were heard, performance levels did not change very much, or employers' opinions about the residents did not significantly change. Of course, if the program director had already made up his or her mind about the resident, then perhaps no report would be interpreted as a real change in the resident. It would be more accurate to test evaluations from two different employers to measure the effects of the environment and of the esprit de corps on the residents' behavior/performance.

Program directors were most likely to hear follow-up reports on the residents who went into the same specialty at another institution. We assume that the professional grapevine facilitates communication of this kind. Program directors also heard reports about residents who switched specialties within the same institution. There were no other significant differences for any other practice setting.

We know that there is a correlation between race and practice setting and the likelihood of hearing a report, but in testing the accuracy of the follow-up report, we wanted to test to see what other characteristics were associated with hearing a report. The only other associations were the number of times program faculty spoke to the resident prior to termination and whether or not the program director had made a call of reference for the resident. These two effects explain our race effect. Recall that program faculty were significantly less likely to speak with non-white residents about their poor performance and program directors were less likely to make calls of reference for non-whites even after controlling for rank.

Summary

What do we know about terminated residents from this analysis? We know that according to program faculty there are a number of reoccurring problems among the resident pool. These problems tend to involve poor preparation for the field, a poor fit within the department and within the culture of surgery, an inability to handle stress, outside interests and events, and a handful of bizarre and unprofessional behaviors. We also know that faculty and residents tend to attribute their poor performance to different factors. With a subsample of cases, we found an average agreement rate of only 40%.

Program faculty tend to note problems early in the residents' tour and programs appear restricted in their ability to rectify the more benign problems, like needing to review the medical curriculum or helping poor test-takers. There is also a lack of flextime opportunities that would allow residents dealing with family crises to take a leave of absence and rejoin the program once other social obligations have been filled. Programs feel they can not be flexible because residents are not only students, but also employees of the institution, providing care on the surgical wards.

We also found that program faculty may not successfully communicate their dissatisfaction with poorly performing residents. There were few attempts at communication made for a number of residents, and a failure to notify the majority in writing about the seriousness of the situation. If the culture is marked in part by constant screaming and badgering by attendings, residents reprimanded in this fashion by their attendings may have felt it was more of the same, the norm, rather than a serious attempt to express dissatisfaction. We also note that non-whites were significantly less likely to be talked to by attendings and that communication between chief residents and white male residents was far more common. And regarding the number of times program faculty spoke with residents, non-white males had the fewest conversations before termination.

We found more race and gender effects in our analysis of the kind of help program directors gave terminated residents. Program directors were more likely to help male residents than female residents even after controlling for overall rank. Program directors were also more likely to make calls of reference for white residents than for non-white residents.

After leaving the program, the majority of these residents either entered a similar program at another institution or entered a different specialty at another institution. Those residents considered the most personable were more likely to find another residency post within the same institution. Twenty percent of these residents did not pursue any additional training (at least not immediately follow-ing termination) but tended to take positions in community hospital emergency rooms. Except for the residents who entered a different specialty at another insti-tution, performance levels remained about the same.

Discussion

Our analysis of the process of termination in these surgical residency pro-grams forces us to have more sympathy for program directors who must handle some bright but disturbed individuals. The public at large and the medical pro-fession entrusts the surgical program faculty with the duty to train competent physicians. In our analysis of residents who resigned, the task seemed simple enough. We could criticize program faculty for failing to reduce the day-to-day stress levels in their programs. We criticized the inflexibility of the training pro-gram which did not allow leave time for residents dealing with family crises. We criticized the medical school curriculum for not providing better exposure to the real demands of surgical training so that residents could have made more in-formed specialty choices. These criticisms were easy to make since the average resident who resigned was performing above-average at the time of his or her resignation. Most of the time there were no doubts about the resigning residents technical competence, or personality. We could lay a heap of blame on the struc-ture and organization of medical education and of the residency program.

The terminated resident, however, represents a different and more compli-cated challenge. Some terminated residents were failures of the selection proc-ess. Due in part to poor or false reporting, program faculty accepted these resi-dents only to find that they could not be trained. Program faculty found them-selves managing the mistakes of a troubled selection process. We can feel sym-pathy for the faculty when they had to deal with bizarre behaviors or poor prepa-ration. We saw cases of truly disturbed behavior and serious drug abuse. We heard claims of poor funds of knowledge. Program directors described physical handicaps that severely hampered residents' ability to perform surgery. These cases underscore the limitation of the current process of selection. The process failed to screen out impaired medical students.

But we also found commonality between problems in both groups, resigna-tions and terminations. For example, we noted a similar lack of communication between faculty and residents based on racial and gender differences. While some residents appear to be victims of poor communication, others are victims of a stressful and unforgiving environment, an untimely personal crisis, or an avoidable clash of personalities. The fact that gender and race continue to be significantly associated with so many of our outcome variables, especially in terms of communication and support, suggest many venues for reform. Even among the poorest performers, the playing field is not level—whites still receive preferential treatment.

We will now turn our attention to our third problem category, the problematic completer. Manifesting many of the same problems as the terminated resident, the problematic completer often just barely avoided being terminated. We will see how these residents avoided the proverbial axe.

VI

Problematic Completers

"He was never bad enough to fire, although some faculty thought so. I don't remember any critical incidents, but at that time, we didn't keep any records."

As we shall see in this chapter, problematic completers shared many of the same problems as the residents who were eventually terminated. Inappropriate behavior, poor preparation, failure to progress and conflicts with staff all plagued a good proportion of the residents who left their programs without the full confidence of the medical faculty behind them. The problematic completer is distinguished from the terminated resident, however, on a number of factors. In some cases, lack of documentation and lack of faculty consensus protected the resident from termination, but the major difference was that program faculty saw potential in the resident despite his or her current poor performance. In program directors' descriptions of the problematic completer, we find repeated comments about potential and good qualities overcoming bad qualities. Program directors felt that there was something redeemable about the problematic completer that they failed to see among the pool of terminated residents. We will explore what factors made these residents appear salvageable. In some of our analyses, we will compare the terminated resident with the problematic completer in order to see what saved the problematic completer from dismissal.

Problematic Completers: A Profile

Like terminated residents, problematic completers were distraught when faculty informed them that their performance fell below acceptable levels. The problematic completer, however, typically received this information with good grace and with promises to do better. About 48% of the problematic completers were married , a greater proportion than the resigners or terminated residents, but not statistically significant. The average medical school rank was 66 on a scale of one to 126. This number is higher than for terminations (71) and a little lower than for resigners (61). The difference between ranks of resigners and terminated residents is significant, but the difference between problematic completers and the other two comparison groups is not. A whopping 80% of problematic completers were from foreign medical schools compared to 12% among the resigners and only 26% among the terminated residents.

Program directors initiated 71% of discussions about problematic performance. Attendings initiated 20%, and chief residents, four percent. Talks began early in the residents' tour, but not as early as among the pool of terminated residents. Residents claimed that a stressful work environment, personality conflicts, marital/family pressures and a self-perceived lack of cognitive knowledge were the main reasons for their poor performance. Program faculty notified in writing only 32% of problematic completers about the program's dissatisfaction with their performance. Faculty ranked problematic completers lowest on their cognitive knowledge, clinical judgment and ability to handle stress. In 61% of cases, faculty considered dismissal since problems were so severe. Overall potential seemed to protect most of the problematic completers from termination.

Sixty percent of the problematic completers sought the program director's help when securing their next position. The highest performing residents were most likely to seek the director's help. Program directors counseled most residents about positions in the same field, and 63% of these residents entered either a group or solo practice in the specialty of their residency program. Twenty-one percent went on for additional training and 16% practiced another specialty.

Only 26% of new employers placed a call of reference to the program directors. Problematic completers' post-residency performance was very much like their residency performance when reports were heard. About 54% of these residents did go on to become board-certified in their specialty.

The Problems

We asked program directors to report any critical incidents that would give some indication of the types of problems the problematic completer had. Of our 210 observations, we have descriptions for 123 (59%) of the problematic completers—about the same as we had for terminations (54%). Recall that we were more likely to have descriptions of critical incidents for white and married residents among the pool of terminated residents. In this section, there are no race or gender effects. The only significant effect is that we are significantly less likely to have descriptions for residents from neurosurgery programs.

Table 6.1 below compares the problems noted by program directors among the terminated residents to the distribution of problems among the problematic completers. Note the significant amount of overlap between the two groups. Below we will discuss the commonalties and important differences between these two groups.

Table 6.1. Types of problems

	Terminations % cases	Problematic Completers % cases
Inappropriate behavior	19%	18%
Poorly prepared/physical problems	14%	9%
Substance abuse	14%	4%
Failure to progress during training	13%	13%
Personal conflicts with staff	8%	13%
Poor fit with the residency staff	8%	7%
Made a grave mistake in patient care	6%	1%
Lost passion or interest in specialty	5%	1%
Defensive response to teaching	4%	1%
Dishonest	4%	1%
Distracted by outside interests/events	3%	13%
Could not follow orders	2%	1%
	n=158	n=123

Inappropriate Behavior

The largest proportion of our problematic completers displayed inappropriate behavior that called into question their overall competency. There are differences within this category between the terminated residents and the problematic completer. As with our analysis of terminations, there was a subsample of residents who shirked their duties:

> "While on call, resident did not respond and took weekend off without call coverage." (white female, plastic surgery)

> "Late for rounds, unprepared for OR, lack of attention to detail." (non-white male, general surgery)

> "Several instances of avoiding patients in the ER." (white male, plastic surgery)

In several other cases, residents demonstrated what program faculty defined as inappropriate sexual behavior. What do not appear among the group of problematic completers, however, are instances of very bizarre behavior that accounted for 20% of the inappropriate behavior we encountered among the terminated residents. There were no cases of outrageous behavior prompting a referral for professional help. The lack of such extreme unconventional behavior among the problematic completers is one sign why program faculty considered these residents more salvageable than some of the terminated residents. It does not help, however, explain the overlap of residents who shirked duties or had sexual episodes and fell into different categories.

The last group of comments is unique to the problematic completer category. In the following cases, it is behavior outside the context of the residency program that casts doubt about the competency of the resident. Faculty caught the resident acting inappropriately outside of the hospital. In our previous analysis of terminated residents, all inappropriate behavior directly affected the resident's work. In these cases, the connection is less direct:

> "Resident arrested for spouse abuse, assault and battery." (non-white male, orthopedic surgery)

> "Walking his dog in the park against rules. Was caught by a policeman who warned him. He said to the policeman, 'OK. Just wait until you have a brain injury and come to the ER!' Subsequently he did write a letter of apology to the policeman." (white male, neurosurgery)

These actions raised doubts in the program faculty's mind about whether the resident had the proper character and morals to assume the responsibilities of doctoring. Spousal abuse by someone in a healing profession is a conundrum since the individual has pledged to "first do no harm." The second case is also striking since the resident threatens to abuse his power as a physician, although most people reading this comment might assume that the resident was blowing off steam. But in none of these cases did the event occur at work or directly involve a patient in the resident's care.

These concerns relate back to our earlier discussion of the difficulty of assessing morals and non-cognitive traits. In professions like medicine where individuals have great responsibility, people hope and demand that medical professionals display good behavior in all his or her social roles and settings. Think of the endless public debate about whether politicians' personal lives are off limits or not when judging their ability to lead. We collectively fear that bad behavior in one realm may spill over into other realms, where it cannot be tolerated or managed. Doctors therefore should be kind and good and compulsive in all situations. We care less if the office worker shouts at a policeman or beats up his or her spouse because that worker's behavior cannot affect others in the same way that a doctor's abuse could affect a patient. The vulnerability of the patient coupled with the directness of the doctor's intervention feeds our need for moral character among our health practitioners. A fragile distinction exists between the public and private in many domains of our social lives.

The fact that the inappropriate behavior occurred outside the work setting may have protected these residents against termination. Program faculty may have felt constrained from using this information about the resident in a dismissal case against him or her. When the inappropriate behavior occurs at the workplace, employers find it easier to use the information against the employee. So although program faculty were concerned about these individuals, they did not force them out of the residency program. In fact, they may not have been legally able to do so no matter what their desire.

Although men were more likely than women to be cited for inappropriate behavior (24% vs. 6%), the difference was not statistically significant.

Poorly Prepared

Program directors identified a smaller percent of the problematic completers than terminated residents as poorly prepared (9% vs. 14%). Faculty's descriptions were very similar to those for the terminated residents—poor fund of knowledge and problems with test-taking:

> "Very deficient in basic knowledge on arrival and did not try to improve. Consistently scored below 5% on ABSITE." (non-white female, general surgery)

> "General lack of basic medical knowledge. He showed steady improvement with an imposed basic service study program." (non-white male, general surgery)

> "Fund of knowledge less than average, in-house exams below average. Resident had a record of very average performance in medical school. We didn't expect to match him." (white male, orthopedic surgery)

On average, program faculty ranked terminated residents significantly lower than problematic completers on cognitive knowledge, manual dexterity and clinical judgment. Terminated residents scored below average on a combination of all these traits while problematic completers scored just average. This helps account for the lower percent of problematic completers identified as poorly prepared. We found no race or gender effects in this category.

Substance Abuse

We also note a much lower percent of residents identified as substance abusers among the pool of problematic completers, but still they appear.

> "Suspicious presence around anesthesia equipment and supplies in hospital. Encouraged to accept back in program if he successfully completed substance abuse program and submitted to random checks." (white male, orthopedic surgery)

"Some irregularities regarding documentation of narcotics use." (white male, neurosurgery)

What distinguishes between the substance abuser that gets fired and the substance abuser that completes his or her program? Residents who suffered from substance abuse and were fired did not significantly differ on any trait, aptitude and characteristic from the problematic completer substance abuser. The only variable that distinguishes these two groups is race. There were no non-whites among the substance abuse problematic completers. In fact, only white males fell into this category. The difference was not statistically significant but the finding raises the question of whether the race and gender of these white male substance abusers offered some protection against termination. The first quote above suggests that the program director required the successful completion of a substance abuse program in order for the resident to remain in the program. We do not have any information on how many of the residents successfully went through a program so we cannot enter this into our analysis.

Failure to Progress

An equal percent of problematic completers and terminated residents fell into the "failure to progress" category. The difference between the problematic completers and terminations in this category appears to be one main component— the willingness and opportunity to extend training. Recall in our previous chapter, program directors had offered some terminated residents an opportunity to repeat years at the junior level, but these residents refused. Among the problematic completers, the residents seized this opportunity. In some cases, the solution to the general failure to progress was specialization. In some ways, this is an ironic solution to the problem of failing to progress—honing in on skills and becoming a specialist—since we typically view specialists as more prestigious than generalists in medicine.

"His clinical and operative skills were poor and his knowledge below average. Was given a chance to extend residency." (non-white male, orthopedic surgery)

"Resident stayed for an extra year of training. Extra year gave resident time to reach necessary levels of cognitive/manual skills." (white male, neurosurgery)

"Difficulty making diagnoses, making clinical decisions using X-ray and lab data. Asked to chose a sub-specialty, become an expert in a narrow field. Completed a spine fellowship and has done very well." (white male, orthopedic surgery)

"This resident's problem was that he was not too smart. I counseled him to do a fellowship and limit his practice to one group of patients that he could master and handle well. Took advice and is doing well." (white male, orthopedic surgery)

Program directors in orthopedic surgery were significantly more likely to offer their residents an opportunity to specialize or extend training. Neurosurgical program directors were least likely to offer this modification. We cannot comment on whether the field of orthopedic surgery lends itself more easily to specialization/extended programs, or whether this solution has been adapted by the community of medical educators in orthopedic programs. Plastic surgery programs were the next most likely to offer these kinds of solutions, with general surgery scoring third (with extended training the most likely offer). A more detailed look at how this works in orthopedic programs might offer some insight into an important area of reform in residency education that could possibly reduce attrition. If this flexible modification becomes the norm, there would be fewer stigmas associated with accepting this training option—a great benefit for residents. It also seems that the acceptance of additional training helped prevent termination in these cases, since the resident was willing to accept responsibility for poor performance and seek the kind of intervention that could help correct the deficiencies.

Personal Conflicts

Our group of problematic completers was actually more likely to be cited as having personal conflicts with members of the staff than the terminated residents (13% vs. 8%). This may seem counterintuitive, since group harmony is such an important and desired aspect of the residency culture. The quotes below suggest that the conflicts experienced by the problematic completers were not as extreme as in the cases of terminations. In one case, the program director described the resident's actions as aggressive, but we do not find descriptions of residents who "got into fights" with staff members, actions associated with terminated residents.

"This resident was very aloof, making personal interaction difficult at times." (white male, general surgery)

"Aggressive actions towards patients and staff." (white male, general surgery)

"The problem was principally with two staff people." (white male, neurosurgery)

"Excessive criticism and attempts to show up senior residents. Resident was a precocious surgical pupil with personality that tended to be arrogant. He was devastated by loss of wife who died of cancer in his third year of training. He took it out on his fellow residents. I stayed with this resident because of his underlying abilities and he has by all reports become a successful, well-regarded practicing neurosurgeon." (white male, neurosurgery)

Note in the last description, the program director states that he stayed with this resident because of his underlying abilities, and the director gives a context in which to interpret this resident's interpersonal conflicts. This program director made allowances for the resident's interpersonal problems because of both his unique abilities and the unique tragedy.

In what other ways do terminated residents that had personal conflicts with staff members differ from problematic completers displaying the same problem? Program directors were significantly more likely to acknowledge that personal conflicts were indeed the residents' problems in the case of problematic completers than among the pool of terminated residents (67% vs. 31%). The faculty ranked these problematic completers as more mature than their terminated counterparts, as well as higher on overall relationships with staff members and with patients. There was no difference in how these two groups of residents fared on their cognitive knowledge, manual dexterity or clinical judgment. So it appears that program faculty did not terminate the problematic completers who had personal conflicts with some staff members for a variety of reasons: 1) their interpersonal conflicts were not as severe as the conflicts occurring between terminated residents and staff members, 2) program directors far more often agreed with the resident that interpersonal conflicts were part of the problem, and 3), program faculty considered problematic completers more mature and having better relationships with staff and patients. The program faculty did not have to expel the resident in order to maintain group harmony.

Poor fit

Program faculty identified a similar percent of problematic completers as not fitting well into the residency setting either due to language difficulties, antagonistic behavior, or just standing out like a sore thumb:

> "If you said it was a nice day, he'd reply that it was a terrible day. He wore combat boots to work at our county hospital. Nice people didn't like him." (white male, neurosurgery)

Although the description above is from the file of a white male resident, nonwhites were significantly more likely to fall into this category. The problem non-white residents typically faced was language difficulties.

Response to Teaching

Since program directors identified less than one percent of problematic completers as making a grave mistake in patient care, of losing passion, or charging them with dishonest behavior, we cannot provide any detailed comparative analyses for these categories of problems. We can, however, contrast a series of comments about response to teaching that we found on the survey with the defensive stance displayed by some of the terminated residents. Based on these comments, problematic completers appear fairly responsive to criticism and evaluation. While 69% of problematic completers responded appropriately to instruction by program faculty, only 44% of the terminated residents did. The difference is highly statistically significant. Here are some quotes which demonstrate these residents' willingness to try to correct the shortcomings outlined by their instructors:

> "Said he would try harder at strengthening his weak points," (white male, general surgery)

> "Understood and accepted criticisms well." (white female, general surgery)

> "Positively, tried to correct deficiencies." (white male, general surgery)

> "Concerned, would try harder and spend more time." (white male, general surgery)

Instead of challenging the faculty's assessment of their performance, these residents agreed to work harder, to accept responsibility, and to find ways to "correct their deficiencies." This accepting attitude played a significant role in protecting these poor performers from termination. Not every problematic completer, however, was so complacent and accepting:

> "Did not accept criticisms well, denied accusations and judgments." (non-white male, general surgery)

> "Reacted as though they were someone else's problems." (white male, general surgery)

Men were significantly less likely to respond appropriately. We will analyze this finding in the next chapter.

Distracted by Outside Events

A larger percent of residents distracted by outside events appear among our pool of problematic completers than among our terminated residents (13% vs. 3%). The most common distraction among the problematic completers were marital and family pressures:

"He had eight children, alimony to support. He had to moonlight and this kept him from reading of surgery. Poor in-house exam scores, wrong judgment about type of operation needed." (white male, general surgery)

"Described personal family pressures, unscheduled time away, crying episodes." (white female, general surgery)

"She left residency after 2 years of clinical training although both she and I agreed that she should stay for an additional year. The reason she left was economic, i.e. her husband went to jail for income tax evasion and she had to go to work to support the family." (white female, anesthesiology)

In some cases, we note that the marital/family pressure was simultaneously an economic pressure—mouths to feed and bills to be paid.

Not every case involved marital/family pressures, however:

"Personal life interfered with work. Unreachable at times, left no number where she could be reached." (white female, general surgery)

"He is very bright but had a diversity of medical and non-medical interests which diluted his efforts." (white male, orthopedic surgery)

Program faculty appear to tolerate marital/family pressures better than any other outside event or crisis. Program faculty are more likely to allow residents enduring a family crisis to finish a residency program than residents distracted by other interests and events. We will pick up this analysis in greater detail in the next chapter.

Potential

From our discussion above, we find these important differences between the problematic completer and the terminated resident. Among the poorly prepared, problematic completers were still better prepared. Those residents who failed to progress were offered and accepted opportunities to extend their training or to specialize. Those residents with personal conflicts tended to have less extreme conflicts and to maintain fairly good relationships with the majority of staff and patients. Program directors also tended to recognize as legitimate residents' claims that interpersonal conflicts were impeding their performance. Problematic completers were more likely to respond favorably to criticism and instruction, and residents distracted by outside events tended to be dealing with family crises. All of these factors together translate into potential. Although the problems were real and performance was lacking, these residents showed enough ability, maturity and commitment to render them salvageable in the eyes of the program faculty. The faculty hoped that setbacks would be temporary and that the resident would attempt to do better now and in the future. They placed their hope in these residents' potential:

> "Capable of maturing into a fine physician, good technical skills, hard worker." (white female, general surgery)

> "First three years of program he led his group, scored above 95% on in-service exams, performed at top of his year. Department believed he could resume this level of performance." (non-white male, general surgery)

What Reasons Did Residents Give for Poor Performance?

Program directors were significantly more likely to agree with problematic completers than with terminated residents about the reasons for their poor performance. Overall, the match rate between program directors and problematic completers for all reasons combined is 49%. This compares with an overall match rate of 36% between program directors and terminated residents. The difference is significant.

The reasons problematic completers gave for their poor performance appear in Table 6.2 below. Just as we found for terminated residents, problematic completers cited a stressful work environment, marital/family pressures, and personality conflicts the three top reasons for their poor performance. The percent citing one or more of these reasons is comparable, with a noticeable difference in the greater number of residents citing marital/family pressures. The main differences between this table and Table 5.3 from our previous chapter are the absence of substance abuse as a category and the appearance of economic pressures as a reason cited by more than 5% of problematic completers. Additionally, we note a higher proportion of residents citing any one of the self-perceived incompetence categories: cognitive knowledge, manual dexterity and clinical judgment. Recall that problematic completers were more likely than their terminated colleagues to accept responsibility for their poor performance.

Problematic completers on average cited 1.6 reasons for their poor performance. Again we find that certain reasons were correlated with each other. Residents citing a stressful work environment were more likely to cite having interpersonal problems with some staff members. Residents citing marital/family pressures were more likely to cite economic constraints. Residents citing interpersonal conflicts were less likely to cite some self-perceived incompetence such as deficiencies in cognitive knowledge, manual dexterity or clinical judgment. And residents citing any one of these self-perceived deficiencies were more likely to cite at least one other deficiency.

We note only one race effect in our table above: whites were significantly more likely than non-whites to cite a self-perceived deficiency in clinical judgment.

Table 6.2. Reasons Residents Cited for Poor Performance

Reason	White Males	White Females	Non-White Males	Non-White Females	Total	By Race: Chi2 Prob.	By Gender: Chi2 Prob.
Stressful Work Environment	39.8% (n=41)	33.3% (n=6)	31.8% (n=7)	33.3% (n=1)	37.7% (n=55)	0.491	0.658
Marital/Family Pressures	37.5% (n=39)	42.1% (n=8)	27.3% (n=6)	66.7% (n=2)	37.2% (n=55)	0.558	0.383
Economic Pressures	7.1% (n=7)	0% (n=0)	14.3 (n=3)	0% (n=0)	7.1% (n=10)	0.263	0.168
Personality Conflicts	42.3% (n=44)	36.8% (n=7)	34.8% (n=8)	0% (n=0)	39.6% (n=59)	0.452	0.462
Self-perceived incompetence:							
Cognitive Knowledge	24.2% (n=24)	26.3% (n=5)	14.3% (n=3)	33.3% (n=1)	23.2% (n=33)	0.370	0.626
Manual Dexterity	9.2% (n=9)	10.5% (n=2)	9.1% (n=2)	0% (n=0)	9.2% (n=13)	0.825	0.991
Clinical Judgment	14.1% (n=14)	16.7% (n=3)	0% (n=0)	0% (n=0)	12.1% (n=17)	0.041**	0.734

* $p < 0.10$, ** $p < 0.05$, *** $p < 0.01$, **** $p < 0.001$

Stressful Work Environment

We will examine the variables associated with the likelihood that a resident identifies a stressful work environment as a reason for his or her poor performance and compare the predictor variables against those we found in our analysis of terminations.

Among our terminated residents, the variables associated with the likelihood of citing a stressful work environment were the resident's ranking on honesty, the resident's ranking on ability to handle stress, and the specialty of plastic surgery. Among our problematic completers, the only variable associated with citing a stressful work environment was the resident's ranking on his or her ability to handle stress. The direction of the association is as expected. The lower a program director ranked a resident on this trait, the higher the likelihood of the resident saying he or she is affected by the stress. Again, however, the direction of causality is not clear. We do not know if program directors ranked residents lower on this trait before the residents cited the environment as a cause of their poor performance, or if program faculty had already noted an inability to handle stressful situations.

We do not find a gender effect working indirectly though residents' ranking on stress in this group as we did for the terminated residents. Women were not more likely to be identified as less able to handle stress. The match rate between program directors and residents on citing this reason was quite high, 64%. This is significantly greater than the match rate for all other reasons combined suggesting that in many of these cases, faculty recognized that the resident found it difficult to function in the stressful work environment that defines residency training.

Personality Conflicts

Personality conflicts accounted for the largest percent of respondents among the problematic completers. Among the terminated residents we found that citing this reason was associated with having been confronted by an attending about poor performance, negatively associated with overall staff relations, and more likely in the field of orthopedic surgery.

Table 6.3. Likelihood of citing personal conflicts as a reason for poor performance.

	Probit coefficients
Chief resident involved in evaluation (1=yes)	0.6832 **
	(0.2670)
Ranking on staff relationships	-0.6876 ****
	(0.1393)
Self-identification of deficiencies in cognitive knowledge	-0.8838**
	(0.4120)
Prob > chi2(10)	0.0000
-LL	70.838563
Sample size	148

* $p < 0.10$; ** $p < 0.05$; *** $p < 0.01$; **** $p < 0.005$

We find that the attending from Table 5.6 has been replaced by the chief resident. When chief residents confronted other residents about their poor performance, the likelihood of citing a personal conflict increased. It may be precisely because the conflict tended to be with other residents rather than with attendings that program directors considered these interpersonal conflicts less severe. The problematic completer's conflict was with a member of the staff low enough on the totem pole to make the conflict seem less threatening and less disruptive.

The next variable repeats itself in both analyses—the better the overall relationship with members of the staff, the less likely the resident was to cite personal conflicts as a source of poor performance. And finally, residents who cited this reason were less likely to cite a self-perceived deficiency in cognitive knowledge as a contributing factor.

Marital/Family Pressures

Problematic completers were more likely to be married and significantly more likely to cite marital/family pressures as a reason for poor performance. Concerns about family finances were part of the marital/family pressure. What is different among the problematic completers, however, is that program directors ranked these residents significantly higher on their overall personality than their terminated counterparts. Program directors also appear to have had more sympathy for the types of marital/family pressures borne by the problematic completers. The descriptions program directors offered were richer in detail than those provided for the terminated residents. The match rate between program directors perceptions and residents' perceptions was significantly greater. Sixty-five percent of program directors agreed with the residents who cited marital/family pressures as a reason for poor performance among the problematic completers. The match rate among terminated residents was only 45%.

Self-Perceived Incompetence

Of the various types of self-perceived incompetence, problematic completers were significantly more likely to cite a deficiency in cognitive knowledge than their terminated colleagues. Recall from our last chapter that while the terminated resident tended to see his or her problem as a problem with manual dexterity, program faculty tended to see it as a problem of cognitive knowledge. In Table 6.4. below, we present some data on the match rates for these three categories for our two groups, problematic completers and terminations:

Table 6.4. Match Rates Between Program Directors and Residents on Self-Perceived Deficiencies

Self-Perceived Deficiency	Problematic Completers	Terminations
Cognitive Knowledge	58%	80%
Manual Dexterity	100%	14%
Clinical Judgment	92%	86%

The places where program directors tended to disagree with residents were for problematic completers citing cognitive knowledge and for terminated residents citing manual dexterity, although among the problematic completers citing cognitive knowledge, the match rate is still considerable

In general, although there is ample overlap in the problems presented by the problematic completers and the terminated residents, there are also some important differences. The problematic completers appear to have less severe problems overall, and when faculty noted problems, problematic completers were more likely to accept criticisms and attempts to correct deficiencies through extended training, special tutoring sessions, and specialization. Their personal conflicts were less extreme and there is some evidence that suggests that conflicts were with lower ranking personnel in the department hierarchy. And perhaps most importantly, program directors and program directors were significantly more likely to agree on the source of the poor performance.

Now we will examine the process by which program faculty informed residents about their poor performance.

Poor Evaluation

Program faculty became aware of the problematic completers' poor performance most often at the end of the second year. The problems terminated residents presented were noted significantly earlier. This is another important difference between our problematic completers and our terminated residents. Table 6.5 compares the timing of the two groups:

Table 6.5. When did program faculty become aware of poor
performance?

Time Period	Problematic Completers	Terminations
First six months	23.46%	40.57%
Second six months	13.97%	25.41%
Second year	33.52%	24.59%
Third year	21.23%	6.56%
Fourth year	5.59%	1.64%
Fifth year	2.23%	1.23%
Total	100%	100%

Program faculty identified only 47% of problematic completers within the first year compared to 66% of the terminated residents. Residents whose problem was manual dexterity, program faculty noticed later than residents presenting any other problem. Apparently, program faculty do allow some grace time for manual skills to develop, and the degree of difficulty of tasks changes as residents progress through their training.

Again we find that program directors were most likely to initiate talks about poor performance, initiating talks 71% of the time. The difference among the problematic completers compared to terminations was the greater frequency of talks being initiated by attendings and chief residents. The fact that staff members lower on the hierarchy were able to handle the initial talks with the residents supports our earlier assumption that the faculty saw the problems as less grave and more manageable.

When controlling for race and gender, we found a significant difference in the likelihood that a program director would speak with a non-white problematic completer. While program directors spoke with an average of 74% of the white residents, they spoke with only 55% of the non-white residents. Since the nature of the problems did not differ between white and non-white residents, we conclude that this result is another indication of the poorer quality and frequency of contact between program directors and non-white residents.

Table 6.6. Who initiated talks about poor performance?

Initiator	Problematic Completer	Termination
Program Director	71%	78%
Attending	20%	13%
Chief resident	5%	1%
Resident him/herself	1%	4%

We also gathered information about the types of attempts made to confront the resident about his or her poor performance. The kinds of attempts were very similar as to those we saw for terminated residents. Program directors were very likely to talk to the resident (98%), followed by the attending(s) (76%), the chief resident (27%), followed by written notification (32%), and finally, a change in the residents' program to allow greater supervision (19%). One significant difference was in the amount of contact made by attendings, which was greater among the problematic completers. The other significant difference was in the likelihood of receiving written notification about poor performance. White male problematic completers were the least likely to receive written notification of poor performance, even after controlling for the nature of the problem, the resident's overall rank in the program, and risk of termination. White males may be significantly underrepresented in this group for a variety of reasons. Their absence suggests that there is better communication between white male residents and faculty members in general, a theme we have seen demonstrated over and over again throughout this study. Program faculty may feel less of a need to notify in writing those residents with whom they have had a satisfactory interpersonal contact. Another factor may be reluctance on the part of the program faculty to "sully" the files of the white males with written documentation of poor performance. They may feel less inclined to burden the white male residents with proof of poor evaluations.

On average, about 2.4 attempts were made to communicate with problematic completers about their poor performance. The distribution of attempts did not significantly differ from what we found for the terminated residents. The number of attempts did not vary by race or gender. Program faculty spoke with the problematic completer an average of eight times compared to six times with the terminated resident. The difference is statistically significant and is explained in part by the length of time in the program—since problematic completers by definition completed their programs, they were in programs longer than terminated residents. In both groups, those residents who cited personality conflicts and economic hardships as reasons for their poor performance had a greater number of conversations with program faculty.

Ranking on Character Traits, Aptitudes and Social Skills

Problematic completers scored just slightly above average on the following traits and characteristics: personality, honesty, maturity, manual dexterity, staff relationships and patient relationships. They scored just below average on maturity, ability to handle stress, cognitive knowledge, and clinical judgment. Comparing terminations and problematic completers on the percent that ranked below average yields the following table:

Table 6.7. Percent of Residents Ranked "Below Average" on the Following Traits, Aptitudes, and Characteristics: A Comparison of Problematic Completers and Terminations

Trait, Aptitude, or Characteristic	Problematic Completers	Terminations
Personality	20%	34%
Honesty	23%	34%
Maturity	31%	43%
Ability to handle stress	27%	51%
Cognitive knowledge	37%	47%
Manual dexterity	21%	37%
Clinical judgment	28%	60%
Staff relationships	25%	47%
Patient relationships	15%	33%

Although both problematic completers and terminations presented many of the same problems and cited the same causes for their poor performance, we note a measurable difference in how program directors ranked the residents who fell into each of these groups. Directors considered problematic completers better residents in each category. The difference in the percentages above and in the average ranking on each of these traits was highly significant between the two comparison groups.

Problematic completers scored lowest on cognitive knowledge, as suggested by the percent of residents who fell into this category in the table above. Recall from Chapter III that programs that weighed cognitive knowledge heavily in the admissions process tended to have more problematic completers. Our finding supports our earlier hypothesis that deficiencies in basic fund of knowledge characterize the problematic completer. That they ranked slightly above average on manual dexterity suggests that their problems are not with surgical procedures per se, but with the application of knowledge.

White males scored significantly lower than the other race and gender categories on personality, honesty, cognitive knowledge and patient relationships. Non-white males scored highest on maturity, ability to handle stress, cognitive knowledge, and staff relationships. In the next chapter, we will discuss how being a white male appears to offer protection against termination for the lowest performing white males among the problematic completers. The poorest performing white males in this group drag down the average among the problematic completers.

Did You Ever Consider Dismissal?

We have already established that the problems presented by the problematic completer were not as grave as the problems presented by the terminated residents, but program faculty came very close to terminating some of the problematic completers. In this section, we will examine what proportion of our problematic completers were almost terminated, what factors exposed them to this risk, and for what reasons the faculty decided not to terminate (Table 6.8).

Programs considered dismissal for 61% of the problematic completers. Although we have stressed that the problematic completers were ranked higher than their terminated colleagues, their problems were severe enough in a large percent of cases to make termination a consideration. The later in the resident's tour that faculty noted problems, the lower the likelihood that the faculty considered dismissal. In the cases of late observation, faculty expressed reluctance to terminate the resident "so late in the game." Recall our discussion in Chapter III about the sunk costs associated with medical education. Program faculty are sympathetic to the investment that even the poorer performing residents have made.

The second variable indicates that when an attending confronted the resident about his or her poor performance, the risk of being considered for dismissal increased. Having a written notice of poor performance also increased the risk of being considered for dismissal. Recall that our white males were the least likely to receive written notification about their poor performance, which helps account for the contingent of poor performing white males in our pool of problematic completers. Without that written notification, the white males were less likely to be considered for termination.

The final variable indicates that residents with good staff relationships were also less likely to be considered for dismissal, holding all other variables constant. We measured no difference based on cognitive knowledge, manual dexterity, or clinical judgment between residents considered for dismissal or not considered for dismissal. There was also no difference based on reason for poor performance in the risk for dismissal. These findings suggest that good staff relationships offered protection against dismissal proceedings.

Why did the program faculty decide not to terminate these residents? Program directors offered a variety of reasons why the resident was saved from termination. In some cases, since the problem was limited to one area of performance such as cognitive knowledge, the faculty thought the problem both insufficient for termination and manageable:

> "Good qualities outweighed bad exam scores." (white female, general surgery)

> "Main problem was cognitive, not sufficient to terminate." (white female, general surgery)

Table 6.8. Likelihood of Being Considered for Dismissal

	Probit coefficients
When did someone first talk to resident about problems	-0.2750 **** (0.0987)
Attending involved in evaluation (1=yes)	0.6634** (0.2667)
Written notification of problems (1=yes)	1.0494**** (0.2837)
Ranking on staff relationships	-0.4638**** (0.1374)
Prob > chi2(10) -LL Sample size	0.0000 76.047618 148

* $p < 0.10$; ** $p < 0.05$; *** $p < 0.01$; **** $p < 0.005$

In other cases, the resident "met minimum standards," so although the resident was not a top performer, the program faculty considered the resident a reasonable surgeon:

> "Performance met minimum standards. He honestly tried to do well and he was not dangerous." (white male, general surgery)

> "He met minimum standards and difficulties were in complex and challenging cases. Faculty believed that he would enter a low-key practice, and he has done very successfully." (white male, general surgery)

In one case, the program decided to keep a resident because:

> "Thought he would do general surgery regardless. Was safe and knew his limits. Was cooperative and hard-working. We decided we would make him the best we could. He is liked by patients, he refers cases he cannot do. He is making an excellent income." (white male, general surgery)

The faculty's response to the fear that this resident would become a professional liability was to work with the resident to make him into a competent surgeon.

In a number of cases, we see the failure to provide the resident with written notification comes back to haunt the faculty. In these cases, the faculty's failure to document poor performance prevents them from following through with the dismissal. Fearing litigation and an inability to back-up their decision with proof of poor performance, the faculty keep the poor performer on board:

> "Resident threatened suit, insufficient documentation in record to justify dismissal, felt he was unfairly accused." (non-white male, general surgery)

> "Afraid of lawsuit, inadequate documentation of deficiencies." (white female, general surgery)

In these cases, it was not redeeming characteristics or underlying potential that kept the resident on board.

And finally, a lack of faculty consensus prevented some terminations. In Chapter III we showed that the more people involved in the evaluation process, the less likely a resident would be terminated. We explained that the more people involved, the more likely the resident will find someone who will support him or her. Without consensus, a termination can appear unfair and biased. We certainly find that phenomenon demonstrated in the following excerpts:

> "Surgical department was not in agreement that she should be dismissed." (white female, general surgery)

> "Support from some faculty members." (white male, general surgery)

> "Lack of consensus among faculty." (white male, orthopedic surgery)

Should Have Terminated

In five percent of our cases, unsolicited comments made by the program director on the survey indicated that in retrospect, the program director wished that the resident had been terminated. In some cases, the termination had been blocked by lack of consensus or fears of litigation. Follow-up reports indicated that the resident was a professional liability and the program director expressed remorse at not having demanded that the individual resident be dismissed:

> "Was not dismissed because when I assumed position, resident only had seven months to go. Now I believe I should have done so. After program he went to X but was dismissed from the hospital there within two years. Then he went to Y—didn't last there one year. Had been dismissed from Z before coming to this program." (white male, general surgery)

"I should have [terminated], but he was a very bright resident with good manual skills. I kept believing his personality and psychiatric problems would clear as he matured. I was wrong, but by then he had gone too far in residency to fire him without him doing something horrible which he didn't do as justification for firing him." (white male, neurosurgery)

We also have a few cases of residents sued for malpractice shortly after leaving their programs and of residents accused by peers of performing unnecessary surgery. In all these cases, program directors expressed regret. In the two cases above, the directors were loath to terminate the resident because of issues involving sunk costs, and unrealized potential. But in hindsight, they used different criteria for judging their own decisions.

Life After the Residency Program: Post-Residency Employment

A smaller percent of problematic completers than terminations sought the help of the program director in finding employment after the residency program. While 68% of the terminated resident sought help, only 60% of the problematic completers did—the difference, however, is not statistically significant. The only variable associated with the likelihood of seeking help from the program director is honesty—the more honest the program director ranked the resident, the greater the chance the resident sought the program director's help. Some faculty perceive requests for guidance as displays of honesty. These requests also reflect the quality of the relationship between the program director and the resident.

Program directors offered the following types of help to the problematic completers seeking employment: positions in the same field, positions in other fields, calls of reference to aid in placement, letters of reference, counseling about non-medical careers, and referral to professional help. These categories were not mutually exclusive. On average, program directors offered two forms of assistance to each resident. Despite their misgivings about the resident's overall competence, program directors were reluctant to counsel these residents about positions in fields outside their current training. We also note again that the large majority of residents (71%) walked away with a letter of recommendation in hand. Program director referred five percent of problematic completers to professional help. Those referred to professional counseling tended to be the known or suspected substance abusers. Program faculty may have felt that these residents would continue to need help to stay sober in their next employment settings. There were no other variables that distinguished this group from the others.

We did note some race and gender effects in our analysis of the help offered by program directors. Program directors were significantly more likely to counsel white males about positions in the same field even after controlling for overall rank in the program. The factors which seem to qualify them for a position in

**Table 6.9. Kinds of help offered to problematic
completers by program directors.**

Counseling/Help	Percent
Positions in the same field	61%
Positions in other fields	14%
Calls of reference	37%
Letters of reference	71%
Counseling about non-medical careers	0%
Referral to professional help	5%

their field appear to be precisely their race and gender. Subsequently, directors were less likely to counsel white males about positions in other fields. Program directors made calls of reference disproportionately for white problematic completers than for non-white problematic completers. Even when controlling for only those residents who sought help, program directors placed calls of reference for 44% of white problematic completers in this category and for only 11% of non-white residents. The difference is highly significant. This race effect remains even after we control for the residents' overall ranking in the program. We found no similar race and gender effects when we looked at who got letters of recommendation, but as we have argued throughout our analyses, calls of reference go a much longer way in securing a good post-residency position.

What Did the Resident Do?

The following table shows what these problematic completers did after completing their residency program. As indicated by the table, about twenty-one percent of these residents did pursue additional training even after successfully completing a program. We do not know how many of these residents had always intended to pursue additional training, or how many chose this option at the advice of their program directors. Residents completing general surgery programs were more likely to go into other surgical training programs.

Only white males comprise the seven percent of residents who entered a similar residency program at another institution. We found no other traits, variables or characteristics that distinguished this group from residents who made different post-residency choices. We also failed to find factors that distinguish the next category, different specialty at same institution, from all the other categories. Among those who entered a different specialty at another institution, we have some significant predictors. The residents who chose this training option were more likely to be non-white than white, to have graduated from a general surgery training program, and to have felt that their problems were due to interpersonal conflicts rather than to some self-perceived deficiency. We do not know if these residents entered another residency program because they were having trouble finding employment or whether they had always intended to pursue another specialty.

Table 6.10. What did the problematic completer do after completing his or her program?

Position Held	Percent
Similar program at another institution	7%
Different specialty at the same institution	2%
Different specialty at another institution	12%
Went into solo practice	28%
Joined a group practice	35%
Opened a solo practice in another specialty	2%
Joined a group practice in another specialty	14%

The twenty-eight percent of residents who went into solo practice, a choice frowned upon by the majority of program directors, differed from their colleagues on two variables: general surgery and indication of problems at interview. Those graduating from general surgery programs were less likely to enter a solo practice, but those who had displayed some indication of a problem at the interview were more likely to enter solo practice—a finding that does not speak highly of those in solo practice. The three most common indications were poor medical school performance, prior history of problems either in medical school or in another residency program, and immaturity. These residents may have ended up in solo practice when they failed to be recommended for group practice positions, an unfortunate result of the job search process. Those who need supervision may end up working alone precisely because they have trouble working with other people.

"Reaction" was the one characteristic that separated the problematic completers who joined group practices from the residents choosing any of the other options. If the resident responded appropriately to the faculty's negative evaluations, he or she was more likely to join a group practice. This finding has the expected effect since the resident, by knowing what constitutes an appropriate response and giving that response, has shown both that he or she can get along with other professionals in the culture of medicine, and a willingness to correct any noted deficiencies.

A very small percent of these residents went into a solo practice in another specialty. Although we do not have details about this practice setting, we expect that in these cases, residents who had pursued specialty training opened a general surgery practice. For the remaining residents who joined a group practice in another specialty, the majority of these were specialists who joined a group of general surgeons. The best of the pool of problematic completers did not tend to choose any one of these practice settings over another. Differences in likelihood of choosing different practice settings were affected by aspects of the specialty and personal attributes not captured in a resident's overall ranking.

As we did for our terminated residents, we asked program directors if the residents' new employers ever asked about the residents' performance in the program. New employers inquired about resident performance for 26% of the problematic completers. This compares with a follow-up rate of 29% for the terminated residents—a comparable percent. This low percent could again be a result of the large proportion of residents who left their programs with letters of recommendation. Having a letter of recommendation was significantly associated with a lower chance of new employer follow-up. New employers were more likely to make inquires about the lower ranking problematic completers, but we do not have information that can help interpret this finding. We do not know if program directors shared some sort of "report card" with the new employer, or reported the resident's national tests scores. There was no significant difference based on any particular trait, just on overall ranking. The chance of an inquiry being made was associated with practice setting: employers from group practices were most likely to check with the program about the resident's performance. Program directors overwhelming said that they would feel obligated to be candid about the resident with a prospective employer. The only case in which they felt less obliged to talk about the resident's performance was in the case of residents whose problem in the program had been a lack of cognitive knowledge.

Reports

Program directors reported hearing reports about problematic completers (58%) more often than for resigners (45%) or terminations (39%). This difference results from the fact that a majority of problematic completers stayed within the same field of practice. New employers ranked problematic completers just about average in their new practice setting. New employers ranked white male problematic completers significantly lower than the other race and gender categories, being ranked just below average.

Whether a program director heard a follow-up report was not affected by race or gender. The correlation between the resident's overall ranking in the program and his or her ranking in the new practice setting was not as strong as expected, measuring at about 0.40. There was also no statistically significant difference in the likelihood of hearing a report based on practice setting although we should note that program faculty heard reports on every resident who switched specialties within the same institution. There was some difference based on the resident's ranking on some traits, aptitudes and characteristics while in the program. Program directors more often heard reports on the residents who ranked higher on personality, maturity, clinical judgement and patient relationships. This effect was separate from a practice setting effect.

Board-Certification

A measure of how problematic the problematic completer's performance remained can be obtained by asking whether or not the residents became board-certified, passed a national exam administered by the National Board of his or her chosen specialty meant to measure cognitive knowledge and, in some cases, competence in practice. Fifty-four percent of these residents went on to become board-certified. Among our problematic completers, white males were significantly more likely to become board-certified than any other race and gender category. This finding is not unique to our data sample, but pervades medicine across specialties and across time. Female and racial minority physicians sit for the exam at a much lower rate than their white male colleagues. The chance of becoming board-certified among our problematic completers was not associated with their overall ranking in the program or with their ranking in their post-residency position. The chance was significantly associated with the resident's ranking on cognitive knowledge. Cognitive knowledge and test-taking are positively correlated. This correlation illustrates a limit of the board-certification exam. Fifty-four percent of the residents that program directors identified as problematic completers, physicians whose competence was questioned by those who trained them, passed the exam. This finding suggests that the judgments that program faculty make about a resident's competency are not necessarily captured by the board-certification exam except in the assessment of cognitive knowledge. But as we discussed in the very first chapters, program faculty consider residents' non-cognitive traits far more important in determining a physician's ultimate competency. A resident can pass a board-certification exam without being thought of as a good overall performer by the program director who trained him or her.

Summary

The problematic completer presents many of the same problems as his or her terminated colleague, though faculty judge the problematic completers' problems as less severe. The problematic completer is significantly more likely than the terminated resident to accept faculty criticisms, and to attempt to correct deficiencies through extended training, special tutoring sessions, and specialization. Program directors are also significantly more likely to agree with problematic completers' assessments of the nature and cause of poor performance. Problems also are noticed later so problematic completers experience a longer honeymoon period.

Although program faculty did consider dismissal for a large proportion of the problematic completers, overall potential saved the majority of these residents from termination. However, we also noted a number of cases where the only thing that protected the resident from termination was the program faculty's failure to adequately document poor performance. Some problematic completers left their programs only to become professional liabilities who faced malpractice suits and who were denied admitting privileges.

Most problematic completers did go into their chosen specialty but their performance remained just about average. Over half of the residents became board-certified, but this was a limited measure of competency.

We again noted a number of race and gender effects among the problematic completers that suggest preferential treatment for whites, and for white males in particular. Program directors were more likely to speak with white residents than with non-white residents. White males were significantly less likely to get written notification about their poor performance, suggesting both better oral communication and unsullied files. Poor performing white males seemed disproportionately represented among the pool of problematic completers. Program directors were more likely to counsel these white males about positions in the same field. And finally, program directors were more likely to make calls of reference for white residents.

Discussion

The key to understanding the difference between problematic completers and the terminated residents comes down to two main differences—program faculty judge the problematic completers' problems as less severe, and problematic completers demonstrate better interpersonal skills. Program faculty's more lenient judgment of problems may result precisely from better interpersonal relationships. The faculty may judge the problematic completers' problems less harshly because they like these residents, or the severity of the problems may be qualitatively different. We cannot disentangle these effects with this data, but the analysis of program director comments suggests areas for future research.

Problematic completers' better interpersonal skills are demonstrated by their response to criticism. They show a willingness to correct deficiencies, to extend training, and to specialize. Problematic completers also differed from the terminated residents in the quality of interaction and level of agreement with program faculty. As we showed in Chapter III, the more evaluators involved in the process of resident evaluation, the greater the chance that residents will garner some support and make some friends. Interpersonal connections protect a poor performer from termination, more evidence that success in a surgical residency program depends on more than cognitive intelligence or manual dexterity. Non-cognitive skills are important for survival, especially if a resident is not a maverick whose manual skills are so unique that faculty are willing to tolerate great misconduct.

The effect of marital and family pressures on residents' ability to meet program requirements again suggests the need for greater flex-time in the training schedule to help residents trying to meet other life demands successfully complete their training. No matter how much faculty try to deny it, residents do have outside obligations that occasionally draw attention away from their medical training. Permanent attrition might actually be decreased if residents were provided with some time away to take care of family matters. Release time would have to be balanced against fears of skill atrophy. Before recommendations are made, more research on skill loss would have to be done. As more and more women enter the field of medicine, the need for flexible scheduling may grow unless we see a change in childcare responsibility at a broader societal level. If more and more men assume some responsibility for childcare, flexible schedules in any particular setting could be shared by all employment sectors and not just those with large proportions of female employees.

The prevailing race and gender effects on the possibility of termination and problematic completion continue to demonstrate the power of the male idiom of surgical work and the power of race and gender similarity in overriding measures of performance. Being white and being male apparently qualify someone for the field of surgery despite performance on a number of quantifiable traits. Being white and being male override measures of competency and maturity to give an edge to white male residents over their female and racial minority colleagues. Faculty may claim that their protection of white males actually results in more homogenous, and therefore more harmonious, work settings, but discrimination cannot be justified by claims of work harmony. These findings require a self-conscious re-evaluation of the priorities of medical education, and the forms and processes of resident evaluation.

And finally, the fact that so many problematic completers became board-certified illustrates the inadequacy of exams in determining physician competence since program directors had little confidence in so many of those eventually certified.

VII

Evaluating Honesty

"Honesty is one of the most important things. Dr. X. specifically is very dramatic and doesn't like excuses or round-about explanations." (R31)

"What is dishonesty? Failing to own up to your mistakes." (A32)

When we asked what is the most important quality of a good resident, program directors in surgical residency programs quickly identified honesty. In this chapter, we will analyze how program faculty define and measure it within the residency program culture. Although the most important trait, faculty lament that honesty is the hardest to measure. Table 7.1 shows how program directors ranked honesty against a host of other traits, aptitudes and characteristics (1= unimportant, 5=very important). Honesty was deemed vital, significantly outranking every other characteristic. The importance of honesty is not unique to physicians. We seek honesty in many occupational and personal relationships (Salovey and Mayer: 1989-90:188), but as we will note below, physician's fiduciary role makes it especially vital in our physicians.

We all share a cultural understanding of what we mean when we say someone is honest, but how do we measure that kind of quality in a person? What does an honest person do that a dishonest person does not do? And how do we assess and reassess our understanding of an individual's honesty over time? Honesty is not a static quality, but a aspect of a person's character that can change with the setting. We assess an individual's honesty over time, through repeated interactions with him or her. We usually assume that the person we are dealing with is honest until he or she proves us wrong. Program directors admit that they assume residents are honest when filling out their applications (Zaslau 1994:36). Once labeled dishonest, a tainted individual must work hard to regain others' trust.

Table 7.1. Assessment of Traits

Trait, Aptitude or Characteristic	Percent of Program Directors who ranked as "very important"	95% Confidence Interval for the Mean
Honesty	94%	4.90-4.95
Patient Relationships	55%	4.40-4.52
Maturity	54%	4.39-4.50
Personality	49%	4.26-4.39
Ability to Handle Stress	49%	4.30-4.42
Staff Relationships	42%	4.24-4.35
Clinical Judgement	41%	4.17-4.30
Cognitive Knowledge	39%	4.17-4.29
Manual Dexterity	19%	3.56-3.71

A person is supposed to be honest with others, to tell the truth. We also, however, have a concept of what it means to be honest with yourself. We judge people as "honest with themselves" when their self-perceptions match the perceptions that we have about them. People with authority typically make this judgment over subordinates. When there is a discrepancy, superiors can claim that their subordinates are "kidding themselves" or "out-of-touch." Shared perceptions create a shared reality, a stable context in which interactions can occur.

When surgical program directors use the term, they mean both types of "honesty." They do mean honesty in its most basic sense of telling the truth. Residents should be truthful when they say that they have seen Patient X and completed the work up. But honesty also means sharing the attending faculty's perception of the proper role of the surgeon and, more broadly, of the culture of surgery. This broad perception includes everything from having the proper demeanor, to sharing the faculty's view of the surgeon as the head of the medical team. It means assuming responsibility for both your own as well as other's actions or misdeeds. It means demonstrating that you are a team player that can recognize the hierarchical structure of surgical work. These are some of the qualities that a good surgeon displays, so to fill the role honestly, the resident has to display the proper attitude, demonstrating that the resident accepts and validates the many different aspects of the culture of surgery.

Honesty in this latter sense translates to a complete acceptance of responsibility. If an individual decides to pursue training as a surgeon, that individual must accept all aspects of that role, not just the aspects that he or she prefers:

> "Dishonesty...unwillingness to accept the realities of the world in which they lived, that's the major thing. Total lack of realism...somebody who is unwilling to accept the realities of what he has to do." (A12)

"And it can be very serious in medicine if you have an individual who is unreliable who should be doing something and not doing it...when you work with someone like that, you tell your superiors about them. You alert those around you that you are working with someone who is dishonest." (R30)

According to program faculty, to accept the responsibility for a patient's life on the operating table but to fail to make sure that pre-op and post-op care has been managed well is dishonest. Additionally, to not get along with some members of the medical staff may be very human, but it is dishonest. To challenge a faculty member's negative evaluation means that you are denying personal responsibility, and it is dishonest. By looking at the culture of surgery, we'll see why these infractions are both considered dishonest and grave.

In Survey II, we asked for information on the resident's response to faculty criticisms of performance for two of our groups—terminations and problematic completers. No resident gets through a residency program without some criticism at one time or another. No individual goes through any training program without getting some correction from a superior. So the question follows, how does the individual respond to the criticism? In the context of the interaction between teacher and student, much information gets relayed. The teacher asserts authority by identifying an area that needs improvement. The manner and content of the student's response conveys whether or not the student recognizes the authority of the teacher. It also indicates the student's willingness to make the necessary changes, i.e. the acceptance of some personal responsibility. And finally, it reflects the degree to which the student believes that the teacher's perspective on the situation is correct. From the teacher's perspective, there are correct and incorrect responses, which in these residency programs are defined as "honest" and "dishonest." This phenomenon will be the focus of this chapter. We will show that the nature of the reaction has a significant effect on a resident's experience in a residency program. In short, a good response signals an honest resident and can save a poor performer from termination.

For the interaction to be successful, both student and teacher need to know the rules of the game. What should be the tone of the response, how should it be worded? What should be the student's demeanor? Passive? Aggressive? A bit of both? How about the teacher's demeanor? How will the behavior and response be interpreted? How well will a man interpret the response of a woman, and vice-versa? How well will a Caucasian interpret the intonations and body language of the foreign national from India? All of these questions illustrate that a great deal of cultural knowledge and cultural mastery is involved in all human interactions. Female and racial minority residents are at a disadvantage in the "old boys'" culture when it comes to responding to criticism. They face three main obstacles: 1) the quantity and quality of interactions with faculty members, 2) the knowledge of what constitutes a correct response, and 3) a greater intolerance for a wrong response. The effect race and gender have, either directly or indirectly, on the likelihood of responding correctly or being perceived as honest will inform our analyses. The information for this chapter draws primarily on our interviews and on the experiences of 287 terminated residents and 209 problematic completers.

The Fiduciary Role

We have already talked at great length about the culture or surgery and the fiduciary role of the physician in Chapter I, but it is helpful to review some of the points below.

People typically go to physicians in the hope of getting relief from an ailment. Often suffering from an affliction that is disrupting their normal life, the patient is in very vulnerable state. Patients look to physicians to restore order in their lives. In some cases, the patient's very life is at stake.

Given the patient's state of vulnerability and the intimacy of physician-patient contact, the fiduciary role of the physician is central. Patients sometimes literally put their lives into the doctor's hands. The amount of faith that this act requires is substantial. The patient must "trust" that the doctor has his or her best interests in mind. The patient trusts that the doctor will do his or her best, that he or she will not take advantage of the patient's vulnerability. These are some of the reasons why honesty is such an important trait for a physician. With unique privileges come unique responsibilities.

Surgery has been defined as the most hands-on of the medical professions. Surgeons are the epitome of competence (Good 1995:66). The prestige accorded active interventions is reflected in surgeons' median incomes, twice the median net income of general and family practitioners (Weitz 1996: 247). They sit at the top of the medical hierarchy.

Surgeons recognize that with work involving such direct intervention in the body comes a more direct and visible line of responsibility. When something goes wrong during an operation, it is hard for the surgeon to claim that he or she had no hand in the outcome, even if the surgeon was not directly responsible for the bad turn of events. As one resident respondent stated, "you feel like if there is one false move, it's like leaving a trail of blood on the water." (R27) But the trail is not just physical; it is moral as well (Parmer 1982:2), since the mistake may be seen as a failure to fulfill the surgeon's fiduciary role. This more direct level of intervention suggests that a surgeon needs to be even more diligent in his or her work than the internist. Shoddy surgical work risks far greater damage to the integrity of the patient's body than other less invasive medical procedures.

Surgery occurs in a surgical theater, and it is not a one-person show. Although the surgeon may be the head of the operating team, he or she relies on other team members—the anesthesiologist, the scrub nurse, the residents, etc.—to perform successfully. This team aspect necessitates that the members work together and cooperate. Although stories abound of the tyrant surgeon throwing temper tantrums in the operating room, the team must still function as a team, even under oppressive conditions. The ideal is that harmony and cooperation prevail.

Not only must there be harmony among the operating room staff, the ideal is that there will be harmony and cooperation among all the staff members in a hospital department. Sharing patients and call coverage, covering for each other during sicknesses and other personal crises, the medical staff must trust that the care given by any member of the team is comparable to the care given by any other member. Ideally, each medical personnel, including nursing, should be dispensable (Zerubavel 1979:44). Each member must have faith in other members' technical proficiency as well as in their "honesty, compulsion" (R23), and commitment to providing good medical care. Some quotes from our respondents illustrate this point:

> "You have residents whom you sort of, after getting to know them, whom you trust implicitly." (A28)

> "The most important thing, no question, this one thing, actually one ingredient, that is the ability for the residents and the attending staff to work well together...I think the ability for the residents and the attending staff to communicate, particularly when they have disagreements in taking care of patients." (R35)

Group harmony and trust, therefore, are very important.

As noted in Chapter I, women and racial minorities remain underrepresented among the surgical specialties despite their increasing numbers among medical school graduates. White males still overwhelmingly staff surgical residency programs. Although women comprised 43% of the 1997 medical school graduates, only about 17% of new surgical residents were women and only one-tenth of one percent were in surgical subspecialties (Steinhauer 1999). As Kanter (1977) has proposed, proportions have an effect on group processes. We hypothesize that because the surgical residency programs have until very recently been homogenous, this homogeneity has facilitated the harmonious functioning of the resident staff and the engendering of trust. Being very much alike, the residents do not have to spend much time learning to trust, making friends, adapting to differences in speech, dress, mannerisms, styles of communication, etc. The shared context for social and professional interaction is already well in place when a group is as alike as possible. With growing diversity comes a change in the rules governing those interactions and new challenges. As Lorber (1984) notes:

> "...in evaluating the performance of novices and peers, the criteria of judgment are not only how well the person works, but whether or not the person is a trustworthy and loyal colleague. It is here that differences in race, religion, ethnic group, social class, education and gender loom so large." (ibid: 8)

Women and racial minorities have failed to enter the field in significant enough numbers to challenge the basic male idiom of surgical work (Cassell 1998, Conley 1998). They are therefore burdened by the challenge of demonstrating their honesty.

A harmonious department group, however, is an ideal that is rarely achieved, even in departments that are comprised exclusively of white males. The reality is that people have trouble getting along:

> "But if you have a guy who is a bit of a loner, a guy who isn't one of the crowd, but yet may be a really great guy. Guys like that tend to have more trouble. They don't become 'one of the boys'...they (the other residents) may use this guy as the fall guy, faulting him, and they can make his life miserable...that's one unfortunate situation where a guy falls by virtue of some circumstance beyond which he really didn't have a lot of control, but in essence he has to take ultimate responsibility because it was his own makeup which resulted in antagonizing some people...who just won't tolerate a guy who just doesn't fit in." (A27)

Being the "right" race and gender does not assure that you will get along with your peers. The medical faculty and the residents both acknowledge that attendings can be petty and arbitrary when evaluating residents. Personal conflicts do exist between some teachers and students.

> "Ten different attendings...All of them have different superficial expectations and I am always interested in the extent to which a resident lives up to my major expectations for responsibility, maturity, things like that. They get tripped up trying to meet superficial expectations." (A32)

> "Then he [program director] always finds the one he can pick on. Resident X is his new one that he can pick on now. So no matter what goes wrong, it's X's fault. I mean the poor man could be on vacation and it would still be his fault." (N18)

But even in an imperfect world, patients and the medical staff have to decide if they trust the medical resident. The patient must trust that he or she will have the very best care. The members of the medical staff must believe that the resident can fulfill the doctor's fiduciary role whenever necessary. How are honesty and trustworthiness displayed in the setting of the residency program? As these interview quotes illustrate, owning up to a mistake is the mark of honesty.

> "I think the worst residents are dishonest....Each incident in and of itself perhaps has a plausible explanation, but it is the monotonous litany, repetition of never being on target, never quite doing what he is supposed to do, always getting a different story. I think the biggest problem with being dishonest, not only with others but with themselves, is not admitting there is stuff they don't know." (A29)

"The most important thing was that you work hard, that you are honest with what you do. If you make a mistake you are honest with it. You are in a position now where you have to be honest. You're learning. I think what attendings hate the most is someone who isn't honest about their mistakes. When they're not honest about their mistakes when they are learning, they're never going to be honest about what they do. That's what scares attendings the most." (R35)

"The biggest problem with this particular individual as far as I was concerned was his inability to say, 'It was my fault.' I think the single most important factor in my eyes about learning surgery is to be able to understand when you are culpable, otherwise you don't learn from your mistakes and you continue to make them...Unable to state when it was his fault, he always had the ability to point the finger at someone else to blame for his mistakes. I think the patients paid the price for his type of care." (A33)

Honesty is taking full responsibility. No one expects a surgeon-in-training not to make mistakes. Program faculty expect that residents will accept responsibility for the mistake, and express an effort to learn from this mistake. The medical staff fears that if the resident does not recognize his or her hand in the error, how will he or she avoid repeating the error?

Do problem residents really have difficulty engendering trust, getting along with others, and accepting responsibility? Although a certain amount of cognitive intelligence and physical skill is necessary to be a surgeon, the residents in our study did not lack these talents. Less than a quarter of the residents left or were released because of a technical error or technical incompetence. Social and behavioral problems were the impetus behind three-quarters of terminations and problematic performances.

With this definition of honesty in hand, we will explore what effect a good response to criticism, an honest owning up to mistakes, has on a resident's risk of attrition and on his or her ranking on honesty.

Responding to Criticism

What are the rules that govern how a resident should respond to criticisms about his or her performance?

"A good response is, 'We're sorry. I don't know how that slipped by us, but you're absolutely right,' and then they go schedule a test for the patient immediately. A bad response is, 'Well, we were busy all day. Everyone was in the operating room. There was the clinic and it was such a busy clinic, just couldn't get out to see the patient. Those nurses, they never tell us when something goes wrong with the patients.' Making excuses." (A34)

Program faculty defined poor responders this way:

"A resident who is defensive is a real problem. Who, when criticized, can't understand that he isn't being attacked, but rather there is an attempt to teach, can be a problem." (A19)

"Any time something went wrong, she blamed someone else, even though she was the chief resident." (A25)

The responses program directors gave to the survey question, "How did residents respond to criticism?", were often brief qualitative descriptions that we subsequently coded as a dummy variable. Responses were coded as honest/appropriate or as dishonest/inappropriate. A sample of responses appears in Table 7.2.

We have significantly more information about white males on this response than any other race and gender category. While we have responses for about 71% of the white males in our sample, we have similar information for just over 50% of our white females, non-white males, and non-white females. As we noted in previous chapters, communication between program faculty and female and minority residents is less frequent and typically more formal. This finding supports these earlier observations. We have more information about white males since program faculty are significantly more likely to interact with white males.

Table 7.2. Sample of Residents' Responses

Appropriate Responses:

- earnest, aware, contrite, and apologetic with promises to change
- expressed a desire to do better
- receptive, accepting of criticisms, verbal agreement to follow advice
- always with efforts to do better and study harder
- took criticisms well and was aware of short-comings
- acknowledged the problem, apologized
- with aplomb, apology, and increased attention to assignments
- concerned, worried about our opinion

Inappropriate Responses:

- denied problem
- defensive, hostile, not insightful
- always had an excuse
- reacted as though they were someone else's problems
- did not accept criticisms well, denied accusations and judgments
- stubborn, no remorse, brisk
- somewhat shocked or at least affected disbelief
- had difficulty accepting criticisms

A Good and Honest Response

Our hypothesis states that program faculty consider residents who respond well to criticism, who accept responsibility for their poor performance when confronted by program faculty, more honest than their colleagues who respond poorly. We did find a strong association between the kind of reaction residents had when criticized by their attendings and their ranking on honesty. Program directors ranked the appropriate responders above average on honesty. Program directors ranked inappropriate responders below average. The significant effect of "reaction" on a resident's ranking on honesty remained even after we controlled for specialty, reason for poor performance, and ranking on other traits and characteristics, suggesting that the effect is robust and significantly associated with how program faculty assess a resident's honesty.

What are the Benefits of a Good Reaction?

As we noted in the previous chapter, terminated residents and problematic completers present many of the same problems. They share many common perceptions of the stresses and strains of the surgical training programs. They also, however, differ in some very important ways. Qualitative descriptions of the problems suggest that problematic completers' problems are less severe. Their potential for improvement is reflected in their acceptance of faculty criticism. Program faculty consider terminated residents unredeemable within the normal work setting.

In the previous chapter we looked at what factors were associated with a resident's risk of being considered for termination among the problematic completers. Below we compare terminated residents and problematic completers, assessing the factors that distinguish between these two attrition groups.

We have a number of associations in the probit output in Table 7.3. We will first address the effect of race. In a simple bivariate probit equation, being white is significantly associated with a decrease in the likelihood of being terminated. This bivariate finding supports our earlier analysis (Chapter II) of the lower risk of termination for white residents compared to non-white residents. So what explains the effect we note in the first variable listed here, "white," which shows a greater likelihood of being terminated? When we factor in the effect of the second variable, "white IMG" (white international medical graduate), the effect becomes clearer. Note that being a white IMG significantly decreases a resident's risk of being terminated.

In our sample of problem residents, 58% (n=56) of our non-white residents and 47% (n=150) of our white residents are IMGs. Of these, only 33% of the non-white IMGs fall into the problematic completer category while a whopping 84% if the white IMGs are labeled problematic completers. The expected race effect, whites having a lower risk of termination, is still in operation when we

control for the effects of being white and being a white IMG. A greater proportion of white IMGs than non-white IMGs gets slotted as problematic completers.
We will expand our discussion of the separate effect that attendance at an international medical school has on a resident's risk later in the chapter.

**Table 7.3. Factors associated with termination: a comparison of problematic com-
pleters and terminated residents.**

	Probit coefficients
Caucasian resident (1 = white)	0.9731 ****
	(0.3051)
Caucasian IMGs[1]	-2.068 ****
	(0.2825)
Ranking on clinical judgment	-0.5218****
	(0.1318)
Self-identification of deficiencies in cognitive knowledge	-1.2904***
	(0.4733)
Substance abuse (1 = yes)	1.5091**
	(0.7305)
Reaction to criticism (1 = appropriate)	-0.6572
	(0.2384)
Prob > chi2(10)	0.0000
-LL	70.838563
Sample size	148

* p < 0.10; ** p < 0.05; *** p < 0.01; **** p < 0.005

   The next variable, clinical judgment, shows the expected sign. The higher the
problem resident is ranked on clinical judgment, the less likely he or she will be
terminated. The next variable, substance abuse, also has the expected effect.
Residents battling substance abuse are more likely to be terminated rather than
allowed to complete their residency training. As we noted in earlier chapters, the
majority of attempts to rehabilitate the drug abuser were unsuccessful. The resident abusing drugs and alcohol is "unredeemable" in the normal context of the
residency program.
   The next variable, self-perceived incompetence, is negatively associated with
the likelihood of being terminated. This reason for poor performance demonstrates an acceptance of responsibility, which is so important to program directors and which is related to a good response. The resident also cites a shortcom-

---

[1] IMG stands for international medical graduate.

ing that can potentially be remedied. If the resident devotes enough hours over books and reading journals, he or she is likely to overcome the failing and raise performance levels.

And finally, we have the "reaction" variable. Even when we control for all of these other effects, we find that residents who respond appropriately to faculty criticisms of their performance are significantly less likely to be terminated. Therefore, the right reaction has a redeeming effect separate from the effect of the reason for poor performance, race, ranking on clinical judgment, and attendance at a foreign medical school. Now that we know that the reaction has a separate and significant effect, we will pose the question, what traits describe the resident who reacts appropriately?

Who Reacts Appropriately?

The probit model that predicts the residents who react appropriately to criticisms must use only exogenous variables. This restriction limits our right hand variables quite extensively since there cannot be any feedback between the residents' reaction and the independent right-hand side variables. This leaves us with a few demographic traits that the residents possessed prior to residency training. This list of variables includes the residents' gender, age, race, marital status, specialty choice, and medical school. For the medical schools, we have information both on whether the resident attended a foreign medical school and a ranking for all American medical schools. [2] Of these, only two variables were significantly associated with the likelihood that a resident will respond appropriately to criticism: being married and being an international medical graduate.

The Marriage Effect

Why would married residents be more likely to respond appropriately to criticism than unmarried residents? We offer two possible explanations, which, however, do not disentangle what may be a cause-and-effect dilemma.

Residents who are married may possess greater emotional intelligence (Goleman 1995, 1998). We are loosely defining emotional intelligence as an ability to read and respond to a social situation in the best and expected way as defined by a particular cultural system. In this line of thinking, being married itself would be a marker of emotional intelligence. Married people have to be good at getting along with others. They must know how to be in a relationship in which there is a give and take and a need to demonstrate mutual respect. Marriage demands this talent in order for the relationship to work.

Another possibility is that married residents respond more favorably to criticism because they are more concerned with keeping their jobs. They may "say

---

[2] Gourman (1991) ranking system.

the right thing" not because they share the faculty's view of the situation, but because they are concerned about the social and financial impact that losing their residency post may have on their spouse and children. Married residents may feel less mobile than the single resident and therefore they may be less willing to say and do things that could rock the boat. So, the propensity to respond correctly among the married residents may have been there prior to starting residency training, or it may reflect their obligations to their families.

The faculty may interpret the response of the married resident with a different lens than that which they use for the single resident. If the married resident is frazzled because he or she has been up all night with an ill child, the attending may not like the resident's fatigue, but he or she may tolerate the fatigue. The unmarried resident, however, should not come in after his or her night off fatigued and distressed, for they have no other demands on their time. We have some examples of how married residents' problems were related to their family obligations or experiences:

> A married, white male problematic completer: His response to criticism was 'concerned', would try harder and spend more time...He had eight children to support. He had to moonlight and this kept him from his reading of surgery.

> Again, a white male problematic completer who "vowed to try harder" when confronted with his poor performance had "difficulty with work load and cognitive knowledge" was able to "always scrape by." This resident "had a child with a major birth defect born" while in the program. The program director "required that he take an extra fellowship year to have study time."

These quotes remind us that the marriage effect we note above may be about both how the resident responds and the filter through which the information is received by program faculty. Program directors appear to have some sympathy for the residents who have significant family problems like ill children and spouses.

Undoubtedly, though, being married is a double-edged sword for the medical or surgical resident. Being married suggests that the resident has other demands on his or her time that are not part of the training program. The married resident must answer to someone who is not a colleague or patient. Program faculty look unfavorably on this additional obligation in the resident's life. This example illustrates that well:

> A white female problematic completer: "Resident had three pregnancies during her training and had interrupted training due to pregnancy leave-of-absences. Her inservice scores lagged behind where she should have been because of *split loyalties* (italics mine). She always rated satisfactory in CCC, but didn't meet our expectations especially in the area of didactic knowledge...She is bright and had adequate promise...but she never reached her full potential. Initially I

thought she had great potential for an academic career and so did she. Pregnancy altered her career goals and I supported that change."

Being married may cause the resident to have troubles, but, luckily, being married also appears to buffer how those troubles are managed and perceived.

If being married offers some protection against termination, than the white women in our sample would be significantly less likely to reap the benefits, since they were significantly less likely to be married than any other race and gender group. We have examples of women and men struggling with troubled pre-marital relationships, but program directors showed more tolerance for marital hardships than romantic hardships. Since white women were more likely to be in pre-marital relationships, program faculty viewed their relationship troubles more disparagingly.

The International Medical Graduate (IMG) Effect

The other variable associated with the likelihood of giving an appropriate response was having been a graduate of an international medical school (IMG). Why would this factor be significant? It may be that international medical graduates are much more willing than their American-educated colleagues to admit that they are not well prepared for the rigors of residency training. They may be more self-aware than their American-trained colleagues that they are behind in the basics. This self-awareness may make it much easier for these residents to accept fuller responsibility for their poor performance. We have already stated that accepting personal responsibility is a good response. Graduates from American medical schools may feel just the opposite—that they are well prepared. Their self-confidence and accomplishments thus far may make it harder for these residents to admit to holes in their medical knowledge or training. Being one step behind may have its advantages for the IMG.

The medical faculty admits some IMGs fully aware that their training will have been less rigorous and thorough than their American-trained counterparts. This may actually lead the medical faculty to view the problems that the foreign-trained residents have with more forgiveness than they view the same shortcomings displayed by the American graduate. They may tolerate poor basic knowledge from the graduate of Kaosiung Medical College more readily than they will tolerate the same lapse from the Harvard graduate. Here again we note that the issue may not only be one of presentation by the resident but also of perception by the program faculty.

We must also note that among the IMG population we also have a race effect. Of the 152 residents who responded well to criticism, 89 or 58% of the good responders were IMGs. Of those 89 residents, 79 (84%) were white IMGs. Although attendance at a foreign medical school has a significant effect, it probably is also true that being white in a white-dominated professional domain helps these residents to know what constitutes an appropriate response and to give it accordingly. For white residents, familiarity with American professional cultures helps them to know what to say when they are confronted with criticisms. All of these factors together—race, the view and perspective of the medical faculty, and the willingness of the IMG to admit that he/she is behind—probably contribute to increasing the likelihood that the resident gives the right response.

Other Traits of the Good Responder

Although "married" and "IMG" were the only exogenous variables associated with responding appropriately, other associations provide a richer picture of how reactions correlate with perceptions of residents as honest or dishonest.

In Survey II, we asked program directors to rank residents on a variety or traits, aptitudes and characteristics. Since we must assume that there is feedback between how residents are ranked on this items and how they interact with program faculty, we are limited to looking at the association between these attributes and the resident's reaction to criticism. After testing for differences between the good and poor responders, we will see if there are any lingering race and gender effects. Program directors used a five-point scale to rate these items with "1" indicating that the resident was unacceptable compared to his or her peers, and "5" if the resident was considered outstanding. We show the differences in Table 7.4 below.

In only two cases do the residents who gave good responses not significantly differ from the residents who gave poor responses. These two areas are cognitive knowledge and manual dexterity. These findings suggest that interpersonal skills significantly distinguish between the good and poor responders. The most striking differences are between the scores on personality, honesty, maturity, staff relationships and patient relationships.

Also note that the program directors ranked good responders highest on honesty (3.404). These residents score significantly higher on honesty than on any other trait other than patient relationships. This finding supports our belief that program directors judge residents' honesty in part based on the content of their interactions with residents.

We can also compare the reasons good and poor responders gave for their poor performance. We see in Table 7.5 some significant differences. The residents that program directors deemed poor responders tended to offer different explanations from the good responders. The fact that there are these differences suggests that directors consider some reasons poor reasons. Program faculty do not accept some reasons as reasonable explanations for substandard performance even if these reasons might be reasonable in other professional or social settings. The reasons these explanations are not acceptable directly relate to the structure and operation of the surgical culture.

Table 7.4. Differences in Average Ranking on Various Traits, Aptitudes and Characteristics by Whether the Resident Gave a Good or Poor Response

Trait, Aptitude or Characteristic	Good Responders (n=156)	Poor Responders (n=126)	P-value for Difference[3]
Personality	3.212	2.524	0.000
Honesty	3.404	2.500	0.000
Maturity	2.955	2.395	0.000
Ability to handle stress	2.710	2.378	0.004
Cognitive knowledge	2.635	2.724	0.501
Manual dexterity	2.929	2.825	0.412
Clinical judgment	2.613	2.378	0.043
Staff relationships	3.083	2.228	0.000
Patient relationships	3.327	2.595	0.000

Table 7.5. Differences in the Percent of Residents Who Cited the Following Reasons for Poor Performance by Good and Poor Responders.

Reason for Poor Performance	Good Responders	Poor Responders	P-value for difference
Stressful work environment	41.22%	38.53%	0.6735
Marital/family pressures	38.58%	24.04%	0.0184
Economic pressures	6.50%	7.00%	0.8837
Personality conflicts with one or more faculty members	25.38%	60.75%	0.0000
Belief that firing was imminent	5.65%	2.02%	0.1733
Chronic illness	2.44%	5.10%	0.2945
Substance abuse	5.69%	10.10%	0.2212
Self-perceived deficiencies in:			
Cognitive knowledge	18.40%	8.08%	0.0263
Manual dexterity	17.32%	7.00%	0.0207
Clinical judgment	17.46%	7.92%	0.0350
Self-perceived deficiency	30.00%	13.39%	0.0008

The first reason significantly more likely to be offered by the good responder than the poor responder is marital/family pressures. We noted earlier that married residents are more likely to respond appropriately. We also noted that faculty appear to tolerate shortcomings caused by family pressures and commitments.

The next significant difference is the percent of poor responders who cite personality conflicts as a reason for poor performance. A very large percent (almost 61%) of poor responders cite this reason as compared to only about 26% of good responders. In our analysis of residency culture, we noted a need for good working relationships in the department. Personality conflicts threaten the harmony of the department. The staff member who is not getting along, or who uses interpersonal conflicts as an excuse, disrupts the community.

---

[3] Ho: mean(poor responders) – mean (good responders) = 0. T-test was performed on the difference of the means.

We also note a significant difference in the percent of good responders who cite a self-perceived deficiency in cognitive knowledge, manual dexterity or clinical judgment. We also created a fourth variable that tests the effect of citing any one of these as a reason. These reasons directly coincide with our earlier discussion of accepting responsibility. Program faculty encourage the acceptance of responsibility for poor performance, especially the acceptance of correctable deficiencies.

Honest Responses

Some of the reasons residents gave for their poor performance were not only associated with a good or bad response, they were also associated with a resident's ranking on honesty, providing additional strength to our suggestion that program faculty consider some reasons more or less honest, more or less reasonable, within the cultural setting of a surgical residency program. Faculty did not consider residents who cited marital/family pressures as a reason for poor performance more honest than their colleagues who did not cite this reason. We do, however, find very significant relationships between citing personality conflicts and honesty, and citing some self-perceived deficiency and honesty.

Program directors ranked residents who cited personality conflicts as an explanation for poor performance significantly lower on honesty (2.52) than their counterparts, who ranked slightly above average (3.24)[4]. This finding supports our proposition that program directors consider blaming poor performance on bad relations with other staff members less than honest, and not valid. On the flip side, directors ranked residents who cited some self-perceived deficiency as a reason for their poor performance higher on honesty (3.71) than those who did not cite this reason (2.82).

Are there any race and gender effects working indirectly through these findings? We find a race effect for two of our above findings. Whites (42%) were more likely than non-whites (23%) to cite personality conflicts as a reason for poor performance. White males in particular were more likely than any other race and gender group to cite this reason. However, on the flip side, it was true that whites (15%) were more likely than non-whites (5%) to cite self-perceived deficiencies as a reason for their poor performance, especially deficiencies in cognitive knowledge. Whites appear to have some advantage in knowing how to explain their poor performance, even if they are also more likely to challenge the authority of the medical faculty, claiming that poor interpersonal relations were the root of their problem.

---

[4] Scale was 1=unsatisfactory, 2=below average, 3=average, 4=above average, and 5=outstanding.

Tolerating White Males' Poor Responses

In our full probit model predicting the likelihood of termination, we did not see a direct gender effect even though in a simple bivariate equation, white males were significantly less likely to be terminated than the other race and gender categories combined. While the race effect is prevalent in the full model, the gender effect appears to work through other variables such as clinical judgment, a trait where men have historically outperformed women.

A review of the reaction variable, however, also revealed another significant effect. Among the poor responders, white males were significantly less likely to be terminated. This effect held even after we controlled for overall ranking, as well as ranking on two significant variables: ranking on clinical judgment and quality of staff relationships (see Table 7.6). Among the group of poor responders, even after we control for ranking on clinical judgment and staff relationships (or overall ranking), the "white male" effect is still significant. This finding suggests that members of the medical faculty are more likely to tolerate poor responses when white males make them. A subset of white males appears protected against the negative effect of a poor response, a protection not shared by the other three race and gender groups, even those who ranked as high as the white males on clinical judgment and staff relationships. Among the 89 white males who responded poorly to their evaluations, only 61% were eventually terminated. Among the other race and gender groups, 81% of poor responders were eventually terminated, a significant difference. Note the absence of a "white male" effect among the pool of good responders.

What form did this tolerance take? Excerpts from the surveys give more detailed insight into this phenomenon. In some of the cases, program directors appear reluctant to fire some of the white male poor responders because the residents were basically well-liked:

> Resident's reaction was one of "denial" but the "academic committee refused to terminate because resident was 'such a nice guy.'"

> Another white male responded "defensively." He was described as "technically inept, poor fund of knowledge, untruthful, tried to cover incompetence with over subservience." He was not fired because he was a "*pleasant fellow* (italics mine) but slow on the pick-up and lacked talent."

In some cases, consensus could not be reached.

> One white male responded to criticism "as though they were someone else's problems" but he was not terminated because "evaluations were uneven."

> This resident reacted to criticism with "total innocence." He "had no idea that he was offending his peers and he had a perfect excuse for the two or three in-

stances that happened—that gave us some cause for concern. He was always 'blameless.'...Approximately 10% of staff thought he should be terminated."

Table 7.6. Likelihood of termination controlling for poor response.

A. Poor Responders	Probit coefficients
Caucasian males (1 = white male)	-0.6663**
	(0.3007)
Ranking on clinical judgment	-0.4663****
	(0.1457)
Ranking on staff relationships	-0.3609**
	(0.1447)
Prob > chi2(10)	0.0000
-LL	64.535751
Sample size	126

* p < 0.10; ** p < 0.05; *** p < 0.01; **** p < 0.005

B. Good Responders	Probit coefficients
Caucasian males (1 = white male)	0.0896
	(0.2437)
Ranking on clinical judgment	-0.5979****
	(0.1329)
Ranking on staff relationships	-0.2075*
	(0.1153)
Prob > chi2(10)	0.0000
-LL	87.804863
Sample size	155

* p < 0.10; ** p < 0.05; *** p < 0.01; **** p < 0.005

In other cases, program directors sought help for these residents rather than terminate them.

Resident who reacted "defensively" and who had "poor OITE scores:" was sent to "an orthopedic review course to try to help him."

Another reacted "negatively" to correction, and the staff decided to seek "psychiatric help for him. We felt he could continue with counseling."

In some other cases, program faculty kept the resident due to manpower shortages or to a lack of documentation against the resident. Recall from our previous chapter our discussion of the reluctance to give white males written notification of poor performance. Lack of documentation appears to have left the programs open to legal action that residents threatened in a few cases.

> Resident "did not acknowledge problem." He was "impossible to deal with." He was not terminated because program "needed him to finish, no one else in PGY4 year."

> Resident was "arrogant, did not admit problem." He was not terminated because program "did not have replacement for PGY5 year. He was competent...he just had an extremely difficult personality."

> Resident "denied problems" but program faculty was "unable to prove problem."

> The resident was "angry" when confronted with poor reviews of his performance. He was always "arguing with attendings, always had an excuse for everything, denied any wrongdoing when he had complications." (Why not terminate?) "All the facts were not clearly documented. Resident threatened to litigate."

Most disturbing in all these examples are the cases in which the resident appears to "get away" with fairly gross misconduct with little consequence for his misdeed:

> Resident "felt I (program director) was overcritical." Problem was "patient complained of fondling during an exam."

> Another resident "denied" poor performance. His "work was not done and he fabricated information." He was not fired because he had come with "good recommendations."

> This resident responded "very defensively" to criticism. "Resident had poor relationship with some attendings. Antagonized other residents from other specialties. Two weeks before completion of program, he was found to have falsified medical records. "He was not terminated because 'major incident occurred two weeks before the end of residency.'"

In a few instances, the program director expressed "regret" for not having fired the problematically performing resident precisely because the resident ran into trouble soon after leaving the residency program.

> This resident was "somewhat unaware that he had problems, thought he was picked on and not liked." He would "invariably...pick an inappropriate surgical plan for the patient's problem. He also had poor technical judgment—took forever on simple tasks and rushed on difficult cases." "Resident was sued in first six months of practice."

We have far fewer comments for our white female and racial minority male and female residents, but we will include the comments we have for comparison. In the case of one non-white male and one white female, although these residents responded poorly to criticism, there was no consensus for dismissal. In two other cases of non-white males, although they responded poorly, the faculty thought the residents had potential, especially one resident who had for "the first three years, scored in the 95% percentile on his in-house exams." And in another case of a non-white male, the resident was not terminated because of "insufficient documentation" of problems. In no cases for our female residents and racial minority residents do we find cases where the poor responder was not dismissed because he or she was a "nice person" or in which help was sought for the resident in the form of some sort of counseling service. We do, however, have one case of gross misconduct by a white female resident that appears to go unpunished:

> This resident was "counseled and warned regularly. She had difficulty accepting criticism. Inadequate evaluation and failure to recognize problem contributed to death of a patient. Frequently failed to call staff when in trouble. Frequently demonstrated poor equipment selection and preparation. Never seemed to accept the fact that her performance was problematic. Surprisingly, department never thought to dismiss her."

Discussion

Our analysis above shows that a good reaction goes a long way in helping the resident with problems present himself or herself as redeemable. An honest resident, when confronted by claims of substandard performance, apologizes for the poor performance, promises to try harder and to do better, and agrees with the faculty's assessment of the situation. The dishonest resident blames his or her poor performance on interpersonal conflicts, on aspects of the training program, or on the incompetence of other staff members. Dishonest residents challenge the faculty's perception of the mistake and of the source of the poor performance.

What characterizes the good responder? Our data show that the good responder is more likely to be a white international medical graduate, and more likely to be married. The good responder outranks his or her colleagues on a number of interpersonal traits including personality, honesty, maturity, ability to handle stress, and staff and patient relationships. The good responder is more likely to cite marital/family pressures and some self-perceived deficiency in cognitive knowledge, manual dexterity and clinical judgment as a reason for his or her poor performance. The good responder is less likely to cite interpersonal conflicts as an excuse for poor performance.

As we hypothesized in the beginning of this analysis, knowing what constitutes a "good" response involves knowing a bit about the culture and what denotes an acceptable exchange. Our description of a good responder certainly shows a race effect. Whites are better at responding appropriately and knowing what constitutes a valid and acceptable explanation for poor performance than their non-white colleagues. They are, however, also more likely to cite interpersonal conflicts, an unacceptable excuse. White males are uniquely protected against the consequences of a poor response since we have shown that program faculty are more likely to tolerate poor responses when made by white males. Whites in general have an advantage, and white males have an advantage whether they respond appropriately or not.

In order to benefit from a good response, the resident has to have some kind of contact with the medical faculty. We have repeatedly shown throughout our analyses that women and racial minorities were less likely than their white male counterparts to interact with the medical faculty. If these contacts do not happen, the benefit cannot be reaped.

In light of these race and gender effects, is the medical faculty's assessment of such an elusive quality as honesty fair and just? We can all agree with program directors that given the tremendous amount of privilege and responsibility physicians have, a goodly amount of honesty is vital. We can also agree that evaluating honesty is a difficult process. We rely heavily on the quality of our interactions with people to judge their honesty—diversity undoubtedly makes this process more challenging. The hope of the medical faculty is that if the resident accepts blame for poor performance, he or she will always be able to proactively improve his or her performance. The acceptance of responsibility suggests that the resident will be able, now and after he or she leaves the residency program, to work with different staff members, at different institutions, with incomplete medical knowledge, etc.—in short, in the uncertain and ever-changing world of medicine and surgery—and still find a way to get the job done. The resident will always strive to fulfill his or her fiduciary obligations. This is a high and admirable standard, but it discounts some real and formidable challenges that a resident can face in training.

We noted that many of our respondents acknowledged that the ideal residency setting does not exist. Our respondents recognized that interpersonal conflicts do exist, that lack of support can hamper performance, and negative evaluations may just be wrong. These were not rare insights, but realities recognized by many of those we interviewed. Abuse, arbitrariness, and personality contests are a part of the reality of the world of surgical residency programs.

An inappropriate response may very well signal that a resident does not have what it takes to become a competent surgeon. Denial and defense do signal an unwillingness to accept responsibility, to learn from mistakes, and to accept instruction. But the data has repeatedly shown that residents' race and gender help determine the failures of these subjective evaluations. The fact that race and gender remain significant even after we control for a variety of intervening factors suggests that program directors are not effectively weeding out the morally deficient and incompetent from their ranks, they are practicing discrimination. A little less tolerance for the misconduct of the white male residents could be balanced out with greater attempts to interact with the women and racial minorities who are undertaking surgical training in an environment in which they remain largely underrepresented.

VIII

Conclusion

When an individual seeks to join a group or organization, how do the members of that organization measure the individual's goodness of fit? And how does the individual assess whether or not he or she made the right choice in seeking membership? When a resident joins a program, what factors predict whether or not he or she will be judged a "good fit" and successfully complete the program? What predicts whether that individual will be disenchanted and decide to leave to pursue another path of training? These are some of the questions we raised in our study of surgical residency programs.

As the questions above demonstrate, the decision to stay or go involves a complicated interplay between the members of the group and the initiate. Both must decide whether to begin and complete the process of initiation. As we have shown in our analysis of the three different study groups, residents can chose to end the process, or faculty can force residents to leave.

In order to understand this interplay, we need to analyze the culture and structure of the organization that a new member wishes to join. This analysis provides information as to why an individual succeeds or fails. It also provides us with information on what traits and characteristics established group members desire in a newcomer as we study the process of selection. In our analysis of the culture of surgery, we noted many factors that would make it hard for any individual to complete the training program. Doctors in general and surgeons in particular work long and hard. The period of training can span a decade when both medical school and residency training are counted. Medical educators look for total commitment from residents and consider outside distractions problematic. It is hard for anyone to commit himself or herself exclusively to one social or occupational role over such a long time period. The demand for total commitment and dedication is one way in which the residency program is like a total institution. Residency programs become changing houses, immersing the resident into the new role of physician. Despite legal restrictions on working more than 100 hours a week, many residents find that they rarely leave the hospital setting. Residents find maintaining the momentum to work these long and hard hours difficult. The timing of this arduous tour occurs during these young men and women's peak childbearing years, presenting great challenges to residents who want to try to start their families during this time.

The long and hard hours are not the only challenging aspects of surgical residency programs. Physicians also assume a great level of responsibility by the very nature of their work. Cutting into flesh, literally taking lives into your hands, requires not only a great deal of self-confidence on the part of the surgeon, but also a great deal of personal responsibility. We grant physicians access to our bodies when we are at some of our most vulnerable states. We expect that in exchange for this great trust, our physicians will do everything possible to help us and will not abuse their positions of power. Accepting this level of responsibility day after day, even in the face of tragedy, requires great stamina.

All physicians have a fiduciary role, but the surgeon is granted the most direct access to our bodies. As we discussed in Chapter I, maleness has traditionally characterized the idiom of surgical work. It is bantered about in the literature (and in modern medical tales on television) that the surgeon must be a highly aggressive, stoic, self-confident individual in order to cut into and rearrange the human body. The desired traits and characteristics of the surgeon have been the traditional traits and characteristics of men. In many ways, the current idiom of surgical work remains quite male. This idiom poses unique challenges to females entering the profession.

But long hours, great responsibility, and maleness themselves do not compete the picture. The way that a medical or surgical department functions in a hospital also requires great camaraderie and trust in order for the hospital team to work effectively together. Patients must trust their doctors, but doctors must also trust each other, especially when coordinating care in a hospital-based medical or surgical department where physicians constantly call upon each other for assistance and patient coverage. We made the argument that homogeneous groups find it easier to develop friendships and trust. Diversity among the medical school population necessitates that these residency programs will eventually become more diversified, but even today, program directors find that they can feed their appetite for white males in the selection of surgical residents. White males have a much higher match rate than any other race and gender group among the surgical specialties and women and minorities remain underrepresented among the ranks.

Given this description of the culture of surgical residency programs, we can look at how newcomers both chose and are chosen into these communities. As we covered in Chapter II, residents often choose a specialty before having extensive exposure to the nature of the work. This imperfect knowledge already creates a potential for disappointment once the resident actually undertakes the work. But imperfect or not, medical school students do make choices and apply for positions in various residency programs. We found little information on how these medical students make their choices, but like other occupational settings, tradition seems to have some effect. Females are more likely to enter specialties where there are more women, and men tend to choose specialties still dominated by men.

We did find and gather more information on what program faculty looks for when choosing residents to join their programs. First and foremost, they make choices about potential candidates from grade point averages and test scores. They cull the stack by choosing the brightest of the group as measured by standardized test scores. But intelligence is a necessary but insufficient trait. Program directors stated that non-cognitive traits were far more important than cognitive knowledge, manual dexterity and clinical judgment in making a good physician. But how do program faculty assess these non-cognitive traits from standard application packets and misleading letters of recommendation? Faculty members hope that they will be able to assess these traits during the interview.

Why are non-cognitive traits so vital? As noted above, the department needs to work as a team, both on the floor and in the operating theater. Members of the faculty want to choose newcomers who will fit in with the people that already staff the department and this is a matter of interpersonal relations. The process of choosing the next cohort of residents is akin to matching the new residents' personalities with the department's personality—not an easy task, and one that is terribly resistant to standardization. How can the spirit of the community, the myriad of relationships both among and between attendings, residents, nurses, and other support personnel be described, enumerated or characterized, and how can faculty assess whether the newcomer will fit into that myriad of relationships?

From this process of choosing newcomers, we already see potential challenges to some candidates. The first challenge is that poor test takers may not be considered. This criteria for making the first cut unfairly taxes the poor test taker which seems unwarranted given that study after study has failed to find an association between test performance and eventual performance as a practicing physician. Some of the best candidates in terms of potential may never be considered, especially minority students who on average and across areas of study perform less well than their white colleagues on standardized tests. Our study also suggests that poor test-takers are at greater risk for attrition because program's ranking is based in part on resident's scores on standardized tests.

The next challenge is in matching the newcomer to the intangible personality of the department. As described in detail in Chapter II, programs typically have one day to share with a prospective resident. Each member of the faculty only has about 30 minutes to speak with the candidate. In this short amount of time, the faculty finds the task of assessing whether or not the candidate will fit in almost impossible.

But choose they do and each year, a new cohort of residents takes their positions in residency programs across the country, but not all these residents finish their tours. In the surgical residency programs, about ten percent of that new cohort will not complete the program, most of whom either leave or are dismissed within the first year. As noted before, white women and racial minority residents' risk of attrition is far greater than that faced by the white male resident.

Why do these chosen fail to complete the training program? We noted in Chapter III that some attrition is the outcome of the particular structure of the program. For example, larger programs have greater attrition even after controlling for social activities, hospital size, specialty, etc. The number and type of evaluators also had different effects on the type of outcome observed. The more people involved in the process, the greater the chance of identifying problematic completers and the less chance of termination. There was also a specialty effect that suggested some interaction among knowledge and experience prior to beginning residency training, the actual experience of surgical work, and attrition.

Program directors in general were surprised that the residents who resigned or were terminated had problems since, according to their recall, there noted no indication during matriculation that there would be problems. Among the pool of problem residents in our study, program directors suspected that about 13% might have problems meeting the challenges of residency training due to poor preparation, outside interests or conflicts, or a lack of fit within the department. In other words, they were surprised by the 87% who seemed to present no problems during the screening process.

Why did the residents in this study have problems meeting the demands of the residency program when few of them showed any signs of potential problems during the selection process? Among the resigners, the majority of residents left because they found their surgical residency program to be too stressful. These residents either had a misconception of the pressures involved or they overestimated their ability to handle the stress. The other most cited reason for resigning from their posts was marital/family pressures. Although these residents performed above average at the time of their resignation, program faculty could not convince them to stay. These residents decided to choose another medical specialty and from follow-up reports, the choice appeared to be reasonable.

A significant number of terminated residents cited a stressful work environment as a source of their poor performance. Terminated residents faced marital/family pressures and personal conflicts with members of the medical staff. Problematic completers, too, cited a stressful work environment, marital/family pressures, and personal conflicts as reasons for their poor performance. The fact that so many of the residents in this study—resignations, terminations, and problematic completers—cited a stressful work environment, marital/family pres-

sures, and personal conflicts as reasons for their poor performance was anticipated given our description of the culture and organization of surgical residency
programs. This work setting is stressful and demanding and requires the harmonious interplay of personalities among staff members. These residents are at an
age where outside life events such as marriage, divorce, and childbearing are
likely to happen. And given the difficulty of matching the personalities of individuals and organizations, it is not surprising to find that some matches were
unsuccessful.

From the faculty's perspective, however, these were not the only problems
that the terminated resident and problematic completers in particular presented.
The faculty described many of these residents' behaviors as inappropriate—
everything from shirking duty, to unconventional acts, to bizarre displays that
led to referrals to professional help. These residents also suffered from poor
preparation for their posts and failure to progress. There was little agreement
between residents and faculty on the source of poor performance among the pool
of terminated residents. There was more agreement between faculty and residents among our problematic completers. Problematic completers also differed
from their terminated colleagues on a number of points. First, the problems they
presented were on average less severe or troubling whether that problem was a
lack of cognitive knowledge or an interpersonal conflict with staff members.
Secondly, the problematic completer was more likely to accept faculty criticisms
of performance, and attempt to correct deficiencies through extended training or
specialization. And finally, troubling performance was noted later in the residents' tour.

Differences of opinion between faculty and residents on the source of poor
performance help illustrate a couple of important findings about the process of
evaluation in these residency programs. In assessing a resident's non-cognitive
traits, faculty use social cues to judge the presence or absence of honesty, integrity, personality, ability to handle stress, the right surgical personality, maturity,
etc. Their assessments cannot be anything other than subjective, since what they
are assessing are non-quantifiable traits and attributes. Familiarity and friendship
can influence subjective assessments. Respondent after respondent described the
evaluation process as capricious and uneven. Residents learn not to trust evaluations that they describe as personality contests rather than accurate assessments
of performance and potential. Subjective evaluations result in differing opinions.
The resident who sees his or her problem as the bullying intolerance of a faculty
member will not agree that the problem lies with his or her own lack of preparation. Many of our respondents agreed and cited cases in which faculty assessments were just wrong. Residents judged incompetent went on to become successful practicing physicians.

We do not claim, however, that the faculty members in this study were always
wrong and the residents were always right in identifying the source of their
troubles. For example, we do not believe that every resident who was terminated

was the victim of a nasty attending. What we do argue, however, is that in some cases, residents were very likely the victims of biased evaluations. But we also recognize that some residents who began their programs were incapable of becoming competent physicians either due to a lack of technical skills, an inability to be a team player, drug addiction, or other serious behavioral problems. Some residents were untrainable in the normal context of the residency program.

Our analyses suggest some ways in which resident evaluation is biased. We have numerous examples of how race and gender negatively effected a resident's experience in the program and increased his or her risk of attrition among our various study groups. We noted above some ways in which the culture already presents some challenges to women and minorities. The idiom of surgical work is quite male. Camaraderie among department members is facilitated by homogeneity and since white men have historically staffed surgery departments, there is some impetus behind repeating history. Once female and minority residents have overcome these obstacles and have been chosen to join a program, they face other substantial hurdles. We will review those hurdles for each of our groups.

Among the residents who resigned, we found a greater risk for leaving for marital/family reasons among our female residents even after controlling for marital status. This finding is not unique to women entering medicine but is a trend among all professional fields. Women remain more likely to interrupt training and professional pursuits to address marital and family issues like childbearing. We also noted that program directors appeared more sympathetic to the family pressures faced by male residents as opposed to female residents, suggesting that the relationships between program directors and male residents were better. We also found that non-white residents were more likely to be asked to resign (resign under duress) than their white colleagues. Non-whites were also more likely to be encouraged to leave when they discussed the possibility of resigning with program directors. These race effects held even after we controlled for the resident's ranking in the program. This finding suggests that somehow the resident's race itself disqualified him or her from remaining in the program. Given our discussion of camaraderie and homogeneity, we suspected that non-whiteness would increase a resident's risk for attrition.

Among the terminated residents, we found that although faculty apparently failed to communicate their dissatisfaction with a large proportion of terminated residents, non-white residents were particularly lacking in communication. Non-white males in particular had the fewest conversations with program faculty before being dismissed. Similarly among the problematic completers we found that program faculty were significantly more likely to speak with white residents, and that white males were least likely to receive written notification about their poor performance. All of these findings suggest that the day-to-day contact between program faculty and white residents, and white male residents in particular, is better. If dissatisfaction is not adequately communicated to the resi-

dent, how can he or she implement the changes necessary to improve performance?

Race and gender effects did not just affect the resident's experience during the
residency program. They also affected the resident's search for a new position
after leaving his or her post. Among the residents who resigned, whites were
more likely to transfer to another specialty within the same institution. Program
directors were also less likely to know the post-residency plans of the non-white
residents reinforcing our sense that relationships between program directors and
non-white residents were poorer. Among the terminated residents we found that
program directors were more likely to help male residents secure new positions
even after controlling for overall rank. And program directors were more likely
to make calls of reference for white residents than for non-white residents. Program directors made calls of reference more often for white residents among the
problematic completers.

We also saw a significant advantage for white male residents in program faculty's greater tolerance for their poor behavior in responding to faculty criticisms. We found in our analysis of honesty and reaction that although responding poorly greatly increased the risk of being terminated among women and
minorities, it carried a much smaller risk for white males. Being white and male
offered some protection for the poorly behaving resident.

Although these race and gender effects are troubling, we anticipated their significance within the culture of surgical residency programs. A white male program director will find it harder to establish good relationships with female and
minority residents. He will also find it more difficult to assess those vital non-
cognitive traits in residents who are less like him. He will have to be aware of
his own biases in what traits and characteristics he deems necessary to get the
job of surgery done. Our intention throughout this study was not to portray the
surgical program director as a bad guy, setting out to exclude women and minorities from the upper echelons of surgical practice. We recognize that the program director faces a daunting task. He or she must first decide if the new residents who join his or her program will fit into the organization. He or she must
then decide whether the individuals who pass through his or her program will be
granted the right to take other people's lives into their hands, to make critical
decisions about the health and welfare of vulnerable and ill individuals. We give
program directors the task of assessing whether these individuals have the moral
character to adequately assume the responsibility associated with the work of
doctoring. This is not an enviable task. Diversity among the residents makes the
task all the harder for the white male program director.

What we have tried to do is illustrate the direct and indirect ways that women
and minorities are hampered in the residency program setting. We want to call
attention to the fact that program faculty are less likely to interact with female
and minority residents, suggesting that their participation in informal networks
at work must suffer. We want to show that program directors are inclined to

encourage minority residents to resign, even when they are objectively performing as well as their white colleagues. We want to illustrate the tendency to provide more help and assistance to white residents in securing new positions and the subsequent lack of information of the post-residency plans of non-whites. And we want to show that faculty tend to tolerate poor behavior if made by white males. These are some of the reasons women and minorities face a greater risk of attrition after joining a surgical residency program.

Since assessing non-cognitive traits introduces potential for biased evaluations and subsequently discrimination based on race and gender, should this basis for judging physician competency be abolished? We do want our physicians to be of high moral character. Program directors want to train physicians who will always strive to improve their performance, and who will always strive to fulfill their fiduciary obligations. So we cannot advocate a totally objective measure of physician competency. What qualifies an individual to have that kind of authority is not an objectifiable quality. We can, however, advocate a greater awareness of how differences between teacher and student, program director and resident, can negatively bias evaluations, and we can suggest ways to bridge the distance between evaluators and residents.

We showed in Chapter III a significant association between the number of social functions coordinated by a residency program and programs' attrition rates. In short, the more programs in place, the lower the attrition. We speculated that these programs provide forums for the transfer of information that every resident needs to succeed in a residency program—information beyond cognitive knowledge, manual dexterity and clinical judgment. The kind of knowledge that can transfer over a cup of coffee helps newcomers cope with various staff members—they learn about the pet peeves of certain attendings and how to avoid antagonizing the nursing staff. This informal information relays the interworkings of the organization that can be vital for the resident's survival so he or she can prove to be a team player. We also noted that functions like coffee hours, journal clubs, department parties provide a formal opportunity for residents to meet under less stressful conditions. This may be very important for diverse resident groups who may be less inclined to socialize with each other outside of the workplace. And these functions can provide a forum for blowing off stream and reducing work-related stress. Less than ten percent of the programs in our study offered our full range of social activities: coffee hours, resident lunches, resident dinners, journal club, and staff parties. There appears to be ample opportunity for most programs to both increase the number of formal department functions and the quality of their current functions.

We also demonstrated a lack of knowledge among the residents we interviewed about the criteria used for evaluation. Residents we interviewed did not appear to know how evaluations were done, whether forms were used and filled out, how often they occurred, and whether reports were placed in their files. We also showed repeatedly a lack of communication between faculty members and female and minority residents. Few attempts were typically made to make sure that residents knew that faculty were concerned about their performance, since in some cases only one faculty member addressed the resident. More formal mechanisms can be developed to assure, especially in cases where informal networks are not well-established, that residents clearly understand the faculty's misgivings about their current levels of performance. Forms need to be filled out, regular meetings need to be scheduled, and residents need to be able to see and to respond to the evaluations. This formalization could help assure good communication despite diversity, provide an opportunity for addressing concerns and improving performance, and avoid horrible surprises. We also learned from our analysis that the orthopedic programs provide a greater flexibility in addressing resident shortcomings. These programs appear much more likely to implement tutoring sessions or to encourage specialization to help problem residents achieve competency. A more focused look at this trend might open up new possibilities for other surgical specialties.

No matter what changes medical educators make in the selection of residents, or in the organization of residency programs, some attrition will always occur among the programs. Given the number and nature of problems outlined in this analysis, it is in some ways remarkable that the attrition rates are not higher in these programs, mirroring the 40% attrition rate for other graduate training programs. Happily for these programs, these are not the attrition statistics they are dealing with. But greater standardization will not address some central concerns. It cannot address the very important fact that each group of individuals and each organization has a unique personality that their current members account for when taking on new individuals. People within all different occupations have found that they can work better with one group than another even when performing the same job. More variables are involved in the creation of friendship, trust, and camaraderie than can be counted and tested in any selection process. And a person can never really know if he or she will enjoy a job that they have never done before no matter what level of anticipatory socialization that person has had. No person can know what it will be like to be a surgeon before he or she has held the scalpel and cut into living flesh. Some people will inevitably have made the wrong choice and only discover that after joining a program.

This study has looked at the associations between the organization of the program, the criteria to judge performance, and the unique problems of residents to provide a detailed look at the process of attrition in surgical residency programs. It has demonstrated factors that affect attrition that are not necessarily unique to residency programs but extend even beyond medical settings, especially the need for trust and camaraderie among group members and the problems inherent in the analysis of non-cognitive traits. It has raised again the need in attrition studies to look at the structure and culture of an organization and not merely lay the blame at the foot of the individual who fails to complete a program. The absence of the resident's voice hampers this study. Program directors filled out the surveys, and although we asked program directors to report on the resident's perspective, this study is limited by the dominance of the program director's voice. Future work in this area should try to collect the resident's own perspective, without having it filtered through the program director.

The other shortcoming of this analysis as stated in our description of the research population is the lack of data on the successes. Although the survey compared the residents who resigned, were terminated, or who problematically completed training against their successful peers in the program, our analysis could be greatly expanded with similar data collected on those who are never identified by program faculty as dissatisfied or problematic. Our current findings, however, suggest many avenues for future research.

We want to end with questions left unanswered by our analyses. In the name of producing high quality physicians, would the members of the medical profession and the society at large be willing to sacrifice fairness? Does the evidence of discrimination bother us? Or would we tolerate some discrimination in the name of group harmony? If so, how much discrimination will we accept? How do program faculty in these residency programs manage the contradictory demands of creating a harmonious residency program and ensuring fairness in selection and retention?

Should we change the way we screen potential candidates for medical school and residency posts? Would we tolerate more and more tests as a way to screen for excellence, even if we know that those tests promote discrimination? How can medical educators help promote the diversification of the medical community when they cannot erase the effects of discrimination accumulated since birth. How can medical educators level the playing field for young men and · women in their 20s and 30s?

Can medical educators reduce the stress levels in their training environments, or does the stress actual help create competent, focused, stoic surgeons? Can medical faculty produce invincible surgeons without subjecting them to 120+ hour weeks? Are there other methods for transforming neophytes into surgeons that are less toxic? Or is immersion in a harsh environment vital to that social transformation? Do we see the demands placed on the surgical resident as a form of abuse, or are we willing to tolerate these harsh conditions in the name of excellence?

In the name of reducing attrition, where should medical educators devote their energies? In revamping the selection process, or in creating a more supportive training environment? Our analyses suggest that reductions could be achieved through reforms in both arenas. Some reforms would require extensive revisions in the current system of selection and orientation, but some other reforms are as simple as making sure that programs provide scheduled times for residents to share a cup of coffee and exchange stories and anecdotes.

We acknowledged from the very start that we give physicians a huge amount of responsibility. Perhaps we would be willing to tolerate some discrimination, even more stringent selection criteria, and the maintenance of a harsh residency environment in order to produce the best surgeons possible. We might even enthusiastically support these measures if evidence suggested that these conditions were necessary to achieve our goals, but the evidence is contradictory if available at all. We do have evidence that intelligence is a necessary but insufficient trait for doctoring. We know that good test scores are not positively correlated with actual performance as a physician. What we do not know is can we develop a less harsh training program and still produce competent surgeons? Can residents take leaves and not experience skill atrophy? Can people share residency slots and still develop their surgical skills? Medical educators will not know until they try.

Appendix 1: Variables in Survey I

Variable	Description	Mean	SD	Min-Max
University	Is program university affiliated?	0.71	0.46	0 – 1
Beds	How many beds in hospital?	826	975	140 - 13,000
Male	Is program director a male?	0.81	0.39	0 – 1
Job	How many years has program director been on job?	8.71	7.19	0 – 35
Personality	How important is having information about the following traits, aptitudes and skills prior to admission?	4.33	0.75	1 – 5
Honesty		4.93	0.30	1 – 5
Maturity		4.45	0.65	1 – 5
Ability to handle stress		4.36	0.72	1 – 5
Cognitive knowledge		4.23	0.70	1 – 5
Manual dexterity		3.64	0.88	1 – 5
Clinical judgment		4.24	0.75	1 – 5
Staff relationships		4.29	0.69	1 – 5
Patient relationships		4.46	0.69	1 – 5
Information:	Is any information sent to residents prior to matriculation about the hospital, department, and/or the community?	2.24	0.94	0 – 3
Assistance:	Is any assistance provided to new residents in the following forms: housing, child-care, education, community resources, and/or employment for spouse?	2.81	1.64	0 – 5
Social:	Are any of the following social activities organized by the department: coffee hours, lunches, dinners, journal clubs, staff parties?	2.83	1.20	0 – 5
Evaluation form	Standard evaluation form used?	0.95	0.22	0 – 1

Evaluation fre-quency	How often are evaluations done?	2.79	1.57	monthly, quarterly, bi-yearly, yearly1
# of evaluators	How many different categories of people are involved: program director, attendings, chief resident, nurses?	2.22	0.76	0 – 4
Program director		0.81	0.39	0 – 1
Attendings		0.98	0.11	0 – 1
Chief resident		0.36	0.48	0 – 1
Nurses		0.06	0.24	0 – 1
Teach	Do residents evaluate teaching?	0.74	0.44	0 – 1
Merit raises	Are merit raises given?	0.08	0.27	0 – 1
Moonlighting	Is moonlighting allowed?	0.41	0.49	0 – 1
Restrictions	If moonlighting allowed, are there restrictions?	0.60	1.20	0 – 1

1. 1=monthly, 2=quarterly, 3=bi-yearly, and 4=yearly

Bibliography

Adler, Robert, MD, and Keith L. Gladstien, MD, PhD, "The First-Year Resident Selection Process," in Donald G. Langsley, MD, editor, *How To Select Residents* (American Board of Medical Specialties, Evanston, 1988)

Albo, Dominic, Jr., MD, et al, "Multifactor Evaluations of Surgical Trainees and Teaching Services," *Surgery*, Vol. 80, No. 1, pp 115-121, July 1976

AMA, *Directory of Medical Education Programs 1989-90*, AMA Copyright, 1989, Chicago

AMA, "Residency Program Requirements," American Medical Association, Internal Medicine Graduates Section, Promoting Diversity in Medicine

Anderson, Peggy, *Nurse* (Berkley Books, New York, 1978)

Anspach, Renee R., "Notes on the Sociology of Medical Discourse: The Language of Case Presentation," *Journal of Health and Social Behavior*, Vol. 29:357-375, 1988

Anwar, Rebecca A. H., PhD, Charles L. Bosk, PhD, and A. Gerson Greenburg, MD, PhD, "Resident Evaluation: Is It, Can It, Should It Be Objective?" *Journal of Surgical Research*, Vol. 30, No. 1, January 1981

Argetsinger, Amy, "Test of Character: US Naval Academy Analyzes Personality Types to Slow Dropout Rate," *The Washington Post,* Monday, October 25, 1999, Section B

Arnold, Louise, PhD, T. Lee Willoughby, and E. Virginia Calkins, "Self Evaluation in Undergraduate Medical Education: A Longitudinal Perspective," *Journal of Medical Education*, Vol. 60, January 1985

Babbott, David, MD, Dewitt C. Baldwin, Jr., MD, Charles D. Killian, MA, and Shelia O'Leary Weaver, MS, "Racial-Ethnic Background and Specialty Choice: A Study of US Medical Graduates in 1987," Academic Medicine, October 1989, Vol. 64, pp: 595-599

Babbott, David, MD, Shelia O. Weaver, MS, and Dewitt C. Baldwin, Jr., MD, "Primary Care by Desire or by Default? Specialty Choices of Minority Graduates of US Medical Schools in 1983," *Journal of the National Medical Association*, Vol. 86, No. 7

Baldwin, Dewitt C., Jr., MD, Steven R. Daugherty, PhD, and Beverly D. Rowly, PhD, "Unethical and Unprofessional Conduct Observed by Residents During Their First Year of Training," *Academic Medicine,* Vol. 73, No. 11, November 1998
————."Emotional Impact of Medical School and Residency: Racial and Ethnic Discrimination During Residency: Results of a National Survey," *Academic Medicine,* Vol. 69, No. 10, October Supplement, 1994

Baldwin, Dewitt C., Jr., MD, Beverly D. Rowley, PhD, Steven R. Daugherty, PhD, and R. Curtis Ray, PhD, "Withdrawal and Extended Leave During Residency Training: Results of a National Survey," *Academic Medicine,* Vol. 70, No. 12, December, 1995

Barondess, Jeremiah A., MD, "Are Women Different? Some trends in the Assimilation of Women in Medicine," *JAMWA,* Vol. 36, No. 3, March 1981:95-104

Bartky, Sandra Lee, "Foucault, Femininity and the Modernization of Patriarchal Power," in Rose Weitz, editor, The Politics of Women's Bodies: Sexuality, Appearance and Behavior, (Oxford University Press, New York, 1998)

Becker, Howard S. et al, *Boys in White: Student Culture in Medical School* (The University of Chicago Press, Chicago, 1961)

Blurton, Richard R., PhD, and Ernest L. Mazzaferri, MD, "Assessment of Interpersonal Skills and Humanizing Qualities in Medical Residents," in John S. Lloyd, PhD, and Donald G. Langsley, MD, editors, *How To Evaluate Residents* (American Board of Medical Specialties, Chicago, 1986)

Boggs, H. Whitney, Jr., MD, and Norman A. Dolch, PhD, "The Contribution of Program Director Evaluations to Colon and Rectal Surgery Board Certification," in John S. Lloyd, PhD, editor, *Residency Director's Role in Specialty Certification* (American Board of Medical Specialties, Chicago, 1985)

Borlase, Bradley C., MD, Edward J. Bartle, MD, and Ernest E. Moore, MD, "Does the In-Service Training Examination Correlate with Clinical Performance in Surgery?" in John S. Lloyd, PhD, and Donald G. Langsley, MD, editors, *How To Evaluate Residents* (American Board of Medical Specialties, Chicago, 1986)

Bosk, Charles L., *Forgive and Remember: Managing Medical Failure* (University of Chicago Press, Chicago, 1979)

————. "Forgive and Remember Revisited," The Eleventh Wiese Lecture in Medical Humanities, The Brigham and Women's Medical Center, October 30, 1997

————. "Superior Surgical Residents: Who Are They?" *Bulletin of the American College of Surgeons*, 68:3: 11-14, 1984

————."Resident Evaluation: A Sociological Perspective," in John S. Lloyd, PhD, editor, *Residency Director's Role in Specialty Certification* (American Board of Medical Specialties, Chicago, 1985)

————. "Mistaking Identity: Medical Errors, Physicians, and Plaintiff's Attorneys," *Transactions & Studies of the College of Physicians of Philadelphia*, Ser.5, Vol. 13, No. 3, 1991, pp 249-261

————. "Reflections on 'The Surgical Personality,'" submitted, *American Journal of Ethics and Medicine*, 1997

Bowen, William G., and Neil L. Rudenstine, *In Pursuit of the PhD* (Princeton University Press, Princeton, 1992)

Boyd, Monica, Mary Ann Mulvihill, and John Myles, "Gender, Power, and Postindustrialism," in Jacobs, Jerry A., editor, *Gender Inequality at Work* (Sage Publications, Thousand Oaks, 1995)

Bragg, Rick, "Quest for Beauty Went Awry at Hands of Fake Surgeon, Miami Police Say," *The New York Times,* National Report, October 7, 1999

Broadhead, Robert S., *The Private Lives and Professional Identity of Medical Students* (Transaction Books, New Brunswick, 1983)

Bucher, Rue, and Joan G. Stelling, *Becoming Professional* (Sage Publications, Beverly Hills, 1977)

Burg, Fredric D., MD, "Deciding What to Evaluate: A Program Director's Checklist for Evaluation of Housestaff," in John S. Lloyd, PhD, and Donald G. Langsley, MD, editors, *How To Evaluate Residents* (American Board of Medical Specialties, Chicago, 1986)

Burkett, Gary and Kathleen Knafl, "Judgment and Decision-Making in a Medical Specialty," *Sociology of Work and Occupations*, Vol. 1. No. 1., February 1974.

Carothers, Suzanne C. and Peggy Crull, "Contrasting Sexual Harrassment in Female- and Male-Dominated Occupations" in *My Troubles are Going to Have Trouble with Me*, Karen Brodkin Sacks and Dorothy Remy, editors (Rutgers University Press, New Brunswick, 1984)

Carter, Michael J., and Susan Boslego Carter, "Women's Recent Progress in the Professions or, Women Get a Ticket To Ride After the Gravy Train Has Left the Station." *Feminist Studies* 7(3):1981

Cassell, Joan, "On Control, Certitude, and the 'Paranoia' of Surgeons," *Culture, Medicine and Psychiatry* 11(1987):229-249
————.*Expected Miracles: Surgeons At Work* (Temple University Press, Philadelphia, 1991)
————.*The Woman in the Surgeon's Body* (Harvard University Press, Cambridge, 1998)

Chapman, Carleton B., "What is a Good Doctor?" in Swazey, Judith P., and Stephen R. Scher,editors, *Social Controls and the Medical Profession* (Oelgeschlager, Gunn and Hain, Boston, 1985)

Cassileth, Barrie R., *The Cancer Patient: Social and Medical Aspects of Care*, (Lea and Ferbiger, Philadelphia, 1979)

Clarke, John R., MD, and Robert S. Wigton, MD, "Development of an Objective Rating System for Residency Applications," *Surgery*, Vol. 96, No. 2, August 1984

Cloutier, Charlotte B., "Formal Controls on Impaired Physicians," in Swazey, Judith P., and Stephen R. Scher,editors, *Social Controls and the Medical Profession* (Oelgeschlager, Gunn and Hain, Boston, 1985)

Cockburn, Cynthia, *In The Way of Women: Men's Resistance to Sex Equality in Organizations* (IRL Press, Ithaca, 1991)

Conley, Frances K., *Walking Out On the Boys* (Farrar, Straus and Giroux, New York, 1998)

Cooke, Donna K., Randi L. Sims, and Joseph Peyrefitte, "The Relationship Between Graduate Student Attitudes and Attrition," *Journal of Psychology*, 129(6):677-688, 1995

Conrad, Peter, "Learning to Doctor: Reflections on Recent Accounts of the Medical School Years," *Journal of Health and Social Behavior*, Vol. 29:323-332, 1988

Cope, R., and Hannah, W., *Revolving College Doors*, (John Wiley and Sons, New York, 1975)

Cousins, Norman, MD, "Internship: Preparation or Hazing," *JAMA*, Jan. 23/30, 1981

(COGME) Council on Graduate Medical Education, "The Underrepresentation of Minorities in Medicine," February 1991, Supplement, US Dept of Health and Human Services

Crandall, Rick, "The Assimilation of Newcomers Into Groups," *Small Group Behavior*, 9(3):331-335, 1978

Cruft, George E., MD, "Peer Review," in John S. Llody, PhD, editor, *Evaluation of Non-cognitive Skills and Clinical Performance* (American Board of Medical Specialties, Chicago, 1982)
————."Suggestions for Evaluating Residents for Specialty Boards: What should be evaluated," in John S. Lloyd, PhD, editor, *Residency Director's Role in Specialty Certification* (American Board of Medical Specialties, Chicago, 1985)

Daniels, Norman, Bruce Kennedy, and Ichiro Kawachi, *Is Inequality Bad for Our Health?* (Beacon Press, Boston, 2000)

David, John S., MD, "The Evaluation Process," in John S. Lloyd, PhD, and Donald G. Langsley, MD, editors, *How To Evaluate Residents* (American Board of Medical Specialties, Chicago, 1986)

Daugherty, Steven R,., Dewitt C. Baldwin, Jr., MD, and Beverly C. Rowley, PhD., "Learning, Satisfaction and Mistreatment During Medical Internship: A National Survey of Working Conditions," *JAMA*, April 15, 1998, Vol. 279, No. 15

Daugherty, Steven R., and Dewitt C. Baldwin, Jr,. MD, "Sleep Deprivation in Senior Medical Students and First-Year Residents," *Academic Medicine*, Vol. 71, No. 1, January Supplement, 1996

Dubos, Rene, *Mirage of Health: Utopias, Progress and Biological Change* (Harper and Brothers, New York, 1959)

Dunn, Marvin R and Rebecca S. Miller, "US Graduate Medical Education, 1996-1997," *JAMA* 1997, 278: 750-754

Eaton, Shevawn Bogdan and John P. Bean, "An Approach/Avoidance
    Behavioral Model of College Student Attrition," *Research in Higher Education*
    36(6):617-645, 1995

Elliott, Rogers, A. Christopher Strenta, Russell Adair et al, "The Role of
    Ethnicity in Choosing and Leaving Science in Highly Selective Institutions," *Research in Higher Education* 37(6):681-709, 1996

Evans, Mariah D., and Edward O. Lauman, "Professional Commitment: Myth or
    Reality?" *Research in Social Stratification and Mobility*, Vol. 2., 1983: 3-40

Fox, Nicholas J.,*The Social Meaning of Surgery* (Open University Press,
    Philadelphia, 1992)

Fox, Renee C., *The Sociology of Medicine: a participant observer's view*,
    Chapter 1, "The Social and Cultural Significance of Health and Illness," pp. 1-37
    (Prentice-Hall, Englewood Cliffs, 1989)
    ————.*Experiment Perilous*, (University of Pennsylvania Press, Philadelphia,
    1974)

Freidson, Eliot, *The Profession of Medicine: A Study of the Sociology of Applied
    Knowledge* (Dodd, Mead and Company, New York, 1970)
    ————.*Professional Powers: A Study of the Institutionalization of Formal
    Knowledge* (The University of Chicago Press, Chicago, 1986)
    ————.*Doctoring Together: A Study of Professional Social Control* (University
    of Chicago Press, Chicago, 1975)

Friedman, Charles P., PhD, William C. Trier, MD, and Colin G. Thomas, Jr.,
    MD, "Evaluation and Redesign of a System to Rank Applicants for Surgical
    Residencies," *Journal of Medical Education*, Vol 62, November 1987: 886-894
    ————."Restructuring a Surgical House Officer Applicant Ranking System," in
    Donald G. Langsley, MD, editor, *How To Select Residents* (American Board of
    Medical Specialties, Evanston, 1988)

Galanti, Geri-Ann, *Caring for Patients From Different Cultures: Case Studies
    from American Hospitals* (University of Pennsylvania Press, Philadelphia, 1991)

Gerber, Lane A., *Married to Their Careers: Career and Family Dilemmas in
    Doctor's Lives* (Tavistock Publications, New York, 1983)

Glantz, Leonard H., "Becoming a Lawyer: Education and Socialization," in
    Swazey, Judith P., and Stephen R. Scher,editors, *Social Controls and the Medical*

Profession (Oelgeschlager, Gunn and Hain, Boston, 1985)

Glaser, Ronald J., *Ward 402*, (George Braziler, Inc., New York, 1973)

Goffman, Erving, *Asylums: Essays on the Social Situation of Mental Patients and Other Inmates* (Anchor Books, Doubleday & Company, Inc., Garden City, NYT, 1961)

Goldstein, Beth L., "Little Brown Spots on the Notebook Paper: Women as Law School Students," *Kentucky Law Journal*, 84(4):983-1025, 1995-1996

Goleman, Daniel, *Emotional Intelligence*, (Bantam Books, New York, 1995)
————.*Working With Emotional Intelligence*, (Bantam Books, New York, 1998)

Gong, H., Jr., N. H. Parker, F. A. Apgar, and Candace Shank, "Influence of the Interview on Ranking in the Residency Selection Process," in Donald G. Langsley, MD, editor, *How To Select Residents* (American Board of Medical Specialties, Evanston, 1988)

Good, Mary-Jo DelVecchio, *American Medicine: The Quest for Competence* (University of California Press, Berkeley, 1995)

Gordon, Noel L., MD, "A System for Evaluating and Counseling Marginal Students During Clinical Clerkships," *Journal of Medical Education,* Vol. 62, April 1987: 353-355

Gough, Malcolm, "Opening Remarks," *Personality Assessment Techniques and Aptitude Testing as Aids to the Selection of Surgical Trainees,* Symposium at the Royal College of Surgeons of England, November 18, 1987

Gourman, J., *The Gourman Report: Undergraduate and Professional Programs in America and International Universities* (Princeton Review, Princeton, 1991)

Greenberg, Gerson, "The Evaluation Process," in Anwar, Rebecca A. H., PhD, Charles L. Bosk, PhD, and A. Gerson Greenburg, MD, PhD, "Resident Evaluation: Is It, Can It, Should It Be Objective?" *Journal of Surgical Research*, Vol. 30, No. 1, January 1981

Greene, Jay, "Residents Say Long Hours Hurt Patient Care," *American Medical News,* Vol. 42, No. 1, March 1, 1999

Griffen, Ward O., Jr., MD, PhD, "Medical Education: A Continuum in

Disarray," *The American Journal of Surgery* 154:255-260, September 1987

Griner, "The Need for Practice Standards," in Langsley, D.G., Dockery, J. Lee and Peyton Weary, *Health Policy Issues Affecting Graduate Medical Education*, (American Board of Medical Specialties, Evanston, 1992)

Groopman, Leonard C., "Medical Internship as Moral Education: An Essay on the System of Training Physicians," *Culture, Medicine and Psychiatry* 11:207-227, 1987

Gutek, Barbara A., and Bruce Morash, "Sex-Ratios, Sex-Role Spillover, and Sexual Harrassment of Women at Work," *Journal of Social Issues,* Vol. 38, No. 4, 1982: 55-74

Haas, Jack and William Shaffir, *Becoming Doctors: The Adoption of a Cloak of Confidence* (Jai Press, Inc., Greenwich, 1987)

Hafferty, Frederic W., *Into the Valley: Death and the Socialization of Medical Students* (Yale University Press, New Haven, 1991)

Hall, Stephen S., "Lethal Chemistry at Harvard," *The New York Times Magazine*, November 29, 1998

Harrison, Michelle, *A Woman in Residence* (Fawcett Crest, New York, 1982)

Hayward, Richard MD, "The Shadow Line in Surgery," *The Lancet*, February 14, 1987: 375-376

Heimbach, David M., MD, and Kaj Johnson, MD, PhD, You Want To Be A Surgeon: A Medical Student's Guide to Surgery Residencies (University of Washington School of Medicine, Seattle, 1986)

Herman, Mary W., PhD, J. Jon Velsoki, and Mohammadreza Hojat, PhD, "Validity and Importance of Low Ratings Given Medical Graduates in Noncognitive Areas," *Journal of Medical Education,* Vol. 58, November 1983, pp. 837-843

Holdsworth, Roger F., "Objective Assessment—the state of the art," *Personality Assessment Techniques and Aptitude Testing as Aids to the Selection of Surgical Trainees,* Symposium at the Royal College of Surgeons of England, November 18, 1987

Hook, Edward W., MD, "The Role of Program Directors in the Evaluation of Noncognitive Skills and Clinical Performance of Residents in Internal Medicine," in John S. Llody, PhD, editor, *Evaluation of Noncognitive Skills and Clinical Performance* (American Board of Medical Specialties, Chicago, 1982)

Hughes, E., *The Sociological Eye*, (Aldine-Atherton, Chicago, 1971)

Illich, Ivan, *Limits to Medicine: Medical Nemesis: The Expropriation of Health* (Penguin Books, New York, 1976)

Iverson, Kenneth V., MD, MBA, FACEP, *Getting Into a Residency: A Guide for Medical Students* (Galen Press, Ltd., Tucson, 1996)

Jacobs, Jerry, *Professional Women at Work: Interactions, Tacit Understandings, and the Non-Trivial Nature of Trivia in Bureaucratic Settings* (Bergin & Garvey, Westport, 1994)

Jacobs, Jerry A., editor, *Gender Inequality at Work* (Sage Publications, Thousand Oaks, 1995)
————."Women's Entry Into Management: Trends in Earnings, Authority, and Values Among Salaried Managers," in Jacobs, Jerry A., editor, *Gender Inequality at Work* (Sage Publications, Thousand Oaks, 1995)
————.*Revolving Doors: Sex Segregation and Women's Careers* (Stanford University Press, Stanford, 1989)

Johnson, Henry C., PhD, "Minority and Nonminority Medical Students' Perceptions of the Medical School Environment," *Journal of Medical Education,* Vol. 53, February 1978

Jonas, Harry S., MD, Sylvia I. Etzel, and Barbara Barzansky, PhD, "Educational Programs in US Medical Schools," *JAMA*, August 21, 1991, Vol. 266, No. 7

Kanter, R.M., *Men and Women of the Corporation* (Basic Books, New York, 1977)

Kapp, Marshall B., "Legal Issues in Faculty Evaluation of Student Clinical Performance," Journal of Medical Education, Vol. 56, July 1981, pp 559-564

Kastner, Laura, PhD, Edmond Gore, MS, Alvin H. Novack, MD, "Pediatric Residents' Attitudes and Cognitive Knowledge, and Faculty Ratings," in John S. Lloyd, PhD, and Donald G. Langsley, MD, editors, *How To Evaluate Residents* (American Board of Medical Specialties, Chicago, 1986)

Kaufman, H. H., R. L. Weingard and R. H. Tunick, "Teaching Surgeons to Operate: Principles of Psychomotor Skills Training," *Acta Neurochir* (Wien) 1987: 1-7

Keck, Jonathan W., PhD, Louise Arnold, PhD, Lee Willoughby, and Virginia Calkins, "Efficacy of Cognitive/Noncognitive Measures in Predicting Resident-Physician Performance," *Journal of Medical Education*, Vol. 54, October 1979

King, Robert B., MD, "Resident Selection: 'What's the Problem?'" in Donald G. Langsley, MD, editor, *How To Select Residents* (American Board of Medical Specialties, Evanston, 1988)
————. "Selection Methods and Entry Criteria for Graduate Medical Education in Neurological Surgery," in Donald G. Langsley, MD, editor, *How To Select Residents* (American Board of Medical Specialties, Evanston, 1988)

Klass, Perri, *A Not Entirely Benign Process* (Signet Books, New York, 1988)

Klineberg, James R., MD, "Problems Evaluating Medical Residents," in John S. Lloyd, PhD, editor, *Residency Director's Role in Specialty Certification* (American Board of Medical Specialties, Chicago, 1985)

Komives, Eugene, Scott T. Weiss, MD, and Robert M. Rosa, MD, "The Applicant Interview as a Predictor of Resident Performance," *Journal of Medical Education*, Vol. 59, May 1984

Konner, Melvin , M.D., *Becoming A Doctor: A Journey of Initiation in Medical School* (Elisabeth Sifton Books, New York, 1987)

Konrad, Alison M., and Jeffrey Pfeffer, "Understanding the Hiring of Women and Minorities in Educational Institutions," *Sociology of Education*, 64 (July): 141-157, 1991

Koran, L. M., "The reliability of clinical methods, data and judgments," *New England Journal of Medicine*, 1975: 293: 642-701

Kuczynski, Alex, "Why Are So Few Plastic Surgeons Women?" *The New York Times*, Sunday Styles, Sunday, July 12, 1998, Section 9

Ladd, John, "Philosophy and the Moral Professions," in Judith P. Swazey and Stephen R. Scher, eds., *Social Controls and the Medical Profession*, (Oelgeschlager, Gunn and Hain, Publsihers, Inc., Boston, 1985)

Landau, Carol, PhD, Stephanie Hall, MD, Steven A. Wartman, MD, PhD, and Michael B. Macko, MD, "Stress in Social and Family Relationships During the Medical Residency," *Journal of Medical Education*, Vol. 61, August 1986: 654-659

Langsley, Donald G., MD, "Evaluation During Residency," in John S. Lloyd, PhD, and Donald G. Langsley, MD, editors, *How To Evaluate Residents* (American Board of Medical Specialties, Chicago, 1986)
————.editor, *How To Select Residents* (American Board of Medical Specialties, Evanston, 1988)
————."Selection of Residents for Graduate Medical Education," in *How To Select Residents* (American Board of Medical Specialties, Evanston, 1988)

Leonard, Arthur, MD and Ilene Harris, "An Approach for Defining Selection Criteria of Applicants for Medical Residency Training," *Journal of Medical Education*, Vol. 55, January, 1980

Levinson, Daniel J., "Medical Education and the Theory of Adult Socialization," Journal of Health and Social Behavior, Vol. 8, Issue 4, Dec. 1967: 253-265

Light, Donald W., *Becoming Psychiatrists: The Professional Transformation of Self* (WW Morton and Company, 1980)
————."Toward a New Sociology of Medical Education," *Journal of Health and Social Behavior*, Vol. 29:307-322, 1988

Linn, L. S., PhD, J. Yager, and D. Cope, et al., "Health Habits and Coping Behaviors among Practicing Physicians," *Western Journal of Medicine*, April 1986, Vol . 144:484-489

Linn, L. S., PhD, Robert K. Oye, MD, Dennis W. Cope, MD, Robin M. DiMatteo, PhD, "Use of Non-Physician Staff to Evaluate Humanistic Behavior of Internal Medicine Residents and Faculty Members," *Journal of Medical Education*, Vol. 61, November 1986: 918-920

Linn, L. S., PhD, D. W. Cope MD, A. Robbins, MD, "Sociodemographic and Premedical School Factors Related to Postgraduate Physicians' Humanistic Performance," *The Western Journal of Medicine,* July 1987, 147:99-103

Littlefield, John H., PhD, "Developing and Maintaining a Resident Rating System," in John S. Lloyd, PhD, and Donald G. Langsley, MD, editors, *How To Evaluate Residents* (American Board of Medical Specialties, Chicago, 1986)

Lloyd, John S., PhD, editor, *Evaluation of Noncogtive Skills and Clinical Performance* (American Board of Medical Specialties, Chicago, 1982) ————.editor, *Residency Director's Role in Specialty Certification* (American Board of Medical Specialties, Chicago, 1985)

Lloyd, John S., PhD, and Donald G. Langsley, MD, editors, *How To Evaluate Residents* (American Board of Medical Specialties, Chicago, 1986)

Lorber, Judith, *Women Physicians: Career, Status and Power* (Tavistock Publications, New York, 1984)

Lowenstein, Leah M., "The Structure and Function of Graduate Medical Education," in Shapiro, Ellen C. and Leah M. Lowenstein, MD, D. Phil, editors, *Becoming a Physician: Development of Values and Attitudes in Medicine* (Ballinger Publishing Co, Cambridge, 1979)

Ludmerer, Kenneth, *Learning to Heal: The Development of American Medical Education* (Basic Books, New York, 1985)

Mankin, Dr., "Audience Discussion of Suggestions," John S. Lloyd, editor, *Residency Director's Role in Specialty Certification*, (American Board of Medical Specialists, Chicago, 1985)

Martin, Emily, "Premenstrual Syndrome, Work Discipline and Anger," in RoseWeitz, editor, The Politics of Women's Bodies: Sexuality, Appearance and Behavior, (Oxford University Press, New York, 1998)

Martin, Steven C., Robert M. Arnold, and Ruth M. Parker, "Gender and Medical Socialization," *Journal of Health and Social Behavior*, Vol. 29:333-343, 1988

Merton, Robert K. et al, *The Student-Physician: Introductory Studies in the Sociology of Medical Education* (Harvard University Press, Cambridge, 1957)

Milkman, R, *Gender at Work: The dynamics of job segregation by sex during WWII*, (University of Illinois Press, Urbana, 1987)

Miller, Elliott V., MD, "Performance Checklist to Evaluate Anesthesia Skills,"\ in John S. Llody, PhD, editor, *Evaluation of Noncognitive Skills and Clinical Performance* (American Board of Medical Specialties, Chicago, 1982)

Miller, Lee T., MD, and Leigh G. Donowitz, MD, *1997-1998 Medical Student's*

Guide to Successful Residency Matching (Williams and Wilkins, Philadelphia, 1997)

Millman, Marcia, *The Unkindest Cut*, (William Morrow & Company, Inc. New York, 1977)

Mitchell, Karen J., PhD, "Use of MCAT Data in Admissions," Association of American Medical Colleges, 1987, Washington, DC

Mizrahi, Terry, *Getting Rid of Patients: Contradictions in the Socialization of Physicians* (Rutgers University Press, New Brunswick, 1986)

Mogul, Kathleen M., "Doctor's Dilemmas: Complexities in the Causes of Physicians' Mental Disorders and Some Treatment Implications," in Swazey, Judith P., and Stephen R. Scher,editors, *Social Controls and the Medical Profession* (Oelgeschlager, Gunn and Hain, Boston, 1985)

Morgan, Elizabeth, *The Making of a Woman Surgeon* (G.P. Putnam's, New York, 1980)

Morrow, Carol Klaperman, "The Medicalization of Professional Self Governance: A Sociological Assessment," in Swazey, Judith P., and Stephen R. Scher,editors, *Social Controls and the Medical Profession* (Oelgeschlager, Gunn and Hain, Boston, 1985)

Mumford, Emily, *Interns: From Students to Physicians* (Harvard University Press, Cambridge, 1970)

Nolen, William A., *The Making of a Surgeon* (Random House, New York, 1968)

Norman, Geoffrey R., PhD, David A. Davis, MD, Sheliah Lamb, MD, Eileen Hanna, BscN, Paul Caulford, MD, Tina Kaigas, MD, "Competency Assessment of Primary Care Physicians as Part of a Peer Review Program," *JAMA*, September 1, 1993, Vol. 270, No.9: 1046-1051

Parmer, Michael A., "Ethics of a Professional Surgeon," *American College of Surgeons Bulletin*, July 1982, pp 2-5

Parsons, Talcott, "Social Structure and Dynamic Process: The Case of Modern Medical Practice," *The Social System* (The Free Press, Glencoe, 1951)

Parmer, Michael A., "Maintaining Competence in Solo Practice," in Swazey,

Judith P., and Stephen R. Scher,editors, *Social Controls and the Medical Profession* (Oelgeschlager, Gunn and Hain, Boston, 1985)

Perkoff, Gerald, "On the Horizon: Regulation of Physician Training Programs, Proceedings of the Conference," Ira Singer, editor, *Medical Education Group of the American Medical Association*, March 2-4, 1989

Piel, Gerard, "Concluding observations," in John S. Lloyd, PhD, editor, *Evaluation of Noncognitive Skills and Clinical Performance* (American Board of Medical Specialties, Chicago, 1982)

Piller, Charles, "The Gender Gap Goes High Tech," *Los Angeles Times*, August 25, 1998

Polk, H. C., Jr., MD, "The evaluation of residents." *American College of Surgeons Bulletin*, March 1983

Preston, Jo Anne, "Gender and the Formation of a Women's Profession: The Case of Public School Teaching," in Jacobs, Jerry A., editor, *Gender Inequality at Work* (Sage Publications, Thousand Oaks, 1995)

Reskin, Barbara F. and Patricia A. Roos, *Job Queues, Gender Queues: Explaining Women's Inroads into Male Occupations.* (Temple University Press, Philadelphia, 1990)

Rhoden, Nancy K., "Litigating Life and Death," *Harvard Law Review*, Vol. 102, 1988

Robinowitz, Carolyn B., MD, "Discussion/Implications," in John S. Lloyd, PhD, editor, *Residency Director's Role in Specialty Certification* (American Board of Medical Specialties, Chicago, 1985)

Rolph, John E., Albert P. Williams, and A. Lee Lanier, *Predicting Minority and Majority Medical Student Performance on the National Board Exams* (Rand Corporation, Santa Monica, 1978)

Roos, Patricia A., and Katherine W. Jones, "Shifting Gender Boundaries: Women's Inroads Into Academic Sociology," in Jacobs, Jerry A., editor, *Gender Inequality at Work* (Sage Publications, Thousand Oaks, 1995)

Rootman, Irving, "Voluntary Withdrawal from a Total Adult Socializing Organization: A Model," *Sociology of Education*, 1972, Vol.45:258-270

Rosenberg, Charles E., *Explaining Epidemics and Other Studies in the History of Medicine* (Cambridge University Press, New York, 1992)

Ross, Colin A., MD, and Pierre Leichner, MD, "Criteria for Selecting Residents: A Reassessment," in Donald G. Langsley, MD, editor, *How To Select Residents* (American Board of Medical Specialties, Evanston, 1988)

Ruddick, William, "'Tough Love,' Physician Advocacy and Moral Diffidence: Philosophical Reflections," in Judith P. Swazey and Stephen R. Scher, eds., *Social Controls and the Medical Profession*, (Oelgeschlager, Gunn and Hain, Publsihers, Inc., Boston, 1985)

Salovey, P., and Mayer, J.D., "Emotional Intelligence," *Imagination, Cognition and Personality,* 9: 185-211

Schaffer, William A., MD, F. David Rollo, MD, PhD, and Carol A. Holt, RN, "Falsification of Clinical Credentials by Physicians Applying of Ambulatory-Staff Privileges," *The New England Journal of Medicine*, Feb. 11, 1988, Vol. 318, No. 6

Schueneman, Arthur L., PhD, "Neuropsychologic Predictors of Operative Skill Among General Surgery Residents," in Donald G. Langsley, MD, editor, *How To Select Residents* (American Board of Medical Specialties, Evanston, 1988)

Schwarz, M. Roy, "Residency Working Conditions," in Langsley, D.G., Dockery, J. Lee and Peyton Weary, *Health Policy Issues Affecting Graduate Medical Education*, (American Board of Medical Specialties, Evanston, 1992)

Scott, Catherine, Alisa Burns and George Cooney, "Reasons for Discontinuing Study: The case of mature age female students with children," *Higher Education* 31:233-253, 1996

Scotti, Rita A., *Cradle Song* (Donald I. Fine, Inc., New York, 1988)

Shapiro, Ellen C. and Leah M. Lowenstein, MD, D. Phil, editors, *Becoming a Physician: Development of Values and Attitudes in Medicine* (Ballinger Publishing Co, Cambridge, 1979)

Shapiro, Ellen C. and Shirley G. Driscoll, "'Training for Commitment:' Effects of Time-Intensive Nature of Graduate Medical Education," in Shapiro, Ellen C. and Leah M. Lowenstein, MD, PhD, editors, *Becoming a Physician: Develop-*

ment of Values and Attitudes in Medicine (Ballinger Publishing Co, Cambridge, 1979)

Shem, Samuel , M.D., Ph.D., *The House of God* (Dell Publishing, New York, 1978)

Singer, Ira, PhD, *On The Horizon: Regulation of Physician Training Programs*, Proceedings of the Conference (Medical Education Group of the AMA, March 2-4, 1989)

Smith, David Barton, "The Racial Integration of Medical and Nursing Associations in the United States," *Hospital and Health Service Administration*, January 7, 1992

Spencer, Frank C., "On the Horizon: Regulation of Physician Training Programs, Proceedings of the Conference," Ira Singer, editor, *Medical Education Group of the American Medical Association*, March 2-4, 1989

Spenner, Kenneth and Rachel A. Rosenfeld, "Occupational Sex Segregation and Women's Early Career Job Shifts" Jerry A. Jacobs, editor, *Gender inequality at work*, (Thousand Oaks, Sage Publications, 1995)

Stanton, Bruce C., A. G. Burstein, and J.C. Kobos, "The Dean's Letter of Recommendation and Resident Performance," *Journal of Medical Education* 54(10):812-813, 1979

Starr, Paul, *The Social Transformation of American Medicine*, (Basic Books, New York, 1982), pp. 30-145

Steinhauer, Jennifer, "For Women in Medicine, A Road to Compromise, Not Perks," *The New York Times,* Monday, March 1, 1999

Swazey, Judith P., and Stephen R. Scher,editors, *Social Controls and the Medical Profession* (Oelgeschlager, Gunn and Hain, Boston, 1985)

Thomas, Barbara J., "Women's Gains in Insurance Sales: Increased Supply, Uncertain Demand," in *Job Queues, Gender Queues: Explaining Women's Inroads into Male Occupations*, (Temple University Press, Philadelphia, 1990)

Tinto, Vincent, Leaving College: *Rethinking the Causes and Cures of Student Attrition* (University of Chicago Press, Chicago, 1993)

Tobin, J, "Estimation of relationships for limited dependent variables," *Ecomometrica* 26: 24-36

Trier, William C., MD, "How Residency Directors View Specialty Boards' Requirements," in John S. Lloyd, PhD, editor, *Residency Director's Role in Specialty Certification* (American Board of Medical Specialties, Chicago, 1985)

Vaillant, George E., MD, Nancy Corbin Sobowale, AB, and Charles McArthur, PhD, "Some Psychologic Vulnerabilities of Physicians," *The New England Journal of Medicine*, August 24 1979, Vol. 287, No. 8

Velsoki, J., Mary W. Herman, PhD, Joseph S. Gonnella, MD, et al, "Relationships Between Performance in Medical School and First Postgraduate Year," *Journal of Medical Education*, Vol. 54:909-916, 1979

Voytovich, Anthony E., MD, Robert M. Rippey, PhD, and Dale A. Matthews, MD, "Deciding How To Evaluate Performance," in John S. Lloyd, PhD, and Donald G. Langsley, MD, editors, *How To Evaluate Residents* (American Board of Medical Specialties, Chicago, 1986)

Wagoner, Norma E., PhD, "Traditional Methods Used in Resident Selection: Valid, Valuable, in Need of Change?" in Donald G. Langsley, MD, editor, *How To Select Residents* (American Board of Medical Specialties, Evanston, 1988)

Wagoner, Norma E., PhD, Robert Suriano, PhD, and Joseph A. Stoner, "Factors Used by Program Directors to Select Residents," in Donald G. Langsley, MD, editor, *How To Select Residents* (American Board of Medical Specialties, Evanston, 1988)

Warnecke, Richard B., "Non-intellectual Factors Related to Attrition from a Collegiate Nursing Program," *Journal of Health and Social Behavior* 14(June):153-167, 1973

Weber, Max, *The Protestant Ethic and the Spirit of Capitalism*, (Routledge, New York, 1993)

Weitz, Rose, *The Politics of Women's Bodies: Sexuality, Appearance and Behavior* (Oxford University Press, New York, 1998)
———.*The Sociology of Health, Illness, and Heath Care: A Critical Approach* (Wadsworth Publishing Company, 1996)

Welch, Claude E., "Laying Down the Scalpel: Reflections on Competence in a

Surgeon's Career," in Swazey, Judith P., and Stephen R. Scher,editors, *Social Controls and the Medical Profession* (Oelgeschlager, Gunn and Hain, Boston, 1985)

Werner, Edwenna R., and Barbara M. Korsch, "Professionalization During Pediatric Internship: Attitudes, Adaptation, and Interpersonal Skills," in Shapiro, Ellen C. and Leah M. Lowenstein, MD, PhD, editors, *Becoming a Physician: Development of Values and Attitudes in Medicine* (Ballinger Publishing Co, Cambridge, 1979)

West, Candace and Don H. Zimmerman, "Doing Gender," *Gender & Society*, Vol. 1, No. 2, June 1987 125-151.

Wilson, Frank C., MD, "Problems in the Evaluation of Surgical House Officers by Program Directors," in John S. Lloyd, PhD, editor, *Residency Director's Role in Specialty Certification* (American Board of Medical Specialties, Chicago, 1985)

Wingard, John R., and John W. Williamson, MD, "Grades as Predictors of Phsyicians' Career Performance: An Evaluative Literature Review," *Journal of Medical Education*, Vol. 48, April 1973

Wong, Edward, "Hospital Met With Doctor it Had Suspended on Project at Clinic," *The New York Times Metro,* Tuesday, February 1, 2000

Yager, Joel, MD, Gordon D. Strauss, MD, and Kenneth Tardiff, MD, "The Quality of Dean's Letters from Medical Schools," in Donald G. Langsley, MD, editor, *How To Select Residents* (American Board of Medical Specialties, Evanston, 1988)

Young, Elizabeth H., Dr.P.H., "Relationship of Residents' Emotional Problems, Coping Behaviors, and Gender," *Journal of Medical Education*, Vol. 62, No. 8, August 1987: 642

Zaslau, Stanley, MD, Match Success: *A "Student-to-Student" Strategy Guide for Applying to Residency Training Programs in the United States* (FMSG, Inc., Freeport, 1994)

Zborowski, Mark, "Cultural Components in Responses to Pain," *Journal of Social Issues*, 8, no. 4 (1969)

Zerubavel, Evitar, *Patterns of Time in Hospital Life* (The University of Chicago

Press, Chicago, 1979)

About the Author

After receiving her Ph.D. from the University of Pennsylvania in 2001, Virginia Adams O'Connell joined the faculty at Swarthmore College in Swarthmore, Pennsylvania where she is currently a Visiting Assistant Professor in the Department of Sociology and Anthropology. Before attending graduate school, she worked as a medical "head hunter" and became intrigued by the way doctors chose new associates. She was fortunate to be able to systematically study this phenomenon in her graduate program. She currently teaches a number of courses about population demographics, bioethics and the socialization of medical professionals. Her publications address issues such as the lay etiology of childhood cancers, physician burnout, alternative medicine, and her more recent work on the experiences of premedical students.

Subject Index